Breast Imaging

Editor

SARAH M. FRIEDEWALD

RADIOLOGIC CLINICS OF NORTH AMERICA

www.radiologic.theclinics.com

Consulting Editor
FRANK H. MILLER

May 2017 • Volume 55 • Number 3

ELSEVIER

1600 John F. Kennedy Boulevard • Suite 1800 • Philadelphia, Pennsylvania, 19103-2899

http://www.theclinics.com

RADIOLOGIC CLINICS OF NORTH AMERICA Volume 55, Number 3
May 2017 ISSN 0033-8389, ISBN 13: 978-0-323-52858-0

Editor: John Vassallo (j.vassallo@elsevier.com)
Developmental Editor: Donald Mumford

Radiologic Clinics of North America (ISSN 0033-8389) is published bimonthly by Elsevier Inc., 360 Park Avenue South, New York, NY 10010-1710. Months of issue are January, March, May, July, September, and November. Periodicals postage paid at New York, NY and additional mailing offices. Subscription prices are USD 474 per year for US individuals, USD 831 per year for US institutions, USD 100 per year for US students and residents, USD 551 per year for Canadian individuals, USD 1062 per year for Canadian institutions, USD 680 per year for international individuals, USD 1062 per year for international institutions, and USD 315 per year for Canadian and international students/residents. To receive student and resident rate, orders must be accompanied by name of affiliated institution, date of term and the signature of program/residency coordinatior on institution letterhead. Orders will be billed at individual rate until proof of status is received. Foreign air speed delivery is included in all *Clinics* subscription prices. All prices are subject to change without notice. **POSTMASTER:** Send address changes to *Radiologic Clinics of North America*, Elsevier Health Sciences Division, Subscription Customer Service, 3251 Riverport Lane, Maryland Heights, MO63043. **Customer Service: Telephone: 1-800-654-2452** (U.S. and Canada); **1-314-447-8871** (outside U.S. and Canada). **Fax: 1-314-447-8029. E-mail: journalscustomerservice-usa@elsevier.com (for print support); journalsonlinesupport-usa@elsevier.com (for online support).**

Reprints. For copies of 100 or more of articles in this publication, please contact the Commercial Reprints Department, Elsevier Inc., 360 Park Avenue South, New York, New York 10010-1710. Tel.: +1-212-633-3874; Fax: +1-212-633-3820; E-mail: reprints@elsevier.com.

Radiologic Clinics of North America also published in Greek Paschalidis Medical Publications, Athens, Greece.

Radiologic Clinics of North America is covered in *MEDLINE/PubMed (Index Medicus), EMBASE/Excerpta Medica, Current Contents/Life Sciences, Current Contents/Clinical Medicine, RSNA Index to Imaging Literature, BIOSIS, Science Citation Index,* and *ISI/BIOMED*.

Printed in the United States of America.

Contributors

CONSULTING EDITOR

FRANK H. MILLER, MD
Chief, Body Imaging Section and Fellowship
Program; Medical Director of MRI; Professor,
Department of Radiology, Northwestern
University Feinberg School of Medicine,
Chicago, Illinois

EDITOR

SARAH M. FRIEDEWALD, MD
Assistant Professor, Feinberg School of
Medicine, Northwestern University, Lynn Sage
Comprehensive Breast Center, Chicago,
Illinois

AUTHORS

LORA D. BARKE, DO
Division of Breast Imaging, Radiology
Imaging Associates and Invision Sally Jobe,
Englewood, Colorado

LAURA BILLADELLO, MD
Assistant Professor, Department of Radiology,
Saint Louis University, St Louis, Missouri

MELISSA A. DURAND, MD, MS
Department of Diagnostic Radiology and
Biomedical Imaging, Yale University School of
Medicine, New Haven, Connecticut

PETER R. EBY, MD
Chief of Breast Imaging, Department of
Radiology, Virginia Mason Medical Center,
Seattle, Washington

PHOEBE E. FREER, MD
Associate Professor of Radiology, Department
of Radiology and Imaging Sciences, University
of Utah Hospital and Huntsman Cancer
Institute, Salt Lake City, Utah

MARY E. FREIVOGEL, MS, CGC
Division of Breast Imaging, Radiology Imaging
Associates and Invision Sally Jobe,
Englewood, Colorado

SARAH M. FRIEDEWALD, MD
Assistant Professor, Feinberg School of
Medicine, Northwestern University, Lynn Sage
Comprehensive Breast Center, Chicago,
Illinois

DIPTI GUPTA, MD
Assistant Professor, Department of Radiology,
Feinberg School of Medicine, Northwestern
University, Chicago, Illinois

MARY K. HAYES, MD
Chief, Women's Imaging, Radiology
Associates of Hollywood-Sheridan,
Department of Radiology, Memorial
Healthcare System, Hollywood, Florida

REGINA J. HOOLEY, MD
Associate Professor, Vice Chair for Clinical
Affairs, Department of Radiology and
Biomedical Imaging, Yale University School of
Medicine, New Haven, Connecticut

BONNIE N. JOE, MD, PhD
Chief, Breast Imaging Section, Professor,
Department of Radiology and Biomedical
Imaging, University of California, San
Francisco, San Francisco, California

AMY MELSAETHER, MD
Assistant Professor, Department of Radiology,
New York University School of Medicine,
New York, New York

LINDA MOY, MD
Professor, Department of Radiology, Center for
Advanced Imaging Innovation and Research
(CAI(2)R), New York University School of
Medicine, New York, New York

STEVEN POPLACK, MD
Professor of Radiology, Breast Imaging
Section, Mallinckrodt Institute of Radiology,
Washington University School of Medicine,
St Louis, Missouri

ELISSA R. PRICE, MD
Assistant Professor of Clinical
Radiology, Department of Radiology
and Biomedical Imaging, University of
California, San Francisco, San Francisco,
California

KIMBERLY M. RAY, MD
Assistant Professor of Clinical
Radiology, Department of Radiology
and Biomedical Imaging, University of
California, San Francisco, San Francisco,
California

LILIAN C. WANG, MD
Assistant Professor, Department of Radiology,
Prentice Women's Hospital, Northwestern
University Feinberg School of Medicine,
Chicago, Illinois

NICOLE WINKLER, MD
Assistant Professor of Radiology,
Department of Radiology and Imaging
Sciences, University of Utah Hospital and
Huntsman Cancer Institute, Salt Lake City,
Utah

Contents

A large body of evidence demonstrates a 30% to 50% mortality benefit of screening mammography for women aged 40 to 49. Because of more rapid cancer growth rates in younger women, annual screening is more effective than biennial. Studies indicate that selective screening of women aged 40 to 49 would miss the majority of breast cancers. If implemented, recent US Preventive Services Task Force breast cancer screening guidelines, which recommend against routine screening of women in their 40s, could result in thousands of preventable breast cancer deaths per year. Vigilance is needed to safeguard younger women's access to screening mammography.

The American College of Radiology, American Cancer Society, and US Preventive Services Task Force agree that mammography screening beginning at age 40 saves more lives than any other strategy. Despite these seemingly concordant summaries of the benefits of screening mammography, there are persistent debates regarding when to start and how often women should participate. Costs of screening, both monetary and personal, comprise the foundation of arguments against screening. This article specifically explores the evidence related to screening intervals and attempts to answer the question: should women be screened annually or biennially?

It is important to recognize that patients at high risk for breast cancer may benefit by following breast cancer screening paradigms that are more robust than those recommended for the average-risk population. Assessing individual cancer risk and using guidelines to determine if a patient is a candidate for genetic counseling and possibly genetic testing are essential components to comprehensive breast cancer screening.

In the last 20 years, there has been rapid evolution of the clinical research on digital breast tomosynthesis supporting its adoption in clinical breast imaging practice. Beginning with proof of principle pilot observational studies and culminating in prospective population-based screening trials and outcome reporting from clinical practice, there is a wealth of data on the DBT technology. This article catalogs the scientific and clinical evidence of DBT, highlighting some of the most important studies that have been reported to date.

Video content accompanies this article at http://www.radiologic.theclinics.com/.

Digital breast tomosynthesis (DBT) is rapidly becoming the new standard of care for breast cancer screening. DBT has improved on the limitations of traditional digital mammography by increasing cancer detection and decreasing false-positive examinations. Interpretation of DBT is slightly different than digital mammography and therefore experience with the technology is paramount to achieve best performance. Examples of malignancies that should be recalled and benign findings that are safely called as benign are provided in this article. Additionally, practical interpretation methods and implementation protocols are explained.

 Video content accompanies this article at http://www.radiologic.theclinics.com/.

Synthesized mammography (SM) is a new imaging technique similar to digital mammography constructed from an acquired digital breast tomosynthesis (DBT) examination. SM allows for widespread screening using DBT, maintaining the benefits of DBT while decreasing the radiation of DBT by nearly half. This article reviews studies evaluating SM, most of which suggest that SM may be appropriate to use clinically to replace an actual acquired conventional 2-dimensional full-field digital mammogram (FFDM) when using DBT for breast cancer screening. These results should be interpreted with caution because there are inherent differences between SM and FFDM image quality and lesion visibility and larger, more robust studies still need to be performed.

Breast density inform legislation is widely accepted in the United States and has fueled research regarding the clinical significance of dense breast tissue present on mammography and the value of supplemental screening. This article reviews the origins and current status of breast density inform laws and strategies for optimal breast density determination. Clinical evidence that dense breast tissue is associated with increased breast cancer risk is presented, together with a review of relative risk compared with other risk factors. Finally, there is in-depth analysis regarding the rationale, benefits, and risks of supplemental screening modalities, including ultrasound, tomosynthesis, and MRI.

Whole-breast screening ultrasonography is being increasingly implemented in breast imaging centers because numerous studies have shown the benefit of supplemental screening for women with dense breasts and breast density notification laws are becoming more widespread. This article reviews the numerous considerations involved in integrating a screening ultrasonography program into a busy practice.

The role of breast MR imaging in preoperative evaluation of disease extent remains controversial. MR imaging increases detection of mammographically occult ipsilateral and contralateral disease, but the clinical impact of these incidental cancers in unknown. There are no randomized trials of recurrence or mortality as the primary end point. This missing evidence is needed before the role of extent of disease MR imaging can be outlined. There are specific clinical scenarios in which breast MR imaging plays a clear role. In most cases, the decision to obtain MR imaging depends on physician practice style and patient preference.

Breast MR imaging is the most sensitive modality for breast cancer detection. This high sensitivity has led to widespread adoption of this technique, particularly in screening women at elevated risk for breast cancer. Despite its high sensitivity, standard breast MR imaging protocols are limited by moderate specificity and relative higher cost, longer examination time, longer interpretation time, and lower availability compared with mammography and ultrasound. As such, new techniques in MR imaging, including abbreviated breast MR imaging, pharmacokinetic modeling, and diffusion-weighted imaging, are active areas of research. This article discusses the rationale, current evidence, and limitations of these new MR imaging techniques.

Breast and whole-body PET/MR imaging is being used to detect local and metastatic disease and is being investigated for potential imaging biomarkers, which may eventually help personalize treatments and prognoses. This article provides an overview of breast and whole-body PET/MR exam techniques, summarizes PET and MR breast imaging for lesion detection, outlines investigations into multi-parametric breast PET/MR, looks at breast PET/MR in the setting of neo-adjuvant chemotherapy, and reviews the pros and cons of whole-body PET/MR in the setting of metastatic or suspected metastatic breast cancer.

▶ Video content accompanies this article at http://www.radiologic.theclinics.com.

The radiologist plays an important role in detection, diagnosis, localization, pathologic correlation, and follow-up imaging of breast cancer. A successful breast surgical treatment program relies on the image guidance tools and skills of the radiologist and surgeon. This article reviews the evolving tools available for preoperative localization. Non–wire devices provide a safe, efficient, noninferior alternative to wire localization and can be placed 0 to 30 days before scheduled surgery. This technology may evolve to other longer-term, efficient, and cost-effective applications for patients who require neoadjuvant treatment or who have findings visible only at MR imaging.

PROGRAM OBJECTIVE

The objective of the *Radiologic Clinics of North America* is to keep practicing radiologists and radiology residents up to date with current clinical practice in radiology by providing timely articles reviewing the state of the art in patient care.

TARGET AUDIENCE

Practicing radiologists, radiology residents, and other health care professionals who provide patient care utilizing radiologic findings.

LEARNING OBJECTIVES

Upon completion of this activity, participants will be able to:
1. Review evidence supporting routine breast cancer screening.
2. Discuss evolving topics in breast PET/MRI.
3. Recognize current and developing imaging techniques in breast cancer screening.

ACCREDITATION

The Elsevier Office of Continuing Medical Education (EOCME) is accredited by the Accreditation Council for Continuing Medical Education (ACCME) to provide continuing medical education for physicians.

The EOCME designates this enduring material for a maximum of 15 *AMA PRA Category 1 Credit*(s)™. Physicians should claim only the credit commensurate with the extent of their participation in the activity.

All other health care professionals requesting continuing education credit for this enduring material will be issued a certificate of participation.

DISCLOSURE OF CONFLICTS OF INTEREST

The EOCME assesses conflict of interest with its instructors, faculty, planners, and other individuals who are in a position to control the content of CME activities. All relevant conflicts of interest that are identified are thoroughly vetted by EOCME for fair balance, scientific objectivity, and patient care recommendations. EOCME is committed to providing its learners with CME activities that promote improvements or quality in healthcare and not a specific proprietary business or a commercial interest.

The planning committee, staff, authors and editors listed below have identified no financial relationships or relationships to products or devices they or their spouse/life partner have with commercial interest related to the content of this CME activity:

Lora D. Barke, DO; Laura Billadello, MD; Anjali Fortna; Phoebe E. Freer, MD; Mary E. Freivogel, MS, CGC; Dipti Gupta, MD; Mary K. Hayes, MD; Bonnie N. Joe, MD, PhD; Amy Melsaether, MD; Linda Moy, MD; Steven Poplack, MD; Elissa R. Price, MD; Kimberly M. Ray, MD; Karthik Subramaniam; John Vassallo; Lillian C. Wang, MD; Katie Widmeier; Amy Williams; Nicole Winkler, MD.

The planning committee, staff, authors and editors listed below have identified financial relationships or relationships to products or devices they or their spouse/life partner have with commercial interest related to the content of this CME activity:

Melissa A. Durand, MD, MS has research support from Hologic, Inc.
Peter R. Eby, MD is a consultant/advisor for Leica Biosystems Nussloch GmbH.
Sarah M. Friedewald, MD is a consultant/advisor for, and has research support from Hologic, Inc., and her spouse/partner is a consultant/advisor for Creative Group, Inc; Novartis AG; Sanofi; and Transplant Genomics, and has stock ownership in Transplant Genomics.
Regina J. Hooley, MD is a consultant/advisor for Hologic, Inc.

UNAPPROVED/OFF-LABEL USE DISCLOSURE

The EOCME requires CME faculty to disclose to the participants:
1. When products or procedures being discussed are off-label, unlabelled, experimental, and/or investigational (not US Food and Drug Administration [FDA] approved); and
2. Any limitations on the information presented, such as data that are preliminary or that represent ongoing research, interim analyses, and/or unsupported opinions. Faculty may discuss information about pharmaceutical agents that is outside of FDA-approved labelling. This information is intended solely for CME and is not intended to promote off-label use of these medications. If you have any questions, contact the medical affairs department of the manufacturer for the most recent prescribing information.

TO ENROLL

To enroll in the PET Clinics Continuing Medical Education program, call customer service at 1-800-654-2452 or sign up online at http://www.theclinics.com/home/cme. The CME program is available to subscribers for an additional annual fee of USD $315.

METHOD OF PARTICIPATION

In order to claim credit, participants must complete the following:

1. Complete enrolment as indicated above.
2. Read the activity.
3. Complete the CME Test and Evaluation. Participants must achieve a score of 70% on the test. All CME Tests and Evaluations must be completed online.

CME INQUIRIES/SPECIAL NEEDS

For all CME inquiries or special needs, please contact elsevierCME@elsevier.com.

RADIOLOGIC CLINICS OF NORTH AMERICA

ISSUE OF RELATED INTEREST

Magnetic Resonance Imaging Clinics of North America
November 2015 (Vol. 23, Issue 4)
MR-Guided Interventions
Clare M.C. Tempany and Tina Kapur, *Editors*
Available at: http://www.mri.theclinics.com

THE CLINICS ARE AVAILABLE ONLINE!
Access your subscription at:
www.theclinics.com

Preface
Breast Imaging

 CrossMark

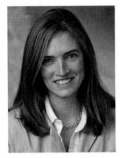

Sarah M. Friedewald, MD
Editor

Breast imaging has increasingly come under scrutiny, not only due to the economic climate of our society and the intense focus on cutting health care costs but also because of the perceived "harms" associated with screening mammography. Faulty assumptions and propagation of misinformation have led some to reach erroneous conclusions. It is unfortunate that an accessible, low-cost, imaging modality that has repeatedly been shown to decrease breast cancer deaths has become controversial.

However, despite these obstacles, the field of breast imaging has accelerated. Rapid adoption of improved technologies such as digital breast tomosynthesis, automated whole breast ultrasound, and abbreviated breast MR will contribute to better patient outcomes. Alternative ways to localize lesions preoperatively will improve patient comfort and satisfaction. Combining modalities such as PET and MR to maximize useful information while minimizing background noise is at the very center of precision medicine.

The resolve of those who know the data to educate and promote breast cancer screening has been indefatigable. It is our duty as researchers, educators, and clinicians to understand the science, teach our colleagues, and be advocates for breast imaging. We are truly lucky to have the life's work of the leaders in our field to be the foundation upon which we build. By promoting early detection, refining current practice, and exploring new technologies, we will ultimately save lives.

Sarah M. Friedewald, MD
Feinberg School of Medicine
Northwestern University
Prentice Women's Hospital
Lynn Sage Comprehensive Breast Center
250 East Superior Street
Room 4-2304
Chicago, IL 60611, USA

E-mail address:
sarah.friedewald@nm.org

Radiol Clin N Am 55 (2017) xi
http://dx.doi.org/10.1016/j.rcl.2017.02.001
0033-8389/17/© 2017 Published by Elsevier Inc.

Evidence to Support Screening Women in Their 40s

Kimberly M. Ray, MD*, Elissa R. Price, MD,
Bonnie N. Joe, MD, PhD

KEYWORDS

• Mammography • Screening • 40 to 49 • Evidence • Controversy

KEY POINTS

- A large body of evidence demonstrates a 30% to 50% mortality benefit of screening mammography for women aged 40 to 49.
- Because of more rapid cancer growth rates in younger women, annual screening is more effective than biennial.
- Selective screening of women aged 40 to 49 based on risk factors to minimize harms would miss the majority of breast cancers.
- If implemented, recent US Preventive Services Task Force (USPSTF) breast cancer screening guidelines, which recommend against routine screening of women in their 40s, could result in thousands of preventable breast cancer deaths per year.

BREAST CANCER DISEASE BURDEN IN WOMEN AGED 40 TO 49

The incidence of breast cancer in the United States increases significantly at approximately age 40 and rises steadily with increasing age thereafter. Based on 2009 to 2013 data from the Surveillance, Epidemiology, and End Results Program of the National Institutes of Health, the annual incidence rises from approximately 0.3 to 0.6 per 1000 women between ages 30 to 39 to 1.2 to 1.9 per 1000 between the ages of 40 and 49, subsequently increasing to 2.2 to 2.6 for women aged 50 to 59 and 3.4 to 4.2 for women aged 60 to 69.[1] In 2015, there were 48,160 women aged 40 to 49 diagnosed with breast cancer in the United States, which accounts for approximately 17%, or 1 in 6, of all breast cancer diagnoses.[2] Moreover, an estimated 40% of the years of life lost to breast cancer can be attributed to women diagnosed while in their 40s.[3] Thus the breast cancer disease burden among women aged 40 to 49 is substantial.

EFFICACY AND EFFECTIVENESS OF SCREENING MAMMOGRAPHY IN WOMEN AGED 40 TO 49

Multiple study types exist to assess the impact of a screening study. The most rigorous and informative studies, randomized controlled trials (RCTs) and observational studies, deserve particular attention.

Randomized Controlled Trials — Overview

The underlying premise of screening is that early detection and treatment can interrupt the natural history of a disease and prevent a patient's death. Early diagnosis per se, however, does not

Disclosures: None of the authors have any interests to disclose.
Department of Radiology and Biomedical Imaging, University of California, San Francisco, 1600 Divisadero Street, Room C250, Mail Box 1667, San Francisco, CA 94115, USA
* Corresponding author.
E-mail address: kimberly.ray@ucsf.edu

Radiol Clin N Am 55 (2017) 429–439
http://dx.doi.org/10.1016/j.rcl.2016.12.002

necessarily guarantee a benefit. Merely finding a cancer earlier may not alter its long-term outcome. A screened patient may seem to have longer survival relative to the unscreened, but this could reflect earlier diagnosis without a corresponding delay in the time of death. Such a phenomenon is referred to as lead-time bias. In addition, screening may preferentially detect some indolent lesions, a phenomenon referred to as length-biased sampling. Because of these potential biases, the only way to prove efficacy of a screening test is to evaluate mortality as an endpoint in the setting of a RCT.

Seven population-based RCTs of screening mammography alone or in combination with physical examination were conducted in the United States and Europe from the 1960s to 1980s, which included women aged 40 to 49 at time of trial entry. In addition, a single non–population-based RCT, the Canadian National Breast Screening Study-1 (CNBSS-1), in which women volunteered to participate, was conducted in the 1980s. Meta-analyses at 10-year to 18-year follow-up have shown statistically significant mortality reductions for women aged 40 to 49 at invitation of 24% in the 7 population-based RCTs, 29% in the 5 Swedish RCTs, and 15% to 18% in all 8 RCTs (including CNBSS-1) (**Table 1**).[4–6] At subsequent 12-year to 13-year follow-up of 2 Swedish trials, statistically significant mortality reductions of 45% and 36%, respectively, were found for women aged 39 to 49 years at randomization in the Gothenburg breast screening trial and for women aged 45 to 49 years at entry in the Malmö mammographic screening program trial (see **Table 1**).[7–9]

Table 1
Randomized controlled trials of screening mammography showing statistically significant breast cancer mortality reduction on long-term follow-up for women aged 40 to 49 years

Trial	Follow-up (y)	Mortality Reduction (%)[a]
All 8 RCTs	10.5–18.0	15–18
7 RCTs (excluding CNBSS-1)	7.0–18.0	24
5 Swedish trials	11.4–15.2	29
Gothenburg, Sweden	12.0	45
Malmö, Sweden	12.7	36

[a] Statistically significant mortality reduction at 95% CI.

Randomized Controlled Trial Controversy

Controversy first arose over screening of women in their 40s when a retrospective subgroup analysis was performed for the first RCT, the Health Insurance Plan (HIP) trial of New York, conducted in the 1960s. Using age 50 as a surrogate for menopause, the investigators evaluated mortality benefit separately for women aged 40 to 49 and 50 to 64. Initial results at 4 years' follow-up (an extremely short follow-up interval) failed to show a statistically significant benefit for women aged 40 to 49 as there was for women aged 50 to 64.[10] At 18 years of follow-up, a 23% mortality reduction was seen for the 40 to 49 age group, the same relative benefit as for women aged 50 to 64; however, the benefit for women aged 40 to 49 remained statistically insignificant.[10]

The lack of a statistically significant benefit for women aged 40 to 49 was due to the fact that there were not enough women in this age group enrolled in the study to provide the statistical power to detect a benefit.[11] A larger study population was needed given the lower incidence of breast cancer in this age group. Unfortunately, the lack of a statistically significant benefit was erroneously interpreted by many as proof that there was no benefit.[12]

None of the RCTs was designed to evaluate the effectiveness of screening for women aged 40 to 49 years. Therefore, early subset analyses for this age group did not find a statistically significant benefit. Longer-term follow-up, however, eventually compensated for the lack of statistical power. In 1997, after 10-year to 18-year follow-up, meta-analysis of 5 Swedish RCTs yielded a statistically significant 29% mortality reduction for women aged 40 to 49, which was the same relative benefit as for older women.[6] Several individual trials also demonstrated a statistically significant mortality reduction for the 40 to 49 age group, ranging from 23% in a reanalysis of the HIP trial at 18 years of follow-up to 36% to 45% for the Swedish Malmö and Gothenburg trials at 12 years to 13 years of follow-up.[7–9]

Canadian National Breast Screening Study

The CNBSS-1 trial warrants particular attention and review. After the HIP trial, CNBSS-1 was launched in 1980, specifically designed to address the efficacy of screening mammography for women in their 40s. The CNBSS-1 allocated (or randomized) 50,430 female volunteers aged 40 to 49 to undergo annual mammography, clinical breast examination, and breast self-examination; or usual care. After 11 to 16 years of follow-up, the investigators reported no reduction in breast cancer mortality.[13]

Analysis of the CNBSS-1 trial revealed serious flaws and deviations from sound scientific methodology. First, although claiming to be an RCT, rather than undergoing blinded randomization, the study volunteers had clinical breast examinations performed by the trial staff. Study organizers were not blinded to the results of physical examination when they assigned women to either the study or control group. There are indications that allocation was likely biased by this information given that there were more women with advanced-stage, node-positive cancers in the screening group than in the control group at trial entry. As a consequence, there were actually more cancer deaths in the screened group compared with the control group.[14,15]

Another major criticism of the CNBSS-1 is that the mammographic technique was poor. No training had been provided for the study technologists or radiologists, and external expert reviewers deemed the examinations technically inadequate.[16] The study's own reference physicist noted that the examinations were "far below state of the art, even for that time (early 1980s)."[17,18]

The combination of these factors severely compromised the CNBSS-1 and help explain why the CNBSS-1 is an outlier as the only RCT that failed to demonstrate any benefit from screening for any age group. Thus, including CNBSS-1 results in RCT analyses diminishes the true benefit of screening.

Age Trial

In 1991, the UK Age trial[19] was undertaken to re-evaluate the impact of screening women in their 40s. A total of 160,921 women aged 39 to 41 were randomized to the treatment group, which consisted of an invitation to undergo annual mammography until the age of 48 or the control group with no invitation to screening. Both the intervention group and the control group then commenced triannual screening at age 50 in accordance with national policy. In contrast to the preceding RCTs, screening in the treatment group was terminated before age 50 so as not to confound the results with benefits accrued from screening after age 50. After a median follow-up of 17.7 years, there was a nonsignificant 12% reduction in mortality.[19]

Although the UK Age trial demonstrated a mortality benefit, the investigators themselves acknowledged that the benefit would likely have been greater if certain conditions had been met.[19] Specifically, single-view mammography

was performed in the trial after the first screen, despite knowledge that 2-view mammography would increase the rate of early cancer detection. Literature from the United Kingom suggests single-view mammography results in 20% to 25% of cancers being missed.[20] Additionally, a lower threshold for biopsy of microcalcifications would have resulted in an increase in cancer detection. An analysis of the false-negative interval cancers during the trial revealed calcifications to be the most common imaging feature. The rate of ductal carcinoma in situ detection was 3 times lower than for the current UK national screening program.

Limitations of Randomized Controlled Trials

RCTs have consistently demonstrated an 18% to 29% mortality reduction related to screening women aged 40 to 49.[4–6] These types of trials, however, still underestimate the mortality benefit of screening for several reasons. Not all women who are invited to be screened actually participate (noncompliance). If any of the invited women who were not screened die from breast cancer, their deaths are counted against the screened group, even though the woman never received the intervention. In addition, some women who are randomized to the control group actually pursue screening outside of the trial (contamination). These women have improved survival because they were screened but are counted in the control group. These effects are substantial; in the screening RCTs, there was a 10% to 39% noncompliance rate and 13% to 25% contamination rate.[21] To avoid selection bias, adjustments cannot be made for noncompliance or contamination. Consequently, the actual benefit of screening is underestimated.

The benefit of screening mammography in the modern era is also likely to exceed that shown in the RCTs because there have been significant improvements in mammographic technique and performance standards since the 1970s. In the RCTs, women were mostly screened with single-view mammography, whereas the current standard is to perform 2 views, which increases cancer detection by up to 20%.[20,22] Improvements in mammographic technique include, for example, the introduction of mammographic grids, newer target materials, and automatic exposure control. Further improvement in performance in younger women with dense breasts was seen with the transition from film screen to digital mammography. Even more recently, improvements in cancer detection have been seen in women who are screened with digital breast tomosynthesis (DBT), which may translate into fewer deaths from breast cancer. Lastly, screening intervals in the RCTs were long, ranging from 24 to 33 months in all except the HIP trial. Annual screening yields a greater benefit, particularly for younger women, whose cancers have faster growth rates.[23–25] According to estimates by Tabar and colleagues,[25] the lead time—defined as the interval during which a cancer remains clinically undetectable—is 1.7 years for women aged 40 to 49. For screening to be effective the screening interval must be shorter than the lead time.

Evidence from Observational Studies

RCTs are the gold standard for showing the benefit of screening mammography. Because of the limitations, discussed previously, however, RCTs underestimate the true benefit of screening. Therefore, observational studies are an alternative approach to determine the true effectiveness of screening. Service screening, where all eligible women receive invitation letters to attend screening, was initiated in Europe and Canada after the RCTs and provide this type of population data on outcomes of screening in women aged 40 to 49.

In Sweden, Tabar and colleagues[26] compared breast cancer mortality rates in 2 counties among women aged 40 to 49 in the 20 years before (1958–77) and 20 years after (1978–97) the introduction of screening. There were mortality reductions of 48% for women aged 40 to 49 years and 44% for all women aged 40 to 69 years. In British Columbia, Coldman and colleagues[27] published a large study documenting outcomes of 7 Canadian screening programs, which encompassed 85% of the Canadian population of more than 2.7 million women. From 1990 through 2009, there was a 39% mortality reduction among women aged 40 to 49 years versus 40% for all women aged 40 to 79 years.

Hellquist and colleagues[28] published a study of service screening that encompassed the entire population of women aged 40 to 49 living in Sweden from 1986 to 2005. Breast cancer mortality rates were compared between counties that invited women to screening and those that did not. After 16 years of follow-up, there was an overall 29% mortality reduction in women who were screened. Because treatment across the country was standardized through the Swedish national health care system, the differences in mortality likely reflected the impact of screening rather than varying treatment regimens.

Taken together, observational studies of screening mammography predict greater mortality reductions for women aged 40 to 49 than the RCTs with similar screening intervals and have demonstrated a similar magnitude of mortality reduction for women age 40 to 49 as for those over age 50.

US PREVENTIVE SERVICES TASK FORCE CONTROVERSY

In November 2009, the USPSTF issued updated guidelines in which they recommended against routine mammographic screening of women aged 40 to 49 years for the average-risk population. The USPSTF argued that the relative benefit of screening for younger women was less than that for women over 50 and did not outweigh the potential harms. They qualified their recommendation, however, by saying if screening were to be initiated prior to age 50, the decision should be an individual one, with discussion about the benefits versus the harms with the referring provider.[29]

Using data from the RCTs, the USPSTF estimated a breast cancer mortality reduction of only 15% for women aged 40 to 59 years compared with a reduction of 32% for women aged 60 to 69 years. The USPSTF estimates of the mortality benefit are low because they included the significantly flawed CNBSS-1 trial, which found no benefit from screening of women aged 40 to 60 years. In addition, they excluded data from service screening, which demonstrated greater mortality benefit on average than the RCTs.

Similarly, the USPSTF dilutes the advantages of screening by citing the number of women needed to be invited (NNI) to screening to prevent 1 breast cancer death. Based on RCT data, they found that NNIs at ages 39 to 49, 50 to 59, and 60 to 69 years were 1904, 1339, and 377, respectively. Because not all women who were invited to screen in the RCTs were actually screened (noncompliance), these numbers underestimate the benefit. When evaluating the efficacy of mammography, the number needed to screen (NNS) is a more appropriate measure of actual performance.[30] Moreover, because of varying life expectancies of different age cohorts, the NNS per life years gained is a more complete measure of screening benefit; in particular, it permits more favorable comparisons of younger versus older women than NNS alone.[30]

The USPSTF also considered the mathematical models of the Cancer Intervention and Surveillance Modeling Network (CISNET), involving 6 independent groups in a project funded by the National Cancer Institute.[30] These models included 20 different mammographic screening protocols beginning and ending at different ages as well as involving annual versus biennial screening intervals. Averaged over the 6 models, annual screening of women aged 40 to 84 years yielded the greatest benefit, a 39.6% mortality reduction. Hendrick and Helvie[31] calculated that this protocol saves 71% more lives or approximately 6500 more lives per year than the USPSTF-recommended protocol of biennial screening of women aged 50 to 74 years, which yielded a 23.2% mortality reduction. Using CISNET modeling, Hendrick and Helvie also calculated that NNSs at ages 40 to 49, 50 to 59, and 60 to 69 years were 746, 351, and 233, respectively. These figures are substantially lower than the NNI declared by the USPSTF, which, in their opinion, were too high to support screening mammography in young women. The NNSs per life years gained in these age groups were even lower, at 28, 17, and 16, respectively.

Additionally, the USPSTF cited higher screening recall rates and false-positive biopsy rates among women aged 40 to 49 to justify their recommendation against screening in this group. Data from the Breast Cancer Surveillance Consortium indicated that the numbers of women recalled from screening to find 1 cancer at ages 40 to 49, 50 to 59, and 60 to 69 years were 47, 22, and 14, respectively. Recall rates, however, for initial prevalence screening examinations are known to be substantially higher than for subsequent incidence examinations, due to lack of prior comparisons.[32] Therefore, it is not younger age per se that is the underlying cause of a higher rate of recall, and delaying screening until age 50 would only transfer the higher recall rates to an older age group.

It is doubtful that the harms of recall outweigh the potential benefit of cancer detection. More than 90% of all recalls do not result in a recommendation for biopsy and merely involve additional mammographic views and/or ultrasound. Even when biopsy is recommended, 99% of American women considered 500 or more false-positive mammograms an acceptable tradeoff for 1 life saved.[33] Furthermore, most women consider the anxiety associated with recall and biopsy minor and short-lived.[34]

2016 UPDATE TO THE US PREVENTIVE SERVICES TASK FORCE GUIDELINES

In February 2016, the USPSTF issued an update to their screening mammography guidelines, but again gave a C rating for screening of women aged 40 to 49, concluding that the net benefit to this cohort was small. They continued to state stated that the decision to undergo screening mammography prior to age 50 should be made individually and should depend on whether a patient places greater importance on the benefits or harms.[35]

In the 2016 guidelines, the USPSTF also labeled DBT an investigational technique and was not recommended for routine screening. The American College of Radiology disputed this assessment, citing the numerous large-scale studies of DBT involving more than 200,000 women that have consistently demonstrated improvements in recall rates and cancer detection rates when DBT is used in conjunction with full-field digital mammography compared with full-field digital mammography alone.[36–41] Kopans[42] has observed the "inconsistency" of the USPSTF position on DBT, given that they would propose to withhold screening mammography from younger women in large part because of false-positive results and yet they do not support the use of DBT, which has been shown to reduce the recall rate in every study to date.

UPDATE OF AMERICAN CANCER SOCIETY GUIDELINES

In October 2015, the American Cancer Society (ACS) updated their guidelines on breast cancer screening for women at average risk.[43] The previous 2003 ACS guidelines recommended annual screening mammography for all women beginning at age 40.[44] In 2015, however, the ACS modified their recommendations for younger women to allow for individualized decision making that takes into account the both benefits and potential harms of screening.[33] For women aged 40 to 44 years, the ACS issued a "qualified recommendation" to provide the opportunity for annual screening mammography, noting that most women would choose this option. They also issued a "strong recommendation" for women to undergo regular screening mammography beginning at age 45.

Contrary to the USPSTF, the ACS cited evidence from the RCTs as well as observational studies showing similar relative benefits of screening mammography among women in their 40s and 50s. They noted, however, that the absolute benefit varies because the incidence of disease differs according to the age group. For example, the ACS noted that the 5-year risk estimates among women aged 45 to 49 years and women aged 50 to 54 years are similar (0.9% vs 1.1%) but exceed that for women aged 40 to 44 years (0.6%). The proportions of person-years of life lost were similar for women aged 45 to 49 years and 50 to 54 years at diagnosis (both approximately 15%). Therefore, the ACS concluded that the burden of disease was very similar among women aged 45 to 49 and those aged 50 to

54, which would justify similar screening regimens for both of these age groups. Because disease incidence was slightly lower for women aged 40 to 45, however, they concluded that a minority of women in this age group might reasonably elect to forego screening due to concerns about harms. The ACS noted, however, that the evidence suggests that a majority of women would still elect to begin screening at age 40. For example, Schwartz and colleagues[33] reported that nearly all (96%) of American women who experienced a false-positive mammogram were glad they underwent the test and remained supportive of screening. Similarly, women involved in the Digital Mammographic Imaging Screening Trial demonstrated only transient, limited anxiety increases after a false-positive mammogram compared with those with a negative mammogram, and there was no difference between the groups' intentions to undergo mammography in the subsequent 2 years.[45]

SCREENING INTERVALS

For screening to reduce breast cancer mortality, there must be sufficiently early detection to enable treatment to alter the course of the disease. The RCTs demonstrated that lives could be saved through the down-staging of disease achieved by earlier detection.[21] A population-based study from the Netherlands reconfirmed that tumor size and nodal status still have a significant influence on overall mortality independent of age and tumor biology, even in the era of modern therapies (2006–2012).[46]

Determination of the appropriate screening interval depends on the lead time for cancer detection, which varies according to patient age. Lead time is defined as the time difference between when a cancer can be detected at screening and when it can be detected clinically. As discussed previously, for screening mammography to be effective, the screening interval must be shorter than the lead time. Moskowitz[24] calculated the lead time in the Cincinnati Breast Cancer Detection Demonstration Project by observing how long it took the cancer detection rate to return to baseline after the cessation of screening. For women aged 35 to 49 years, the lead time was on average 2 years ± 0.5 years, whereas it was 3.5 years ± 0.5 years for women over 50. Similarly, in the Swedish Two-County trial, Tabar and colleagues[25] estimated that the lead time was 1.7 years for women aged 40 to 49 years and 2.6 to 3.8 years for women aged 50 to 74 years. Thus, for the 40 to 49 cohort, the evidence supports annual screening mammography as a 2-

year screening interval would exceed the lead time and, therefore, miss most of the faster growing cancers that tend to predominate in younger women and can be life-threatening.

The ACS examined several lines of evidence regarding the impact of annual versus biennial screening intervals. In a meta-analysis of the RCTs, for women randomized before age 50, only those screened at intervals less than 24 months had a significant reduction in breast cancer mortality.[47] The ACS also commissioned an analysis by the Breast Cancer Surveillance Consortium that found premenopausal women were more likely to have larger tumors and more advanced stage disease at diagnosis with a screening interval of 23 to 26 months compared with an interval of 11 months to 14 months.[48] Finally, the ACS cited the mathematical models of the 2009 CISNET analysis, all of which estimated that more breast cancer deaths could be averted with annual compared with biennial screening for all age groups.[49] Based on the evidence, the ACS acknowledged that annual screening yields the greatest benefit, particularly at younger ages. They noted, however, that more frequent screening is associated with more cumulative false-positive results. Thus, the ACS issued a qualified recommendation for annual screening in all women aged 45 to 54 as well as in those women aged 40 to 44 who choose to initiate screening, noting that some may choose less frequent screening to avoid false-positive results. Meanwhile, the American College of Radiology and the Society of Breast Imaging prioritize saving lives and therefore support annual screening for all women 40 and older because this strategy yields the greatest mortality benefit.[50]

OVERDIAGNOSIS

Among the potential harms of screening, both the ACS and USPSTF rate overdiagnosis as the most significant.[35,43] Overdiagnosis is defined as the identification of cancers that would not have become clinically apparent or impactful in the absence of screening. This may be due to the indolent nature of certain cancers and to a patient's competing comorbidities, which may pose a greater threat to life. Treatment of such cancers would therefore impart greater harm than benefit. Although overdiagnosis is an important conceptual problem, the reality is that in the current medical paradigm, even at the height of scientific understanding, cancers cannot be stratified into which will progress to be potentially life threatening and which will remain harmless.[51]

Estimating overdiagnosis is complex, and lead time and trends in background incidence of disease must be considered when calculating rates. Estimates have been obtained by comparing the cancer incidence during screening to the incidence after the cessation of screening, and those from 13 European service screening studies have varied widely, from 0% to 54%.[52] Puliti and colleagues[52] showed that the studies reporting high estimates of overdiagnosis failed to properly adjust for lead time. Because screening advances the time of cancer detection, there is initially an excess of cancers in the screened population. After screening stops, it takes time for the cancer incidence to return to baseline. Duffy and Parmar[53] showed that a follow-up period of approximately 25 years is necessary to sufficiently adjust for lead time. Thus in the Swedish Two-County trial, Yen and colleagues[54] found that the cumulative incidence of breast cancer was the same in the screened and control groups at 29-year follow-up. There was a nonsignificant excess of cancers among the screened group aged 70 to 74, suggesting that the degree of overdiagnosis is small and more likely to be confined to older women.

In discussing the harms of screening for women in their 40s, the USPSTF cited a high risk of over-diagnosis, estimating that at least 19% of screen detected breast cancers are overdiagnosed.[55,56] Putili and colleagues[52] demonstrated a low level of overdiagnosis (1%–10%) when appropriate adjustments for temporal trends, risk factors, and lead time were considered. Similarly, Helvie and colleagues[57] demonstrated only a small degree of overdiagnosis when required adjustments for background incidence trends are made. Moreover, overdiagnosis is more likely to affect women at the older rather than the younger end of the age spectrum. Finally, earlier initiation of screening at age 40 versus age 50 should not increase the cumulative rate of overdiagnosis because the tumors would eventually be found after screening begins, regardless of age.

RISK-BASED SCREENING

Some groups have called for selective screening of women aged 40 to 49 who are at elevated risk of developing breast cancer, with the ostensible goal of improving the balance of benefits and harms of screening. In their 2009 guidelines, the USPSTF recommended limiting screening of women aged 40 to 49 to those who were considered at "high risk."[29] In the 2016 guidelines, the USPSTF noted that women in their 40s with a history of breast cancer in a first-degree relative have the same relative risk as women aged 50 to 59

without a family history, and thus the USPSTF supported mammographic screening in this subgroup of women aged 40 to 49.[35] Schousboe and colleagues[58] proposed screening only those women aged 40 to 49 with a family history of breast cancer or a history of previous breast biopsy. van Ravesteyn and colleagues[59] recommended that women aged 40 to 49 should be screened biennially if they had a 3-fold increased risk and annually only if they had 4-fold increased risk.[60] The latter investigators suggested that this protocol would achieve the same harm-benefit ratio in women aged 40 to 49 as for women aged 50 to 74 undergoing biennial screening.

Critics of the previously described risk-based screening regimens have highlighted that 80% of women with newly diagnosed breast cancers have no significant previous risk factors.[61,62] Therefore, such regimens would be expected to miss a majority of screen detected breast cancers. Numerous retrospective studies have examined the association between risk factors and the development of breast cancer in women aged 40 to 49. These studies showed that approximately 60% to 80% of women aged 40 to 49 with breast cancer lacked any family history and approximately 80% to 90% lacked a first-degree relative with breast cancer.[63–66]

In a meta-analysis of breast cancer risk factors among women aged 40 to 49, Nelson and colleagues[66] showed that the only risk factors that would confer a 2-fold higher relative risk were a first-degree family history or extremely dense breast tissue. In a recent retrospective study at University of California, San Francisco, Price and colleagues[67] showed that a very strong family history was absent in 88% of screen detected breast cancer cases and extremely dense tissue was absent in 86% of cases. Of all patients with screen-detected malignancies, 76% had neither very strong family history nor extremely dense breasts. In summary, all the studies to date are highly concordant in finding that a majority of breast cancers arise in women without special risk factors; this holds true for women in their 40s and beyond. Therefore, limiting screening to only women aged 40 to 49 at elevated risk would eliminate most of the benefit and endanger many young lives.

COST ANALYSIS

With the adoption of the Affordable Care Act in 2010, there has been increasing interest in reducing national health care expenditures. Analyses of the costs of screening mammography have evaluated the potential savings due to more limited screening strategies. For example, O'Donoghue and colleagues[68] estimated the costs associated with 3 different screening strategies: annual (ages 40–84 years), biennial (ages 50–69 years), and USPSTF (high-risk ages 40–49 years, biennial ages 50–74 years). The annual cost for each of these plans was estimated at $10.1 billion, $2.6 billion, and $3.5 billion, respectively. The investigators failed to acknowledge, however, that screening costs are offset by savings due to down-staging of disease and a concomitant decrease in the need for aggressive treatments, such as extensive surgery and chemotherapy.[69] A recent analysis by Blumen and colleagues[70] evaluated the stage-dependent cost of breast cancer treatment of a commercially insured population of women with newly diagnosed breast cancer. The average cost per patient in the year after diagnosis was 58% greater for stage III ($129,387) than for stage I/II ($82,121) disease, and this cost differential was primarily due to chemotherapy costs.

In a 1994 study, Rosenquist and Lindfors[71] estimated a cost per life year gained of $26,000 for women aged 40 to 49 compared with $20,000 for women aged 60 to 69, assuming a 30% mortality reduction through annual screening mammography. Although the initial costs of screening are higher for younger women, these costs are counterbalanced by the greater life expectancy of younger women compared with their older counterparts. Even when the analysis of Rosenquist and Lindfors is adjusted for the current costs of mammography, the estimates still fall well below the $100,000 per year of life threshold that is commonly accepted for preventive tests.[72]

Finally, continued technological advances show promise to further deliver value-based care. A recent economic modeling study of DBT within a hypothetical US-managed care plan reported an overall $28.53 savings per woman screened.[73] The cost savings were due to the reduction in the number of women recalled for additional imaging and invasive testing as well as the down-staging of disease through earlier detection, leading to reduced treatment costs.

SUMMARY

There is a large body of evidence demonstrating a 30% to 50% mortality benefit of screening mammography for women aged 40 to 49. The magnitude of the mortality benefit is equal to that for women over 50. Because of more rapid cancer growth rates in younger women and shorter average lead-times, annual screening has been shown more effective than biennial screening.

Critics of mammography have overemphasized the potential harms of screening relative to the life-saving benefits. Research has shown that a vast majority of women are highly tolerant of false-positive results, which in most instances merely consist of additional imaging. The best available evidence indicates that fewer than 10% of breast cancers are overdiagnosed. Meanwhile, ample studies indicate that selective screening of women based on risk factors to minimize the harms would miss the majority of breast cancers. Most women find the modest risks of screening acceptable tradeoffs for the far greater benefit of early detection, which means a lesser chance of dying from breast cancer and a reduced need for aggressive and toxic treatments.

If implemented, the recent USPSTF breast cancer screening guidelines, which recommend against routine screening of women in their 40s, could result in thousands of preventable breast cancer deaths per year. The 2015 Congressional Protecting Access to Lifesaving Screenings Act (PALS Act, H.R. 3339) places a 2-year moratorium on implementation of the USPSTF recommendations on breast cancer screening and mandates insurance coverage for mammography for women in their 40s. Continued vigilance is necessary, however, to safeguard women's access to lifesaving technology.

REFERENCES

1. Howlader N, Noone AM, Krapcho M, et al, editors. SEER Cancer Statistics Review, 1975-2013. Bethesda (MD): National Cancer Institute. Available at: http://seer.cancer.gov/csr/1975_2013/. Based on November 2015 SEER data submission, Accessed May 1, 2016.
2. American Cancer Society. Breast cancer facts & figures 2015-2016. 2015. Available at: http://www.cancer.org/acs/groups/content/@research/documents/document/acspc-046381.pdf. Accessed May 1, 2016.
3. Shapiro S, Venet W, Strax P, et al. Periodic screening for breast cancer, the health insurance plan project and its sequelae 1963-1976. Baltimore (MD): Johns Hopkins University Press; 1988.
4. Smart CR, Hendrick RE, Rutledge JH, et al. Benefit of mammography screening in women ages 40 to 49 years: current evidence from randomized controlled trials. Cancer 1995;75:1619–26 [Erratum appears in Cancer 1995;75:2788].
5. Falun Meeting Committee and Collaborators. Breast-cancer screening with mammography in women aged 40-49 years. Swedish Cancer Society and the Swedish National Board of Health and Welfare. Int J Cancer 1996;68:693–9.

6. Hendrick RE, Smith RA, Rutledge JH, et al. Benefit of screening mammography in women aged 40-49: a new meta-analysis of randomized controlled trials. J Natl Cancer Inst Monogr 1997;22:87–92.

7. Andersson I, Janzon L. Reduced breast cancer mortality in women under 50: updated results from the Malmö Mammographic Screening Program. J Natl Cancer Inst Monogr 1997;22:63–8.

8. Bjurstam N, Bjorneld L, Duffy SW, et al. The Gothenburg breast screening trial: first results on mortality, incidence, and mode of detection for women ages 39-49 years at randomization. Cancer 1997;80: 2091–9.

9. Bjurstam J, Bjorneld L, Warwick J, et al. The Gothenburg Breast Screening Trial. Cancer 2003; 97:2387–96.

10. Shapiro S, Venet W, Strax P, et al. Periodic screening for breast cancer, the health insurance plan project and its sequelae 1963-1986. Baltimore (MD): Johns Hopkins University Press; 1988.

11. Kopans DB, Halpern E, Hulka CA. Statistical power in breast cancer screening trials and mortality reduction among women 40–49 with particular emphasis on the National Breast Screening Study of Canada. Cancer 1994;74:1196–203.

12. Fletcher SW, Black W, Harris R, et al. Report of the International Workshop on Screening for Breast Cancer. J Natl Cancer Inst 1993;85:1644–56.

13. Miller AB, To T, Baines CJ, et al. The Canadian National Breast Screening Study-1: breast cancer mortality after 11 to 16 years of follow-up. A randomized screening trial of mammography in women age 40 to 49 years. Ann Intern Med 2002; 137:305–12.

14. Kopans DB, Feig SA. The Canadian National Breast Screening Study: a critical review. AJR Am J Roentgenol 1993;161:755–60.

15. Boyd NF, Jong RA, Yaffe MJ, et al. A critical appraisal of the Canadian National Breast Cancer Screening Study. Radiology 1993;189(3):661–3.

16. Baines CJ, Miller AB, Kopans DB, et al. Canadian National Breast Screening Study: assessment of technical quality by external review. AJR Am J Roentgenol 1990;155(4):743–7 [discussion: 748–9].

17. Yaffe MJ. Correction: Canada study [letter]. J Natl Cancer Inst 1993;85:94.

18. de Koning HJ, Boer R, Warmerdam PG, et al. Quantitative interpretation of age-specific mortality reductions from the Swedish breast cancer-screening trials. J Natl Cancer Inst 1995;87:1217–23.

19. Moss SM, Wale C, Smith R, et al. Effect of mammographic screening from age 40 years on breast cancer mortality in the UK Age trial at 17 years' follow-up: a randomised controlled trial. Lancet Oncol 2015;16:1123–32.

20. Wald NJ, Murphy P, Major P, et al. UKCCCR multicentre randomized controlled trial of one and two view mammography in breast cancer screening. BMJ 1995;311:1189–93.

21. Feig SA. Screening Mammography Benefit Controversies Sorting the Evidence. Radiol Clin North Am 2014;52:455–80.

22. Tabar L, Vitak B, Chem JJ, et al. The Swedish two-county trial twenty years later. Radiol Clin North Am 2000;38:625–52.

23. Feig SA. Determination of mammographic screening intervals with surrogate measures forwomen aged 40-49 years. Radiology 1994;193:311–4.

24. Moskowitz M. Breast cancer: age specific growth rates and screening strategies. Radiology 1986; 161:37–41.

25. Tabar L, Fagerberg G, Day NE, et al. What is the optimum interval between screening examination? An analysis based on the latest results of the Swedish Two-County Breast Cancer Screening trial. Br J Cancer 1987;55:47–51.

26. Tabar L, Yen MF, Vitak B, et al. Mammography service screening and mortality in breast cancer patients: 20-year follow-up before and after introduction of screening. Lancet 2003;361:1405–10.

27. Coldman A, Phillips N, Warren L, et al. Breast cancer mortality after screening mammography in British Columbia women. Int J Cancer 2007;120:1076–80.

28. Hellquist BN, Duffy SW, Abdsaleh S, et al. Effectiveness of populations-based service screening with mammography for women ages 40-49 years: evaluation of the Swedish Mammography Screening in Young Women (SCRY) cohort. Cancer 2011;117: 714–22.

29. US Preventive Services Task Force. Screening for breast cancer: US Preventive Services Task Force recommendation statement. Ann Intern Med 2009; 151:716–26.

30. Mandelblatt JS, Stout NK, Schechter CB, et al. Collaborative Modeling of the Benefits and Harms Associated With Different U.S. Breast Cancer Screening Strategies. Ann Intern Med 2016;164: 215–25.

31. Hendrick RE, Helvie MA. Mammography screening: a new estimate of number needed to screen to prevent one breast cancer death. AJR Am J Roentgenol 2012;198(3):723–8.

32. Frankel SD, Sickles EA, Cupren BN, et al. Initial versus subsequent screening mammography: comparison of findings and their prognostic significance. AJR Am J Roentgenol 1995;164:1107–9.

33. Schwartz LM, Woloshin S, Fowler FJ Jr, et al. Enthusiasm for cancer screening in the United States. JAMA 2004;291(1):71–8.

34. Schwartz LM, Woloshin S, Sox HC, et al. US women's attitudes to false-positive mammography results and detection of ductal carcinoma in situ: cross-sectional survey. West J Med 2000; 173(5):307–12.

35. Siu AL. Screening for Breast Cancer: U.S. Preventive Services Task Force Recommendation Statement. Ann Intern Med 2016;164:279–96.

36. Available at: http://www.acr.org/About-Us/Media-Center/Position-Statements/Position-Statements-Folder/20141124-ACR-Statement-on-Breast-Tomosynthesis. Accessed May 1, 2016.

37. Skaane P, Bandos AI, Gullien R, et al. Comparison of Digital Mammography Alone and Digital Mammography Plus Tomosynthesis in a Population-based Screening Program. Radiology 2013;267(1):47–56.

38. Ciatto S, Houssami N, Bernardi D, et al. Integration of 3D digital mammography with tomosynthesis for population breast-cancer screening (STORM): a prospective comparison study. Lancet Oncol 2013; 14(7):583–9.

39. Haas BM, Kaira V, Geisel J, et al. Comparison of tomosynthesis plus digital mammography and digital mammography alone for breast cancer screening. Radiology 2013;269:694–700.

40. Rose SL, Tidwell AL, Bujnoch LJ, et al. Implementation of breast tomosynthesis in a routine screening practice: an observational study. AJR Am J Roentgenol 2013;200:1401–8.

41. Friedewald SM, Rafferty EA, Rose SL, et al. Breast Cancer Screening Using Tomosynthesis in Combination with Digital Mammography. JAMA 2014; 311(24):2499–507.

42. Kopans DB. The problem with the new breast cancer screening recommendations. Available at: http://www.forbes.com/sites/matthewherper/2016/01/15/the-problem-with-the-new-breast-cancer-screening-recommendations/#114cd3155cbf. Accessed May 1, 2016.

43. Oeffinger KC, Fontham ET, Etzioni R, et al. Breast Cancer Screening for Women at Average Risk 2015 Guideline Update From the American Cancer Society. JAMA 2015;314(15):1599–614.

44. Smith RA, Saslow D, Sawyer KA, et al. American Cancer Society guidelines for breast cancer screening: update 2003. CA Cancer J Clin 2003; 53(3):141–69.

45. Tosteson AN, Fryback DG, Hammond CS, et al. Consequences of false-positive screening mammograms. JAMA Intern Med 2014;174(6):954–61.

46. Saadatmand S, Bretveld R, Siesling S, et al. Influence of tumour stage at breast cancer detection on survival in modern times: population based study in 173,797 patients. BMJ 2015;351:h4901.

47. Tonelli M, Connor Gorber S, Joffres M, et al. Recommendations on screening for breast cancer in average-risk women aged 40-74 years. CMAJ 2011;183(17):1991–2001.

48. Miglioretti DL, Zhu W, Kerlikowske K, et al. Breast tumor prognostic characteristics and biennial vs. annual mammography, age, and menopausal Status. JAMA Oncol 2015;1(8):1069–77.

49. Mandelblatt JS, Cronin KA, Bailey S, et al. Effects of mammography screening under different screening schedules: model estimates of potential benefits and harms. Ann Intern Med 2009;151:738–47.

50. Available at: https://www.sbi-online.org/Portals/0/ACR-SBI%20press%20release%20ACS%20FINAL%20for%20web.pdf. Accessed May 1, 2016.

51. Price ER. Overemphasis on overdiagnosis. Acad Radiol 2015;23(1):125–6.

52. Puliti D, Duffy SW, Miccinesi G, et al. Overdiagnosis in mammographic screening for breast cancer in Europe: a literature review. J Med Screen 2012; 19(Suppl 1):42–56.

53. Duffy SW, Parmar D. Overdiagnosis in breast cancer screening: the importance of length of observation period and lead time. Breast Cancer Res 2013;15: R41.

54. Yen AM, Duffy SW, Chen TH, et al. Long-term incidence of breast cancer by trial arm in one county of the Swedish Two County Trial of Mammography screening. Cancer 2012;118:5728–32.

55. Nelson HD, Cantor A, Humphrey L, et al. Screening for breast cancer: a systematic review to update the 2009 U.S. Preventive services Task Force recommendation. Evidence synthesis No. 124. AHRQ publication No. 14-05201-EF-1. Rockville (MD): Agency for Healthcare Research and Quality; 2015.

56. Nelson HD, Fu R, Cantor A, et al. Effectiveness of breast cancer screening: systematic review and meta-analysis to update the 2009 U.S. Preventive Services Task Force recommendation. Ann Intern Med 2016;164(4):244–55.

57. Helvie MA, Chang JT, Hendrick RE, et al. Reduction in late-stage breast cancer incidence in the mammography era: Implications for overdiagnosis of invasive cancer. Cancer 2014;120(17): 2649–56.

58. Schousboe JT, Kerlikowske K, Loh A, et al. Personalizing mammography by breast density and other risk factors for breast cancer: analysis of health benefits and cost-effectiveness. Ann Intern Med 2011; 155:10–20.

59. van Ravesteyn NT, Miglioretti DL, Stout NK, et al. Tipping the balance of benefits and harms to favor screening mammography starting at age 40 years: a comparative modeling study of risk. Ann Intern Med 2012;156:609–17.

60. Feig SA. Personalized screening for breast cancer: a wolf in sheep's clothing? AJR Am J Roentgenol 2015;205:1365–71.

61. Seidman H, Stellman SD, Mushinski MH. A different perspective on breast cancer risk factors: some implications of nonattributable risk. Cancer 1982;32: 301–13.

62. Solin L, Schwartz G, Feig S, et al. Risk factors as criteria for inclusion in breast cancer screening programs. In: Ames F, Blumenschein O, Montague E,

editors. Current controversies in breast cancer. Austin (TX): University of Texas Press; 1984. p. 565–72.

63. Curpen BN, Sickles EA, Sollitto RA, et al. The comparative value of mammographic screening for women 40-49 years old versus women 50–64 years old. AJR Am J Roentgenol 1995;164:1099–103.

64. Destounis SV, Arieno AL, Morgan RC, et al. Comparison of breast cancers diagnosed in screening patients in their 40s with and without family history of breast cancer in a community outpatient facility. AJR Am J Roentgenol 2014;202:928–32.

65. Arleo EK, Dashevsky BZ, Reichman M, et al. Screening mammography for women in their 40s: a retrospective study of the potential impact of the U.S. Preventive Service Task Force's 2009 breast cancer screening recommendations. AJR Am J Roentgenol 2013;201:1401–6.

66. Nelson HD, Zakher B, Cantor A, et al. Risk factors for breast cancer for women aged 40 to 49 years: a systematic review and meta-analysis. Ann Intern Med 2012;156:635–48.

67. Price ER, Keedy AW, Gidwaney R, et al. The potential impact of risk-based screening mammography in women 40–49 years old. AJR Am J Roentgenol 2015;205(6):1360–4.

68. O'Donoghue C, Eklund M, Ozanne EM, et al. Aggregate cost of mammography screening in the United States: comparison of current practice and advocated guidelines. Ann Intern Med 2014;160:145–53.

69. Feig SA. Cost-effectiveness of mammography, MRI, and ultrasonography for breast cancer screening. Radiol Clin North Am 2010;48(5):879–91.

70. Blumen H, Fitch K, Polkus V. Comparison of treatment costs for breast cancer, by tumor stage and type of service. Am Health Drug Benefits 2016; 9(1):23–32.

71. Rosenquist CJ, Lindfors KK. Screening mammography in women aged 40–49 years: analysis of cost-effectiveness. Radiology 1994;191:647–50.

72. Gold M, Siegel J, Russell L, et al. Cost-effectiveness in health and medicine. New York: Oxford University Press; 1996.

73. Bonafede M, Kalra V, Miller J, et al. Value analysis of digital breast tomosynthesis for breast cancer screening in a commercially-insured US population. Clinicoecon Outcomes Res 2015;7:53–63.

Evidence to Support Screening Women Annually

Peter R. Eby, MD

KEYWORDS

- Mammogram • Screening • Breast cancer • Annual interval • Biennial

KEY POINTS

- Screen-detected cancers are more often smaller, lower stage, node negative, and localized to the breast, resulting in lower morbidity, costs of treatment, and mortality.
- Biennial screening misses the opportunity to detect approximately two-thirds of preclinical cancers because the average sojourn time for breast cancer is less than 24 months.
- Annual screening incurs greater costs in dollars, recalls, and benign biopsies than biennial screening, but also saves more lives while decreasing extent and costs of therapy.
- Despite multiple national recommendations, only 50% of eligible women report having a mammogram in the prior 12 months and 67% in the prior 24 months.
- Since screening became widespread in the 1980s, US breast cancer mortality has decreased 36% and could be further reduced with more regular and frequent participation.

INTRODUCTION

Screening mammography saves lives. Most randomized controlled trials (RCTs) demonstrate a 20% to 30% decrease in mortality from breast cancer when women are invited to screening.[1,2] The true benefit, when measuring the outcomes for women who accept the invitation and participate in screening, ranges from 38% to 49%.[3–5] Multiple US medical organizations recognize this scientific fact. The American College of Radiology (ACR), American Cancer Society (ACS), and US Preventive Services Task Force (USPSTF) agree that annual screening beginning at 40 will save the most lives.[6–8] The ACS recently concluded in their revised guidelines from 2015 that "Screening mammography in women aged 40 to 69 years is associated with a reduction in breast cancer deaths across a range of study designs, and inferential evidence supports breast cancer screening for women 70 years and older who are in good health."[6] The USPSTF has stated that "The USPSTF found adequate evidence that mammography screening reduces breast cancer mortality in women aged 40 to 74 years."[7] Similarly, the ACR advises "screening mammography should be performed annually beginning at age 40 for women at average risk for breast cancer."[8]

Despite these seemingly concordant summaries of the benefits of screening mammography, there are persistent debates regarding when to start and how often women should participate. Although therapy for breast cancer does impact patient outcomes, the primary improvement in morbidity and mortality stems from a shift in presentation from late stage and metastatic disease to early and localized disease facilitated by screening. This article specifically explores the evidence related to screening intervals and attempts to answer the question: should women be screened annually or biennially? The following paragraphs explore the factors impacting the timing

Department of Radiology, Virginia Mason Medical Center, C5-XR, 1100 Ninth Avenue, Seattle, WA 98111, USA
E-mail address: peter.eby@virginiamason.org

Radiol Clin N Am 55 (2017) 441–456
http://dx.doi.org/10.1016/j.rcl.2016.12.003
0033-8389/17/© 2017 Elsevier Inc. All rights reserved.

radiologic.theclinics.com

of screening for breast cancer, such as neoplastic growth rate, sojourn time, impact on staging and mortality, costs, rising incidence, minority and elderly populations, and the difference between recommendations and actual participation.

SCREENING CONCEPTS

For any screening tool to be effective, there must be a window of time between the development of disease and the appearance of clinical manifestations or physical signs or symptoms. Simply stated, there must be a time period after which breast cancer has developed and before the patient or her physician notices anything amiss. The length of this period, known as the sojourn time, impacts the frequency of performing the test (**Fig. 1**).

A screening test, to provide value to the patient, must also offer the opportunity to positively impact prognosis. We strive to detect cancer early (stages 0 or I) to provide patients with the most favorable prognosis, easiest treatment, and minimal psychosocial impact. Larger tumors, local or regional nodal metastases, and distant metastases at the time of diagnosis increase the costs and morbidity of therapy, recovery time, mastectomy rate, and mortality (**Fig. 2**). If detection of breast cancer before it was palpable did not change the outcome for the patients, it would be meaningless.

Biology of Breast Cancer

The timing of screening depends heavily on the opportunity to impact prognosis and/or therapy, which in turn depends upon the rapidity of disease progression. The incidence of breast cancer in the population is slowly increasing 1% to 2% per year; the number of cancers is finite at any given time and they are all growing.[9] If 2 equal size populations of women are screened for breast cancer

for 3 years at 2 different intervals, annual and triennial, for example, the same number of cancers will be discovered in both groups. However, the cancers detected will be larger and later stage at diagnosis in the group that is screened every third year.[10]

Recent research confirms that breast cancer is a heterogeneous disease consisting of multiple phenotypes with correspondingly variable growth rates. How do these revelations inform screening recommendations? Some advanced techniques, such as dynamic contrast-enhanced (DCE) MR imaging and contrast-enhanced digital mammography (CEDM), may predict which tumors are more rapidly progressive using radiomics and radiogenomics.[11,12] However, the monetary cost, time, contraindications, and risks and requirements of contrast injection currently prevent implementation of DCE-MR imaging and CEDM for widespread screening of average risk populations.

Screening and Sojourn Time

A screening mammogram at a single time point reveals very little about the growth rate of an individual cancer. Some highly mitotic tumors may double in weeks, while others may languish for years (**Fig. 3**). The distribution reflects a biologic bell curve. Fortunately, the simplicity and ease of mammography, along with proven lifesaving effects, provide an opportunity to detect cancer in the preclinical sojourn period. The screening strategy depends on the length of that period, and the range of tumor doubling times one hopes to intercept. A short screening interval would capture both the fastest- and the slowest-growing tumors at small sizes. However, as a consequence, this strategy would also subject patients, if they have tumors with protracted growth, to many unnecessary examinations. A long screening interval would spare the population from many tests but would

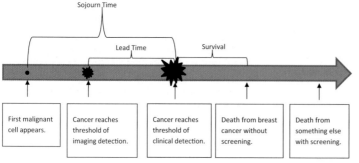

Fig. 1. Diagram of the time between development and clinical presentation (sojourn time), mammographic detectability, and clinical presentation (lead time) and survival (time from detection to death). By screening at the appropriate interval, cancer can be detected during the sojourn time at sizes that are too small to cause symptoms or create physical signs. If the outcome of death is not improved, survival can still appear longer if cancers are detected by imaging because the lead time is added to total survival time. Ideally, early detection eliminates breast cancer as a cause of death and changes the time of death and extends a woman's life.

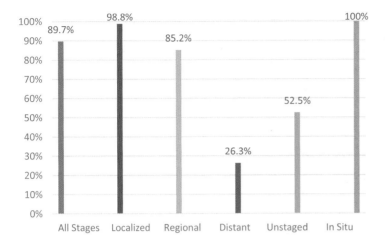

Fig. 2. Five-year relative survival rates from breast cancer as a function of stage at diagnosis. Data are based on the SEER registries from 2006 to 2012. "All Stages" is restricted to invasive carcinoma and does not include pure in situ diagnoses. (*Data from* Howlader N, Noone AM, Krapcho M, et al. SEER cancer statistics review, 1975-2013, National Cancer Institute. In: Cronin KA, editor. Bethesda (MD): 2016. Available at: http://seer.cancer.gov/csr/1975_2013/. Accessed August 8, 2016.)

miss the opportunity to find aggressive cancers at early stages. Therefore, determining the appropriate balance between the 2 approaches is critical. An accurate estimate of the median growth rate of breast cancer is a key factor in determining the appropriate screening interval.

By screening 10,000 women over 10 years of follow-up, prior research estimated an average lead time of 18 months for breast cancer in women less than 50.[13] Eighteen months is relatively short, and lead time does not represent a true improvement in survival time. However, the 18 months suggests the limits of the sojourn time, a period that is clearly shorter than 2 years. In a biennial screening practice, this translates into clinical presentation for all but the slowest growing cancers before the next screening examination. More importantly, with the patient in mind, one should focus on the impact on outcome.

Screening Interval and Stage

Screening is expected to detect early-stage cancers, improve mortality and cosmetic outcomes, and decrease treatment time, morbidity, and costs. The investigation by Moskowitz[13] also found that the stage of breast cancer was significantly higher for women whose last screening mammogram was more than 12 months ago (**Table 1**). The data show that stage 0 and I cancers outnumbered stage II cancers for all ages when the screening interval was 12 months. The data also show the opposite relationship. When women were last screened over 12 months ago, there were more stage II cancers than stage 0 and I combined. Finally, 5-year survival was significantly worse for patients when the cancer was detected more than 12 months since the last mammogram (98% vs 71%).

Modeling Screening and Stage

Michaelson and colleagues[14] gathered data from a retrospective review of positive mammograms to create a mathematical model for predicting doubling time and the probability of metastasis as a function of tumor size. The probability of metastatic disease was then considered in scenarios encountered in routine screening practice with multiple variables: (1) the threshold size (millimeters) of a mammographically detectable cancer; (2) the growth rate (doubling time) of that cancer; and (3) the screening interval. The results indicate that if 12 mm (10^8 cells) is the median size of a detectable cancer, screening intervals of 3, 2, and 1 years will reduce metastatic disease by 7%, 14%, and 33%, respectively (**Table 2**).

A subsequent model, based on 84,812 biennial screening examinations in 33,375 women aged 50 to 59 years old in Finland from 1988 to 2000, corroborates the results of Wu and colleagues.[15] The simulation estimated the mean sojourn time of 2.02 years for localized tumors and 0.82 years for nonlocalized tumors. Stated another way, 39% of cancers transitioned from the preclinical screen-detectable phase to clinical detection in 1 year and 63% transitioned in 2 years, meaning that a biennial strategy will miss the opportunity to detect cancer at smaller size and earlier stage in nearly 2 out of 3 women. The model estimated 28%, 37%, and 53% reductions in advanced breast cancer for triennial, biennial, and annual screening programs, respectively (see **Table 2**).

Stage at Diagnosis: Real Patients

Modeling provides a low-cost method of estimating the effects of an intervention across a large population in a short time. Models can be influenced by the biases of the data and/or creators

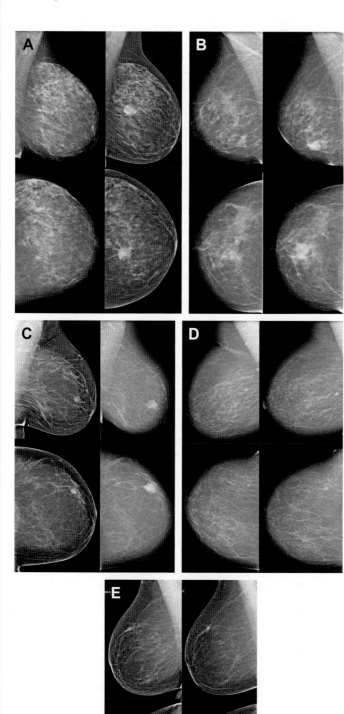

Fig. 3. Five examples of breast cancer at variable growth rates. Baseline images are on the left and follow-up images on the right for each case. (*A*) A cancer in the left breast at 9 o'clock posterior depth presenting as a clinically palpable lump 10 months after a negative screening examination. (*B*) A cancer in an asymptomatic patient in the right breast at 6 o'clock middle depth detected with screening mammography 12 months after a negative screening examination. (*C*) A cancer in an asymptomatic patient in the left breast at 3 o'clock anterior depth present on 2 consecutive screening examinations 17 months apart. (*D*) A cancer in an asymptomatic patient in the right breast at 9 o'clock posterior depth on 2 screening examinations 27 months apart. (*E*) A cancer in an asymptomatic patient in the right breast at 11 o'clock at middle depth on 2 screening examinations 54 months apart. Annual screening is not frequent enough to catch some of the most aggressive cancers (*A*). Biennial screening will allow aggressive cancers (*A–C*) to enlarge and spread to lymph nodes and distant organs. Biennial or even triennial screening may be safe for the most indolent cancers (*D, E*). However, it is not known which women will have which type of cancer until it is found.

Table 1
Cancers detected by stage and time during screening versus more than 12 months since the last screening mammogram from Moskowitz,[13] 1986

	Women Less than 50		Women 50 and Older		All Women	
Stage	Cancers Detected During Screening	Cancers Detected More than 12 mo Since Last Screening	Cancers Detected During Screening	Cancers Detected More than 12 mo Since Last Screening	Cancers Detected During Screening	Cancers Detected More than 12 mo Since Last Screening
0	15	9	19	10	34	19
I	12	23	23	34	35	57
II	5	45[a]	15	45[a]	20	90[a]
Total	32	77	57	89	89	166

[a] Stage II cancers outnumber the combination of stage 0 and I cancers for all ages when the last screening mammogram was more than 12 months ago.

Data from Moskowitz M. Breast cancer: age-specific growth rates and screening strategies. Radiology 1986;161(1):37–41.

upon which they rely. Trials populated by specific patients tied to specific interventions and outcomes help refute or support the model.

Hunt and colleagues[16] retrospectively reviewed the experience of mammography in California from 1985 through 1997 and compared the staging of 40- to 79-year-old women who self-selected annual versus biennial screening. Women who presented for annual screening had lower recall rates, smaller tumors, less node-positive, and lower-stage cancers compared with those selecting biennial examinations.

A meta-analysis including patients from the Swedish Two County trial, Massachusetts General Hospital, and Van Nuys Breast Center (University of Southern California) found invasive tumors detected by screening were significantly smaller than those presenting clinically (**Table 3**).[17]

White and colleagues[18] investigated the impact of annual versus biennial screening through an observational study of 7 US registries and Breast Cancer Surveillance Consortium (BCSC) data.

The study included only 2 rounds of screening mammograms in 40- to 89-year-old women. Across all ages, there was a higher risk of invasive cancer (as opposed to in situ cancer) and a higher risk of estrogen receptor-negative invasive cancer among the biennial screening group. In addition, biennial screening produced a significantly higher incidence of late stage cancer in 40- to 49-year-old women. Mortality and treatment costs are unknown in this short observational trial, and women self-selected their screening intervals. Some allowed 2 years between the first and second mammogram and then returned in 1 year for the third, thus truncating the critical second round.

A review of the entire experience of the Swedish Two County trial in 2007 (**Table 4**), including 10,177,113 person-years and 23,092 cancers, confirmed a significant reduction in node positivity, tumor size, and tumor stage for patients exposed to screening.[19]

Randall and colleagues[20] compared annual and biennial screening in a select population of women

Table 2
Estimated reductions in metastatic or advanced breast cancer as a function of screening interval from modeling or population data

Screening Interval	Estimated Reduction in the Incidence of Distant Metastatic Breast Cancer[a]	Estimated Reduction in the Incidence of Advanced Breast Cancer[b]
Triennial	7%	28%
Biennial	14%	37%
Annual	33%	53%
Biannual	62%	Not estimated

[a] Estimated reduction in the incidence of metastatic disease as a function of various screening strategies if growth is Gompertzian and the median size of a detectable cancer is 12 mm (10^8 cells).[14]
[b] Estimated reduction in advanced breast cancer at presentation for triennial, biennial, and annual screening strategies based on a population of patients screened from 1988 to 2000 in Finland.[15]

Table 3
Mean size of invasive breast cancer detected in screened and unscreened populations

Data Source	Mean Size of Invasive Cancer Detected with Screening Mammography (mm)	Mean Size of Invasive Cancer Presenting Clinically (mm)
Swedish Two County Trial	12.5	20
Massachusetts General Hospital	12	20
Van Nuys Breast Center (University of Southern California)	11	20

Tumors detected by screening are significantly smaller than those presenting through signs or symptoms.

Data from Michaelson JS, Satija S, Kopans D, et al. Gauging the impact of breast carcinoma screening in terms of tumor size and death rate. Cancer 2003;98(10):2114–24.

with at least one first-degree relative with breast cancer aged 50 to 69 in New South Wales, Australia. Annual screening significantly improved the odds of being diagnosed with a cancer smaller than 20 mm, 15 mm, and 10 mm and with normal lymph nodes. This group of women, at increased risk for breast cancer, may not reflect the general population but corroborates the trend of smaller cancers at lower stage detected with annual screening.

Using data from the BCSC, Kerlikowske and colleagues[21] compared tumor size and stage across women who underwent annual versus biennial or triennial screening from 1994 to 2008. Biennial screening increased the odds of advanced stage and larger cancers in 40- to 49-year-old women.

Miglioretti and colleagues[22] also used BCSC data to interrogate the impact of annual versus biennial screening on prognostic characteristics of 15,440 breast cancers in women aged 40 to 85 from 1996 to 2012. Biennial screening, for premenopausal women and postmenopausal women on hormone replacement therapy, was associated with significantly increased risk of stage IIb or higher tumors, tumors larger than 15 mm, and positive lymph nodes.

Actual Reduction in Late-Stage Breast Cancer

Trends in the incidence of invasive breast cancer and metastatic disease in the United States corroborate the estimates from the models by Michaelson and colleagues[14] and Wu and colleagues.[15] Using data from the US population and trends from the Surveillance, Epidemiology, and End Results (SEER) database, Helvie and colleagues[9] compared the incidence of various stages of breast cancer in the pre-mammography era (1977–1979) with the post-mammography era (2007–2009). The investigators concluded that regional breast cancer decreased by 39%, distant disease decreased by 26%, and localized disease increased by 19%. The positive effect on the US population after the introduction of screening confirms what one would expect: a shift of breast cancer from distant to local staging. These data also explain the 36% decrease in mortality observed

Table 4
Combined results for all 6 Swedish counties by age group, endpoint, and exposure category adjusted for missing data and changes in incidence

Age	Endpoint	Exposed RR (95% CI)	Unexposed RR (95% CI)
40–49	Node positive	0.71 (0.59–0.85)	1.12 (0.89–1.42)
	Size >2 cm	0.55 (0.46–0.66)	1.11 (0.88–1.38)
	Stage II plus	0.58 (0.57–0.81)	1.07 (0.88–1.30)
50–69	Node positive	0.84 (0.78–0.90)	1.07 (0.99–1.17)
	Size >2 cm	0.67 (0.62–0.72)	1.00 (0.91–1.09)
	Stage II plus	0.79 (0.74–0.85)	1.00 (0.93–1.07)

Relative risk (RR) is in comparison to the prescreening epoch. Patients exposed to screening have significantly reduced node-positive cancers that are smaller size and earlier stage.

Data from Swedish Organised Service Screening Evaluation Group. Effect of mammographic service screening on stage at presentation of breast cancers in Sweden. Cancer 2007;109(11):2205–12.

in the United States from 1989, when widespread screening was instituted, to 2012.[23]

Summary of Effects of Annual Versus Biennial Screening on Tumor Size and Staging

In summary, the growth rate of breast cancer is variable among patients. One cannot predict who will develop cancer any more than one can predict how fast it will grow. The sojourn time, the window of opportunity to detect cancer before it becomes clinically apparent, averages approximately 18 months. A biennial strategy will miss the opportunity to detect preclinical disease in nearly 2 out of 3 women. Early detection is associated with smaller tumors that have not spread to lymph nodes or distant sites as evidenced by reduction in advanced and metastatic disease in the US population since screening became widespread in the 1980s. The next question to ask is whether early detection improves outcomes for patients, and how often should we do it?

ANNUAL VERSUS BIENNIAL OUTCOMES
Annual Versus Biennial Modeling Outcomes

In 2009 and 2015, the USPSTF considered the data related to screening mammography and updated their recommendations.[7,24–27] The data included estimates of benefits and costs of screening from computer models from the Cancer Intervention Surveillance Modeling Network (CISNET).[28,29]

The CISNET models were derived by a consortium of institutions and investigators sponsored by the National Cancer Institute and charged with estimating the effects of interventions, such as mammography, on mortality and other outcomes in the general population.[30] The USPSTF considered models of screening strategies from 6 institutions from the Breast Cancer Working Group in different geographic locations of the United States. The strategies varied by age to begin screening, age to stop screening, and annual or biennial frequency (Table 5). The primary outcome was impact on mortality. The models also estimated the recalls for additional imaging, deaths averted, life years gained, and benign biopsy procedures generated from screening mammography. The report of the CISNET working group in 2016 confirmed the results in 2009 that found consistent annual screening maximizes the benefits for patients[29] (Table 6). Annual screening, whether begun at 40, 45, or 50, reduces mortality from breast cancer more than any biennial or hybrid strategy.

Hendrick and Helvie[31] used the models and data from CISNET to project, ultimately, how many lives would be saved or lost in the United States from each screening strategy. Annual screening of women aged 40 to 84 provides a 39.6% reduction in mortality from breast cancer. In comparison, biennial screening of women aged 50 to 74 conveys a 23.2% reduction in mortality. Based on US population data for the group of women aged 30

Table 5
Median of 6 CISNET model estimates of the impact of various screening strategies

Screening Strategy	Median of All CISNET Models per 1000 Women Screened vs No Screening[a]					
	Screening Examinations	Mortality Reduction (%)	Deaths Averted	Years of Life Gained	Recalls from Screening	Benign Biopsy Procedures
Biennial						
50–74	11,127	25.8	7	122.4	953	146
45–74	13,212	27.2	8	138.2	1220	176
40–74	16,013	30.4	8	152.0	1529	213
Hybrid						
45–74	15,966	29.5	8	147.7	1520	202
40–74	20,884	32.0	9	164.1	2106	256
Annual						
50–74	21,318	33.0	9	144.8	1798	228
45–74	26,136	35.9	9	166.0	2355	283
40–74	31,037	37.8	10	191.8	2941	338

Hybrid strategies vary annual and biennial intervals during the specified age range. The greatest mortality reductions (33.0%–37.8%) and total number of screening examinations are all found within the annual screening strategies.
[a] The models assume consistent and appropriate therapy for all patients.
Adapted from Mandelblatt JS, Stout NK, Schechter CB, et al. Collaborative modeling of the benefits and harms associated with different U.S. breast cancer screening strategies. Ann Intern Med 2016;164(4):215–25.

Table 6
Lives saved using various strategies and participation rates among the US population of women aged 30 to 39 about to begin screening

	Annual Screening Ages 40–84 (ACR)	Biennial Screening Ages 50–74 (USPSTF)	Increase in Lives Saved for Annual Screening Ages 40–84 Compared with Biennial Screening Ages 50–74
Lives saved per 1000 women screened over a lifetime	12	7	5
Total lives saved over a lifetime with 100% participation of US women aged 30–39[a]	239,592	139,762	99,830
Total lives saved over a lifetime with 65% participation of US women aged 30–39[a]	155,735	90,845	64,890

[a] This assumes 19,965,964 women aged 30 to 39 in 2009 from census data and baseline 3% risk of death from breast cancer, and 65% participation is based on US population reporting data.[51]
  Data from Hendrick RE, Helvie MA. United States Preventive Services Task Force screening mammography recommendations: science ignored. AJR Am J Roentgenol 2011;196(2):W112–6.

to 39, following an annual screening schedule will save 99,829 more lives than a biennial schedule over the course of their lifetimes (see **Table 6**).

Yaffe and colleagues[32] used the CISNET W model to estimate the impact of various screening strategies on women in Canada. Annual screening from ages 40 to 74 saved more life years from breast cancer than any other strategy. More frequent screening created more recalls and benign biopsies but also found more in situ cancer and the lowest number of women needed to screen to save one life.

Annual Versus Biennial Observed Outcomes

In 2003, Smith-Bindman and colleagues[10] published the results of a retrospective comparison between screening strategies in the United States and the United Kingdom. The analysis included 5.5 million mammograms detecting 27,612 breast malignancies in women 50 years old and higher. The UK national service program invited triennial screening for all women aged 50 to 64 during the study period. In contrast, screening in the United States was administered by numerous diverse clinics and hospitals and subject to individual initiative, different insurance plans, and variable physician recommendations. Cancer detection rates were similar and recall rates were lower for the UK program suggesting an advantage to the triennial screening plan. However, there were twice as many cancers larger than 20 mm detected at screening in the UK than in the United States—a clear indicator of the negative impact of prolonged screening intervals. The study was not able to analyze downstream outcomes of mortality, breast conservation surgery, or costs of therapy.

In summary, biennial screening may miss the opportunity to detect cancer during the preclinical sojourn period. Annual screening maximizes the opportunity to detect preclinical cancer at smaller sizes and earlier stages (0 and I) and decreases metastatic disease, thereby improving outcomes for patients. Annual screening starting at age 40 provides the highest gain in life years and deaths averted. Critics of screening will point out that annual attendance strategies also require the highest number of examinations, recalls, and benign biopsy procedures, which fuel the debate about when to start and how often to screen.

COSTS OF SCREENING

Screening incurs many quantifiable costs, such as dollars spent and additional procedures, as well as subjective costs, such as anxiety. The effects of radiation exposure are extrapolated from events such as prior atomic bomb detonation and represent potential but unverifiable risks. Compared with a biennial strategy, annual screening increases the costs of mammography, the time spent on the examination, the radiation exposure, and the frequency and anxiety of recall. However, the decreased downstream costs of treatment, morbidity, and mortality offset the initial investment of more frequent screening. Modeling the impact of digital imaging in place of film, Stout and colleagues[33] concluded that annual screening always increases the cost per life year saved and quality-adjusted life years saved compared with biennial screening. However, switching from biennial to annual screening also saves an additional 2.2 lives per 1000 women screened.

Cost Effectiveness

At first glance, annual screening costs financially twice as much as a biennial regimen. However, a more accurate estimate of the dollars spent is much more complicated. The 6 CISNET models suggest mortality reductions of 32.5% to 43.6% for annual screening of women aged 40 to 74.[29] This wide range of outcomes for a single screening strategy contributes to differing estimates of cost.

O'Donoghue and colleagues[34] conscripted the CISNET, BCSC, and Behavioral Risk Factor Surveillance System 2010 Survey data to create a model of expenses related to different screening strategies of women aged 40 to 85 years old. The costs included downstream recall diagnostic mammograms and subsequent breast biopsies recommended from initial screening. The final estimate for all costs related to screening actually performed in the United States in 2010 was $7.8 billion (Table 7). The cost estimate for biennial screening of women 50 to 69 was considerably lower: $2.6 billion. It should immediately be noted that the investigators maximized the differences in costs by comparing multiple variables: different age ranges (40–85 vs 50–69) and screening strategies (annual vs biennial). The investigators also declined to consider the benefits of screening.

Monetary Costs of Not Screening

The costs of testing are important. O'Donoghue and colleagues did not complete the analysis by weighing them against the benefits of testing and the costs of not testing. Costs for treatment of cancer increase with stage at diagnosis. Montero and colleagues[35] estimated treating a woman with metastatic breast cancer costs $250,000. The cost of a woman dying from breast cancer in her 40s, from lost productivity, is $1.4 million[36] and not covered by medical insurance. Families bear the emotional and financial losses. SEER estimates 246,660 new cases of breast cancer in 2016 and 40,450 deaths.[37] Metastatic cancer represents 6% of all new cases, and 17% of all deaths from breast cancer are in women diagnosed between 40 and 49 years old. Using the estimates from Montero and colleagues[35] and Bradley and colleagues,[36] the annual costs of treating metastatic disease (246,660 new cases × 0.06 metastatic × $250,000 per case = $3.7 billion) and lost productivity for women under age 40 to 49 (40,450 deaths × 0.17 × $1.4 million = $9.6 billion) total $13.3 billion (Table 8). These costs of treatment and lost productivity each year far exceed the cost of the annual screening and additionally do not include the indirect value of the lives that are saved.

Anxiety Related to Recalls from Screening

Critics of annual screening often bemoan the anxiety related to recalls. Tosteson and colleagues[38] surveyed 1226 women with a 6-question anxiety scale and follow-up interview to understand the short- and long-term impact of a recall

---

Table 7
Costs of screening and diagnostic mammography and related reduction in mortality in increase in life years gained associated with various screening strategies

Screening Strategy	Costs of Screening Mammograms (2010, Billions $)	Costs of Screening and Diagnostic Mammograms and Biopsy (2010, Billions $)	Reduction in Breast Cancer Mortality[d]	Years of Life Gained per 1000 Women[d]
Biennial 50–69 Model[a]	2.08	2.61	15%	99
Hybrid 40–84 Model[b]	2.75	3.46	NA	NA
Annual 40–84 Model[a]	8.06	10.14	35%	210
Actual 40–84[c]	6.17	7.80	36%[e]	NA

[a] Biennial and annual plans assume 85% participation.
[b] The hybrid plan is biennial and assumes 20% participation among women 40 to 49, 85% participation among women 50 to 69, and 25% to 37.2% participation among women 70 to 85.
[c] Actual plan varies participation across ages from 61% to 75%. Cancers and years of life lost are based on US SEER population data.[6]
[d] From 2009 CISNET Model S (exemplar model).[28]
[e] From ACS decrease in mortality from breast cancer because widespread screening was implemented in the late 1980s.[23]

Table 8
Estimates of lives lost, saved, and savings in productivity for women 40 to 49 years old for annual versus biennial screening strategies

Lives Lost to Breast Cancer in 2016 (SEER)	Decrease in Mortality[b]	Estimated Lives Lost to Breast Cancer per Year in the United States	Lives Saved per Year with Screening	Women Diagnosed 40–49 y Old Saved by Screening per Year[d]	Annual Savings in Productivity for Women Diagnosed 40–49 y Old[c]	Annual Loss in Productivity for Women Diagnosed 40–49 y Old[c]
No screening	0%	65,032 (40,450/0.622)	0	0	$0	$15.5 billion (65,032 × 0.17 × $1.4 m)
40–74 biennial	30.4%	45,262 (65,032 × 0.696)	19,770	3361 (19,770 × 0.17)	$4.7 billion (3361 × $1.4 m)	$10.8 billion (45,262 × 0.17 × $1.4 m)
40–74 annual	37.8%	40,450[a]	24,582	4179 (24,582 × 0.17)	$5.9 billion (4179 × $1.4 m)	$9.6 billion (40,450 × 0.17 × $1.4 m)
Benefits of annual vs biennial	7.4% additional decrease	4812 more lives saved per year	4812 more lives saved per year	818 more lives saved per year	$1.2 billion saved per year	$1.2 billion saved per year

[a] 40,450 is the SEER estimate for deaths from breast cancer in 2016.[37]
[b] Mortality reduction from 2016 CISNET models.[29]
[c] Estimated $1.4 million lost in productivity from death of a woman diagnosed at 40 to 49 years old.[36]
[d] Women age 40 to 49 years old account for 17% of all breast cancer cases.[37]

examination. Women who were recalled from screening and did not have cancer reported increased anxiety in the short term but not the long term. A recall did not produce any measurable health utility decrement. Unexpectedly, women were twice as likely to undergo future breast cancer screening after a recall, suggesting that there are no lasting negative effects for most women who participate in screening.

Cumulative Risk of Recall from Screening

Winch and colleagues[39] compared recall rates, cancer detection, biopsy recommendation, and tumor size in 231,824 women at a no-cost metropolitan screening program. The standard approach provided biennial screening to women aged 50 and higher. Annual screening was offered for patients at elevated risk of breast cancer, which biased the study population. As expected, the annual screening group had higher risk of recall and biopsy over a 10-year period as well as smaller cancers.

Hendrick and Helvie[31] calculated the incidence of various risks of screening over time. A 40- to 49-year-old woman having annual mammography can expect to have one recall every 10.2 years, additional imaging every 11.9 years, and benign breast biopsy once every 149 years.

Using a meta-analysis to inform the USPSTF recommendations, Nelson and colleagues[26] concluded that 61% and 42% of women would have at least one recall over 10 years for annual and biennial screening, respectively. The likelihood of biopsy is 7% to 9% for annual and 5% to 6% for biennial screening. Although these are important costs of screening, they must be weighed against the advantages of detecting smaller, node-negative tumors that allow less expensive and extensive therapy as well as higher chances of breast conservation. Ultimately, the investigators acknowledged that "...overdiagnosis, anxiety, pain, and radiation exposure...effects on individual women are difficult to estimate and vary widely."

Overdiagnosis

Overdiagnosis, defined as "...breast cancer detected at screening that would not have been diagnosed by usual care or become clinically evident in a woman's lifetime...," is often cited as a major risk of screening by those opposed to mammography. Although overdiagnosis is the most common term, overtreatment is the most significant impact on patients. The true frequency of overdiagnosis from screening mammography is highly debated and very difficult to measure. Numerous estimates, using models and projections of the baseline incidence of disease, range

from 0% to 50%.[9,40–43] This wide range of results testifies to the inexact nature of the models. Autopsy studies estimate overdiagnosis by counting the cancers that had not become "clinically apparent." On average, 1.3% of women had undetected invasive breast cancer and 8.9% had ductal carcinoma in situ at autopsy.[44] The exact frequency of overdiagnosis is unlikely to exceed the incidence of undetected disease in autopsy studies. In addition, as stated above, the number of cancers in the population is finite. Screening more frequently will not create more cancer or increase overdiagnosis. However, it does offer the opportunity to find smaller cancers.

Radiation Risk

The absorbed radiation dose to the breast from a mammogram is very low and noncumulative. There are no confirmed individual cases of cancer caused by a single mammogram. However, there is a theoretic risk of inducing cancer anywhere in the human body from even the smallest radiation dose. All estimates of the risk from radiation-induced death from breast cancer emerge from models subject to bias and speculation. The most recent model estimates 968 lives saved and 16 possible radiation-induced breast cancer deaths from annual screening plus diagnostic workups of 100,000 women aged 40 to 74 years old.[45] Biennial screening of women 40 to 74 is estimated to induce 12 deaths from breast cancer and save 732 lives. The tradeoff of annual versus biennial screening, therefore, is 236 additional lives saved and theoretically 4 lives lost from radiation-induced breast cancer.

SPECIAL CONSIDERATIONS FOR SPECIAL POPULATIONS
Screening Older Populations

US women aged 65 to 84 years account for 36.6% of all new cases and 41.5% of all breast cancer deaths.[37] Women aged 75 and older account for 19.7% of all new cases and 36.7% of deaths (**Table 9**). The RCTs of screening mammography in the 1960s through 1980s confirmed a decrease in mortality for women included in those studies, all of which were between the ages of 40 and 74 years. Recommendations from the ACR, USPSTF, and ACS vary considerably in the absence of RCT data to address the older population, and life expectancy continues to improve. Physicians are frequently asked how often to screen women older than 74 and when to stop.

Sanderson and colleagues[46] used Medicare claims data from multiple regions of the SEER registry to analyze the relationship between screening

Table 9
Age group percentages of new cases and deaths from breast cancer among women from all races in the United States

Age Group	% of New Breast Cancer Cases in the United States	% of Breast Cancer Deaths in the United States
20–34	1.8	0.9
35–44	8.9	5.0
45–54	21.3	14.0
55–64	25.7	22.0
65–74	22.6	21.4
75–84	14.0	20.1
>84	5.7	16.6

The population of women 75 and older was not included in the original RCTs and account for 36.7% of all breast cancer deaths.
Data from Howlader N, Noone AM, Krapcho M, et al. SEER cancer statistics review, 1975-2013, National Cancer Institute. In: Cronin KA, editor. Bethesda (MD): 2016. Available at: http://seer.cancer.gov/csr/1975_2013/. Accessed August 8, 2016.

interval and mortality from breast cancer in 64,384 women. The investigators found the 10-year hazard ratio for mortality from breast cancer is significantly lower for women aged 69 to 84 years old participating in annual screening compared with biennial, and irregular or no screening.

Screening Intervals and Minority Trends

A population-based approach to screening intervals removes bias, offers equal opportunity to all women, and accounts for the most common patterns. However, some minority trends deserve discussion. An analysis of breast cancer incidence and outcome data by DeSantis and colleagues[47] found African American women are 42% more likely to die from breast cancer than non-Hispanic white women in the United States (**Table 10**). The incidence of breast cancer among African American women has historically been lower than non Hispanic white women. However,

the incidence has steadily increased, and in 2012, they equalized.[48]

The combination of rising incidence and significantly higher mortality saddles the African American population with a disproportionate breast cancer burden. The data indicate that African American women are diagnosed with invasive breast cancers that do not display estrogen, progesterone, or her-2-neu surface receptors twice as often (11% vs 22%) as non-Hispanic white women.[47] Such tumors characteristically grow more rapidly and metastasize earlier than other tumors.[49] In addition, African American women are more likely to present with lymph node metastases than non-Hispanic white women. Both factors support annual screening to provide the best opportunities for early detection.

Investigations of other minority populations in the United States have uncovered groups that would benefit from annual screening. A review of data from the BCSC found Hispanic women

Table 10
Comparison of median age at diagnosis and death, tumor surface receptor characteristics, and lymph node metastases at presentation between African American and Non-Hispanic white women in the United States (African American women are 42% more likely to die of breast cancer)

	Non-Hispanic White	African American
Median age at diagnosis	62	58
Median age at death	68	62
Triple negative, %	11	22
ER positive, %	76	62
Lymph node metastases at presentation, %	25.8	33.6

African American women are diagnosed and die younger and have more aggressive tumor profiles (BCSC).
Data from DeSantis CE, Lin CC, Mariotto AB, et al. Cancer treatment and survivorship statistics, 2014. CA Cancer J Clin 2014;64(4):252–71.

aged 50 to 74 have a higher risk of large tumors (odds ratio [OR], 1.6; 95% confidence interval [CI], 1.1–2.4) and late-stage disease (OR, 1.6; 95% CI, 1.0–2.5) when screened biennially versus annually.[50] The same study reported biennial screening increased the risk of lymph node metastases in Asian women aged 40 to 49 years (OR, 3.1; 95% CI, 1.3–7.1). These factors argue heavily in favor of annual screening for all women.

RECOMMENDATIONS VERSUS REALITY IN THE UNITED STATES

Despite previous recommendations for annual screening in the United States, there has been incomplete compliance in annual or biennial screening at all age levels.[51] Close examination of multiple geographic regions as well as anonymous surveys confirms variable and infrequent attendance to screening. According to national survey data, only 67% of eligible women aged 40 years and older report having had a mammogram in the last 2 years.[52,53] The rates are even lower for annual mammography. Despite slow increases in overall utilization, on average, slightly less than 50% of eligible women have had a mammogram in the last 12 months.[54] Importantly, minorities and impoverished women take advantage of screening mammography even less frequently.

Analyzing a multiethnic cohort of 81,722 women in Hawaii and Los Angeles, Edwards and colleagues[55] found that over a 6-year follow-up period, only 36% of women reported regular annual mammography. In addition, attendance at annual or biennial screening was significantly lower for minorities (African American, Hispanic, and Native Hawaiian) compared with white women.

Bhanegaonkar and colleagues[56] report annual and biennial screening rates for women 40 to 64 years old in the West Virginia Medicaid fee-for-service program declined steadily from 1999 to 2008. This decline predates the 2009 USPSTF retreat from initiating screening at 40.

FUTURE OF SCREENING

Digital breast tomosynthesis (DBT) is available throughout the United States and Europe. The most recent estimates suggest 20% to 25% of all mammography units in the United States are capable of DBT examinations. How does this impact the debate over annual versus biennial examination? Opponents of screening cite recall examinations and associated imaging and procedures as a major cost of screening as has been seen. DBT can decrease recalls by 15% to 36% without a decrease in cancer detection.[57–69]

What the Referring Physician Needs to Know

1. Screen-detected cancers are, on average, smaller, localized, node-negative, nonmetastatic cancers.
2. Screen-detected cancers are, on average, associated with lower mortality, morbidity, and treatment costs.
3. The estimated median sojourn time of breast cancer is 18 to 24 months.
4. A biennial screening plan will miss the opportunity to detect preclinical cancer in 63% of patients.
5. A triennial screening plan and an annual screening plan spread over 3 years will detect the same number of cancers, but the cancers in the triennial screening plan will be larger and more often node positive or metastatic at diagnosis.
6. Although most organizations in the United States recommended annual screening beginning at age 40 through the 1990s and early 2000s, only 50% of women report having had a mammogram in the prior 12 months and 70% in the prior 24 months.
7. Since screening became widespread in the late 1980s, mortality from breast cancer in the United States has decreased 36% and could be even greater with more regular and frequent participation.
8. $7.8 billion is one estimate of the amount spent on screening US women aged 40 to 84 in 2010. The estimated lost productivity from just the 40- to 49-year-old women who will die from breast cancer in 2016 is $9.6 billion.
9. Multiple subpopulations of US women have statistically significant improvements in outcomes with annual screening.

SUMMARY

In summary, data clearly show, and major US organizations agree, that annual screening detects breast cancer that is smaller and lower stage compared with biennial screening. Smaller, earlier-stage tumors decrease the monetary and psychosocial impacts of treatment as well as costs for treating metastatic cancer and mortality. Savings in productivity lost to death from breast cancer exceed the costs of additional mammograms and benign biopsies incurred by annual screening. Downstream costs of recalls from screening are expected to decrease as recall rates decrease with DBT. Despite frequent recommendations for annual screening and a mortality reduction of 36% in the United States since the late 1980s, only around 50% of eligible women have had a mammogram in the last year. We have an opportunity to save thousands more lives per year with a consistent annual screening approach beginning at age 40.

REFERENCES

1. Shapiro S. Screening: assessment of current studies. Cancer 1994;74(1 Suppl):231–8.
2. Independent UK Panel on Breast Cancer Screening. The benefits and harms of breast cancer screening: an independent review. Lancet 2012;380(9855):1778–86.
3. Broeders M, Moss S, Nyström L, et al. The impact of mammographic screening on breast cancer mortality in Europe: a review of observational studies. J Med Screen 2012;19(Suppl 1):14–25.
4. Coldman A, Phillips N, Wilson C, et al. Pan-Canadian study of mammography screening and mortality from breast cancer. J Natl Cancer Inst 2014; 106(11):dju261.
5. Nickson C, Mason KE, English DR, et al. Mammographic screening and breast cancer mortality: a case-control study and meta-analysis. Cancer Epidemiol Biomarkers Prev 2012;21(9):1479–88.
6. Oeffinger KC, Fontham ETH, Etzioni R, et al. Breast cancer screening for women at average risk: 2015 guideline update from the American Cancer Society. JAMA 2015;314(15):1599–614.
7. Siu AL, U.S. Preventive Services Task Force. Screening for breast cancer: U.S. preventive services task force recommendation statement. Ann Intern Med 2016;164(4):279–96.
8. Lee CH, Dershaw DD, Kopans D, et al. Breast cancer screening with imaging: recommendations from the Society of Breast Imaging and the ACR on the use of mammography, breast MRI, breast ultrasound, and other technologies for the detection of clinically occult breast cancer. J Am Coll Radiol 2010;7(1):18–27.
9. Helvie MA, Chang JT, Hendrick RE, et al. Reduction in late-stage breast cancer incidence in the mammography era: Implications for overdiagnosis of invasive cancer. Cancer 2014;120(17):2649–56.
10. Smith-Bindman R, Chu PW, Miglioretti DL, et al. Comparison of screening mammography in the United States and the United kingdom. JAMA 2003;290(16):2129–37.
11. Li H, Zhu Y, Burnside ES, et al. MR imaging radiomics signatures for predicting the risk of breast cancer recurrence as given by research versions of MammaPrint, oncotype DX, and PAM50 GENE Assays. Radiology 2016;281(2):382–91.
12. Grimm LJ, Zhang J, Mazurowski MA. Computational approach to radiogenomics of breast cancer: luminal A and luminal B molecular subtypes are associated with imaging features on routine breast MRI extracted using computer vision algorithms. J Magn Reson Imaging 2015;42(4):902–7.
13. Moskowitz M. Breast cancer: age-specific growth rates and screening strategies. Radiology 1986;161(1):37–41.
14. Michaelson JS, Halpern E, Kopans DB. Breast cancer: computer simulation method for estimating optimal intervals for screening. Radiology 1999;212(2):551–60.
15. Wu JC-Y, Hakama M, Anttila A, et al. Estimation of natural history parameters of breast cancer based on non-randomized organized screening data: subsidiary analysis of effects of inter-screening interval, sensitivity, and attendance rate on reduction of advanced cancer. Breast Cancer Res Treat 2010; 122(2):553–66.
16. Hunt KA, Rosen EL, Sickles EA. Outcome analysis for women undergoing annual versus biennial screening mammography: a review of 24,211 examinations. AJR Am J Roentgenol 1999;173(2):285–9.
17. Michaelson JS, Satija S, Kopans D, et al. Gauging the impact of breast carcinoma screening in terms of tumor size and death rate. Cancer 2003;98(10):2114–24.
18. White E, Miglioretti DL, Yankaskas BC, et al. Biennial versus annual mammography and the risk of late-stage breast cancer. J Natl Cancer Inst 2004; 96(24):1832–9.
19. Swedish Organised Service Screening Evaluation Group. Effect of mammographic service screening on stage at presentation of breast cancers in Sweden. Cancer 2007;109(11):2205–12.
20. Randall D, Morrell S, Taylor R, et al. Annual or biennial mammography screening for women at a higher risk with a family history of breast cancer: prognostic indicators of screen-detected cancers in New South Wales, Australia. Cancer Causes Control 2009; 20(5):559–66.
21. Kerlikowske K, Zhu W, Hubbard RA, et al. Outcomes of screening mammography by frequency, breast density, and postmenopausal hormone therapy. JAMA Intern Med 2013;173(9):807–16.
22. Miglioretti DL, Zhu W, Kerlikowske K, et al. Breast tumor prognostic characteristics and biennial vs annual mammography, age, and menopausal status. JAMA Oncol 2015;1(8):1069–77.
23. American Cancer Society. Breast Cancer Facts & Figures 2015–2016. Atlanta: American Cancer Society, Inc; 2015. Available at: http://www.cancer.org/acs/groups/content/@research/documents/document/acspc-046381.pdf.
24. US Preventive Services Task Force. Screening for breast cancer: U.S. Preventive Services Task Force recommendation statement. Ann Intern Med 2009; 151(10):716–26. W–236.
25. Nelson HD, Tyne K, Naik A, et al. Screening for breast cancer: an update for the U.S. Preventive Services Task Force. Ann Intern Med 2009;151(10):727–37. W237–42.
26. Nelson HD, Pappas M, Cantor A, et al. Harms of breast cancer screening: systematic review to update

the 2009 U.S. Preventive Services Task Force recommendation. Ann Intern Med 2016;164(4):256–67.

27. Nelson HD, Cantor A, Humphrey L, et al. Screening for Breast Cancer: A Systematic Review to Update the 2009 U.S. Preventive Services Task Force Recommendation [Internet]. Rockville (MD): Agency for Healthcare Research and Quality (US); 2016. Report No.: 14-05201-EF-1. U.S. Preventive Services Task Force Evidence Syntheses, formerly Systematic Evidence Reviews.

28. Mandelblatt JS, Cronin KA, Bailey S, et al. Effects of mammography screening under different screening schedules: model estimates of potential benefits and harms. Ann Intern Med 2009;151(10):738–47.

29. Mandelblatt JS, Stout NK, Schechter CB, et al. Collaborative modeling of the benefits and harms associated with different U.S. breast cancer screening strategies. Ann Intern Med 2016;164(4):215–25.

30. Berry DA, Cronin KA, Plevritis SK, et al. Effect of screening and adjuvant therapy on mortality from breast cancer. N Engl J Med 2005;353(17):1784–92.

31. Hendrick RE, Helvie MA. United States Preventive Services Task Force screening mammography recommendations: science ignored. AJR Am J Roentgenol 2011;196(2):W112–6.

32. Yaffe MJ, Mittmann N, Lee P, et al. Clinical outcomes of modelling mammography screening strategies. Health Rep 2015;26(12):9–15.

33. Stout NK, Lee SJ, Schechter CB, et al. Benefits, harms, and costs for breast cancer screening after US implementation of digital mammography. J Natl Cancer Inst 2014;106(6):dju092.

34. O'Donoghue C, Eklund M, Ozanne EM, et al. Aggregate cost of mammography screening in the United States: comparison of current practice and advocated guidelines. Ann Intern Med 2014;160(3):145–53.

35. Montero AJ, Eapen S, Gorin B, et al. The economic burden of metastatic breast cancer: a U.S. managed care perspective. Breast Cancer Res Treat 2012;134(2):815–22.

36. Bradley CJ, Yabroff KR, Dahman B, et al. Productivity costs of cancer mortality in the United States: 2000-2020. J Natl Cancer Inst 2008;100(24):1763–70.

37. Howlader N, Noone AM, Krapcho M, et al. SEER cancer statistics review, 1975-2013, National Cancer Institute. In: Cronin KA, editor. Bethesda (MD): 2016. Available at: http://seer.cancer.gov/csr/1975_2013/. Accessed August 8, 2016.

38. Tosteson ANA, Fryback DG, Hammond CS, et al. Consequences of false-positive screening mammograms. JAMA Intern Med 2014;174(6):954–61.

39. Winch CJ, Sherman KA, Boyages J. Toward the breast screening balance sheet: cumulative risk of false positives for annual versus biennial mammograms commencing at age 40 or 50. Breast Cancer Res Treat 2015;149(1):211–21.

40. Kopans DB, Smith RA, Duffy SW. Mammographic screening and "overdiagnosis". Radiology 2011;260(3):616–20.

41. Puliti D, Duffy SW, Miccinesi G, et al. Overdiagnosis in mammographic screening for breast cancer in Europe: a literature review. J Med Screen 2012;19(Suppl 1):42–56.

42. Duffy SW, Agbaje O, Tabár L, et al. Overdiagnosis and overtreatment of breast cancer: estimates of overdiagnosis from two trials of mammographic screening for breast cancer. Breast Cancer Res 2005;7(6):258–65.

43. Bleyer A, Welch HG. Effect of three decades of screening mammography on breast-cancer incidence. N Engl J Med 2012;367(21):1998–2005.

44. Welch HG, Black WC. Using autopsy series to estimate the disease "reservoir" for ductal carcinoma in situ of the breast: how much more breast cancer can we find? Ann Intern Med 1997;127(11):1023–8.

45. Miglioretti DL, Lange J, van den Broek JJ, et al. Radiation-induced breast cancer incidence and mortality from digital mammography screening: a modeling study. Ann Intern Med 2016;164(4):205–14.

46. Sanderson M, Levine RS, Fadden MK, et al. Mammography screening among the elderly: a research challenge. Am J Med 2015;128(12):1362.e7-14.

47. DeSantis CE, Lin CC, Mariotto AB, et al. Cancer treatment and survivorship statistics, 2014. CA Cancer J Clin 2014;64(4):252–71.

48. DeSantis CE, Siegel RL, Sauer AG, et al. Cancer statistics for African Americans, 2016: progress and opportunities in reducing racial disparities. CA Cancer J Clin 2016;66(4):290–308.

49. Parise CA, Caggiano V. Breast cancer survival defined by the ER/PR/HER2 subtypes and a surrogate classification according to tumor grade and immunohistochemical biomarkers. J Cancer Epidemiol 2014;2014(2):469251.

50. O'Meara ES, Zhu W, Hubbard RA, et al. Mammographic screening interval in relation to tumor characteristics and false-positive risk by race/ethnicity and age. Cancer 2013;119(22):3959–67.

51. Wolf AB, Brem RF. Decreased mammography utilization in the United States: why and how can we reverse the trend? AJR Am J Roentgenol 2009;192(2):400–2.

52. Swan J, Breen N, Graubard BI, et al. Data and trends in cancer screening in the United States: results from the 2005 National Health Interview Survey. Cancer 2010;116(20):4872–81.

53. National Center for Health Statistics (US). Health, United States, 2015: With Special Feature on Racial and Ethnic Health Disparities. Hyattsville (MD): National Center for Health Statistics (US); 2016. Report No.: 2016-1232. Health, United States. Available at: https://www.ncbi.nlm.nih.gov/pubmed/27308685. Accessed August 8, 2016.

54. Wharam JF, Landon BE, Xu X, et al. National trends and disparities in mammography among commercially insured women, 2001-2010. J Public Health Manag Pract 2015;21(5):426–32.

55. Edwards QT, Li A, Pike MC, et al. Patterns of regular use of mammography–body weight and ethnicity: the Multiethnic Cohort. J Am Acad Nurse Pract 2010;22(3):162–9.

56. Bhanegaonkar A, Madhavan SS, Khanna R, et al. Declining mammography screening in a state Medicaid Fee-for-Service program: 1999-2008. J Womens Health (Larchmt) 2012;21(8):821–9.

57. Haas BM, Kalra V, Geisel J, et al. Comparison of tomosynthesis plus digital mammography and digital mammography alone for breast cancer screening. Radiology 2013;269(3):694–700.

58. Michell MJ, Iqbal A, Wasan RK, et al. A comparison of the accuracy of film-screen mammography, full-field digital mammography, and digital breast tomosynthesis. Clin Radiol 2012;67(10):976–81.

59. Skaane P, Bandos AI, Gullien R, et al. Comparison of digital mammography alone and digital mammography plus tomosynthesis in a population-based screening program. Radiology 2013;267(1):47–56.

60. Ciatto S, Houssami N, Bernardi D, et al. Integration of 3D digital mammography with tomosynthesis for population breast-cancer screening (STORM): a prospective comparison study. Lancet Oncol 2013; 14(7):583–9.

61. Rafferty EA, Park JM, Philpotts LE, et al. Assessing radiologist performance using combined digital mammography and breast tomosynthesis compared with digital mammography alone: results of a multi-center, multireader trial. Radiology 2013;266(1): 104–13.

62. Greenberg JS, Javitt MC, Katzen J, et al. Clinical performance metrics of 3D digital breast tomosynthesis compared with 2D digital mammography for breast cancer screening in community practice. AJR Am J Roentgenol 2014;203(3):687–93.

63. McCarthy AM, Kontos D, Synnestvedt M, et al. Screening outcomes following implementation of digital breast tomosynthesis in a general-population screening program. J Natl Cancer Inst 2014; 106(11):dju316.

64. Rafferty EA, Park JM, Philpotts LE, et al. Diagnostic accuracy and recall rates for digital mammography and digital mammography combined with one-view and two-view tomosynthesis: results of an enriched reader study. AJR Am J Roentgenol 2014;202(2):273–81.

65. Friedewald SM, Rafferty EA, Rose SL, et al. Breast cancer screening using tomosynthesis in combination with digital mammography. JAMA 2014; 311(24):2499–507.

66. Durand MA, Haas BM, Yao X, et al. Early clinical experience with digital breast tomosynthesis for screening mammography. Radiology 2015;274(1):85–92.

67. Gilbert FJ, Tucker L, Gillan MGC, et al. Accuracy of digital breast tomosynthesis for depicting breast cancer subgroups in a UK retrospective reading study (TOMMY Trial). Radiology 2015;277(3): 697–706.

68. Gilbert FJ, Tucker L, Gillan MG, et al. The TOMMY trial: a comparison of TOMosynthesis with digital MammographY in the UK NHS Breast Screening Programme–a multicentre retrospective reading study comparing the diagnostic performance of digital breast tomosynthesis and digital mammography with digital mammography alone. Health Technol Assess 2015;19(4):i–xxv, 1–136.

69. Conant EF, Beaber EF, Sprague BL, et al. Breast cancer screening using tomosynthesis in combination with digital mammography compared to digital mammography alone: a cohort study within the PROSPR consortium. Breast Cancer Res Treat 2016;156(1):109–16.

Breast Cancer Risk Assessment Models and High-Risk Screening

Lora D. Barke, DO, Mary E. Freivogel, MS, CGC*

KEYWORDS

- Breast cancer screening • High-risk screening • Risk assessment models • Mammography
- Breast MR imaging • Hereditary cancer syndromes

KEY POINTS

- The paradigm has recently shifted from a uniform method of breast cancer screening to an individualized approach that incorporates patient risk factors.
- Assessment of risk can be a complicated process and is greatly enhanced when a genetic counselor is involved to perform a comprehensive evaluation.
- Although the breast imaging center may be the logical location for this triage to occur, many patients with family history and elevated risk may benefit from earlier screening and require intervention before the age at which they present for routine breast screening.
- This article provides a practical approach to the risk assessment process and includes an overview of the risk models paired with recommendations for those at elevated risk for breast cancer.

INTRODUCTION

Significant progress has been made over the past few decades in the fight against breast cancer. Most notably, screening mammography has resulted in mortality reduction. Screening for breast cancer is performed in patients without signs or symptoms of disease with a goal of discovering the disease in an early stage when it is more treatable, less debilitating, and has improved survival rates. In fact, the stage at diagnosis influences overall survival significantly, regardless of advances in therapy.[1] There are, however, limitations to mammography, especially in women with increased risk for breast cancer because many of these women are younger and have dense breasts.

Screening recommendations vary based on patients' risk of developing the disease. Because of many factors, including hereditary risk, the incidence of breast cancer increases. Although mammography is the only imaging test that has proven to decrease breast cancer mortality, supplemental screening with additional imaging tools has shown increased cancer detection in patients particularly with an elevated risk of breast cancer. This finding began a movement to personalize or individualize breast cancer screening based on patient risk factors.

With new scientific evidence available regarding breast MR imaging in 2007, the American Cancer Society (ACS) published breast cancer screening recommendations that specifically included women at high risk for developing breast cancer. The ACS concluded that annual screening mammography and breast MR imaging may be indicated in patients with an elevated of risk of breast cancer.[2] Additionally, patients with elevated risk may also benefit from beginning screening earlier than those with average risk. This conclusion was largely based on research that found an increase in cancer detection with the addition of breast MR imaging or ultrasound to screening mammography.[3]

A thorough evaluation of individual risk factors will help establish personalized screening

Division of Breast Imaging, Radiology Imaging Associates and Invision Sally Jobe, 10700 East Geddes Avenue, Suite 200, Englewood, CO 80112, USA
* Corresponding author.
E-mail address: mary.freivogel@riaco.com

Radiol Clin N Am 55 (2017) 457–474
http://dx.doi.org/10.1016/j.rcl.2016.12.013
0033-8389/17/© 2017 Elsevier Inc. All rights reserved.

protocols. In addition, risk assessment will determine if patients are candidates for genetic testing or may benefit from chemoprevention.

BREAST CANCER RISK ASSESSMENT

Breast cancer risk assessment can be confusing because various tools and models exist. These tools and models can be broken down into 3 categories:

- Genetic counseling referral guidelines: A patient's personal/family history that is suspicious for a hereditary cancer syndrome will trigger a genetic counseling referral. At this point, the genetic counselor can gather a more detailed medical history and determine whether genetic testing is appropriate. Not everyone who is identified for referral to a genetic counselor will be a candidate for genetic testing.
- Genetic testing guidelines: These guidelines, often used by genetic counselors, are primarily designed to determine if genetic testing for a particular hereditary cancer syndrome is indicated.
- Breast cancer risk assessment models: These models are mathematical models that estimate a woman's risk to develop breast cancer over defined time periods. They are used to identify patients who can benefit from interventions, such as chemoprevention for risk reduction and breast MR imaging screening as an adjunct to mammography for increased surveillance. They are often not applicable to patients with a hereditary cancer syndrome,

emphasizing why genetic counseling/testing should be pursued first when indicated.

Genetic Counseling Referral Guidelines

There are many models available to estimate a woman's risk to develop breast cancer over a specific time period. However, it is important to understand that many of these models are not applicable to women who carry a pathogenic variant (also known as a mutation) in a highly penetrant gene, such as *BRCA1* or *BRCA2*. In these situations, the presence of the pathogenic variant is often what defines the woman's risk to develop breast cancer and, depending on which gene is involved, may define her risk for other types of cancer as well. Thus, when embarking on breast cancer risk assessment, the health care provider must first determine whether patients meet the criteria for referral to a genetic counselor and/or discussion of genetic testing for hereditary cancer syndromes (**Fig. 1**).

The National Comprehensive Cancer Network's (NCCN) guidelines are the most commonly used parameters for identifying patients who are candidates for genetic counseling and testing. Their guidelines include criteria for referral to a genetic counselor for consideration of genetic testing.[4] Additional tools exist and are endorsed specifically by the United States Preventive Services Task Force (USPSTF) to determine the need for in-depth cancer genetic counseling for hereditary breast cancer (**Table 1**).[5]

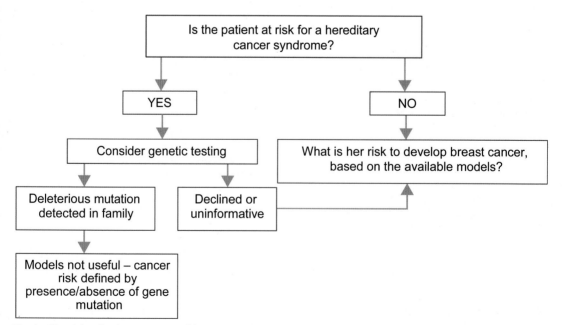

Fig. 1. Algorithm for breast cancer risk assessment.

Table 1
Tools available to guide referral for genetic counseling

Model/Tool	Relatives Included	Cancers Included	Ancestry	Output
Ontario Family History Assessment Tool[10]	First, second, and third degree	Female or male breast, bilateral breast, ovarian, colorectal, prostate, including age at diagnosis; also breast and ovarian in the same individual	Not for use in Ashkenazi Jewish patients	Referral for scoring ≥10
Manchester Scoring System[11]	First, second, and third degree	Breast, ovarian, pancreatic, prostate, including age at diagnosis	Not for use in Ashkenazi Jewish patients	Referral for scoring ≥10 for BRCA-specific or ≥15 combined.
Referral Screening Tool (B-RST)[12,13]	First and second degree	Female breast ≤50 y, male breast at any age, ovarian at any age, ≥2 cases of breast cancer in women ≥50 y on the same side of the family	Accounts for Ashkenazi Jewish ancestry	Checklist of 13 items; referral for ≥2 positive responses
Pedigree Assessment Tool (PAT)[14]	First, second, and third degree	Female breast ≤50 y or >50 y, male breast, ovarian at any age	Accounts for Ashkenazi Jewish ancestry	Referral for scoring ≥8
Family History Screen 7 (FHS-7)[15]	First degree only	Female breast ≤50 y, bilateral breast, breast and ovarian in the same individual, male breast, ≥2 cases of breast and/or ovarian or breast and/or colon	Not for use in Ashkenazi Jewish patients	Checklist of 7 items; referral for ≥1 positive response

Adapted from Moyer VA. Risk assessment, genetic counseling, and genetic testing for BRCA-related cancer in women: U.S. Preventive Services Task Force recommendation statement. Ann Intern Med 2014;160(4):271–81.

General red flags for hereditary breast cancer syndromes include any of the following in patients or their families[6]:

- Ovarian or fallopian tube cancer at any age
- Breast cancer at 50 years of age or younger
- Breast cancer in both breasts at any age
- Both breast and ovarian cancer
- Male breast cancer
- Triple negative breast cancer
- Ashkenazi Jewish heritage and breast cancer at any age
- More than one relative with any of these cancers: breast, ovarian/fallopian tube, prostate, pancreatic, and melanoma

Genetic Testing Guidelines

The NCCN also provides more detailed guidelines for when to offer genetic testing for various types of hereditary cancer syndromes.[4] These guidelines include guidelines for BRCA1/2 gene testing as well as other genes, such as TP53 and PTEN.

In addition to clinical criteria, there are mathematical models that can be used to estimate the chances that a woman carries a BRCA1/2 gene mutation. Myriad Genetics has published extensive prevalence data based on their large dataset of clinical genetic testing samples.[7] There are other models that estimate the likelihood of a woman carrying a BRCA1/2 mutation, including BRCAPRO, Tyrer-Cuzick, and BOADICEA (Breast and Ovarian Analysis of Disease Incidence and Carrier Estimation Algorithm). These models also estimate breast cancer risk and are discussed in detail. Although these models are useful for helping patients understand their chances of testing positive for BRCA1/2 (which is often a very essential part of the genetic counseling process), there are no standard guidelines that designate a specific threshold that justifies genetic testing. Thus, many practitioners rely on clinical criteria from organizations like NCCN versus mathematical models to identify candidates for BRCA1/2 testing.[8]

The Importance of Genetic Counseling

If patients meet the criteria for genetic testing related to cancer risk, they should be offered genetic counseling. If a pathogenic variant is found in a gene related to hereditary breast cancer, this will be factored into patients' cancer risk assessment. If patients are not a candidate for genetic testing, refuse genetic counseling/testing, or test negative for genes related to hereditary breast cancer risk, then the health care provider should proceed with risk assessment using the applicable breast cancer risk assessment models.

It is important to note that a negative genetic test result must be interpreted in the context of patients' family history, other genetic testing that has been completed in relatives. A true-negative result is defined by a patient testing negative for a mutation already identified in the family. However, this differs from an uninformative negative result, when a patient tests negative but a familial mutation has not been identified. This result leaves the possibility of other unknown genetic factors that might be contributing to breast cancer risk in the family. The implications of a negative result can vary, and extreme care should be taken in explaining these results to patients, avoiding a false sense of reassurance about their cancer risk. Additionally, variants of uncertain significance (VUS) are very common, which are alterations in the DNA that do not have adequate evidence to classify them as disease causing (deleterious) or benign. In general, a VUS should not be factored into patients' risk assessment or medical management plan. Many clinicians have been shown to interpret VUSs incorrectly, leading to inappropriate interventions for patients (ie, unnecessary preventive surgeries).[9] To further complicate the matter, different laboratories use different variant classification processes, which may lead to discrepant calls from one laboratory to another. These nuances underscore the importance of involving an expert, such as a genetic counselor, in these cases.

It is important to recognize that there are multiple known single genes that relate to breast cancer risk. Widely available multigene panels allow for simultaneous analysis of many of these genes that relate to patients' risk for breast and other types of cancer. Some of the genes on these panels, such as BRCA1 and BRCA2, are highly penetrant and are typically thought to be associated with a

significantly increased risk for breast cancer. In these cases, there are defined cancer screening protocols, risk reduction strategies, and prevention recommendations that are considered standard of care and significantly differ from what would be offered to those patients based on family history alone. Other genes on these panels are newly discovered, and less is known about the associated cancer risks. They may be considered moderate penetrance, meaning that they increase breast cancer risk but the magnitude of risk is less than that with genes such as BRCA1 and BRCA2. For some of these genes, the magnitude of risk is yet to be determined with statistical significance. Often medical management of patients with these pathogenic variants depends on the strength of the family history. **Table 2** summarizes the genes that are commonly included on multigene panels for hereditary breast cancer including their effect on breast cancer risk and breast cancer screening recommendations. Most of these genes are associated with an increased risk of other types of cancer. Therefore, the identification of a mutation can affect screening and medical management recommendations for these other cancers as well.

Some hereditary breast cancer syndromes are associated with early onset breast cancer; therefore, breast cancer risk assessment must be completed at a young age. Depending on the strength of patients' family history, the age of onset of breast cancer in the relatives, and the results of their genetic testing, regular breast cancer screening may start as early as the mid-20s. Thus, it is important to provide a risk assessment and offer genetic counseling/testing to the appropriate patients in their early 20s. Genetic testing for hereditary cancer syndromes is typically not offered to patients younger than 18 years, unless there is a family history of childhood cancers or very early onset breast cancer or a known hereditary cancer syndrome associated with childhood cancers, such as Li Fraumeni syndrome. It is important to note that patients' family history and other risk assessment-related information should be updated on an annual basis, as risk factors can change over time.

Genetic counseling is an essential part of the process of breast cancer risk assessment and/or genetic testing. Genetic counselors are health care providers with specialized training in genetics and the psychosocial aspects of hereditary diseases. They partner with patients to assist in making an informed choice about genetic testing for patients as well as for their relatives. They educate patients about risks for various types of cancer and, therefore, empower patients to partner with their physicians to create a personalized cancer screening plan with the goal of early detection, if not

Table 2
Genes associated with hereditary breast cancer syndromes

	Gene Name	Breast Imaging Recommendations (as per NCCN)[4,a]	Estimated Breast Cancer Risk	References
High familial penetrance	BRCA1	Begin annual breast MR imaging @ 25 y	Up to 87%	Ashton-Prolla et al,[15] 2009, Ford et al,[46] 1994
	BRCA2	Begin annual mammogram @ 30 y	Up to 84%	Antoniou et al,[47] 2003
	TP53	Begin annual breast MR imaging @ 20 y; Begin annual mammogram @ 30 y	Up to 79%	Ford et al,[48] 1998, Chompret et al,[49] 2000
	PTEN	Begin annual mammogram and breast MR imaging @ 30–35 y	Up to 85%	Bougeard et al,[50] 2015
	PALB2	Begin annual mammogram and consider breast MR imaging @ 30 y	Up to 58%	Tan et al,[51] 2012
	STK11	Begin annual mammogram and consider breast MR imaging @ 25 y	45%–50%	Antoniou et al,[52] 2014
	CDH1	Begin annual mammogram and consider breast MR imaging @ 30 y	39%–52% (lobular)	van Lier et al,[53] 2010; Pharoah et al,[54] 2001; Kaurah et al,[55] 2007
Moderate familial penetrance	CHEK2	Begin annual mammogram and consider breast MR imaging @ 40 y	25%–39%	van der Post et al,[56] 2015; Weischer et al,[57] 2008
	ATM		17%–52%	Cybulski et al,[58] 2011; Ahmed & Rahman,[59] 2006; Swift et al,[60] 1991
Moderate familial penetrance, not as well characterized	NBN	Begin annual mammogram and consider breast MR imaging @ 40 y	Up to 30%	Thompson et al,[61] 2005; Zhang et al,[62] 2011
	NF1	Begin annual mammogram @ 30 y; consider breast MR imaging @ 30–50 y	Elevated	Steffen et al,[63] 2006; Seminog et al,[64] 2013
	BRIP1	No specific recommendations, follow average risk screening	Unknown	Madanikia et al,[65] 2012; Rafnar et al,[66] 2011; Seal et al,[67] 2006
	RAD51C		Unknown	Easton et al,[68] 2016; Le Calvez-Kelm et al,[69] 2012
	RAD51D		Unknown	Coulet et al,[70] 2013
Other novel genes, not well characterized	MUTYH	No specific recommendations, follow average risk screening	Unknown	Loveday et al,[71] 2011; Vogt et al,[72] 2009
	MRE11A		Unknown	Rennert et al,[73] 2012
	RAD50		Up to 30%; unknown	Rennert et al,[73] 2012; Damiola et al,[74] 2014

a Breast cancer screening plans may be individualized and begin earlier based on the earlier known breast cancer in the family; tomosynthesis should be considered: see NCCN's guidelines for details.

prevention, of cancer. Genetic counselors are well suited to guide patients and their relatives to the right genetic test, at the right time, and by the right laboratory, ensuring that health care dollars are used effectively. One can find a genetic counselor in a specified area by visiting www.nsgc.org. Patients at increased risk for breast cancer, whether due to a specific gene mutation or based on family history alone, may have additional unique needs; health care providers should consider referrals to support organizations such as Bright Pink (www.brightpink.org) or Facing Our Risk of Cancer Empowered (www.facingourrisk.org) for assistance.

Breast Cancer Risk Assessment Models

Various mathematical models exist to estimate a woman's risk to develop breast cancer over certain time periods. Some of the most commonly used models are reviewed here, including their benefits, limitations, and other relevant details. Some mammography reporting software packages incorporate risk assessment with various models, and other types of software exist that are designed specifically for risk assessment for breast and other cancers. Some models vary in their accuracy for certain patients (as detailed later in this article, **Table 5**). A summary of the models is included in **Table 3**.

It is important to note that a comprehensive breast cancer risk assessment includes calculation of risk via multiple models, as they will vary in their estimates and applicability to patients, depending on the clinical scenario. Additionally, mathematical models must be supplemented with clinical judgment, as there are certain essential risk factors that may be excluded from the calculation. For example, if a woman was treated with mantle field radiation between 10 and 30 years of age, this will automatically place her in a high-risk category, regardless of risk assessment models.[2,16] Additionally, mammographic density is a significant risk factor. Women with ACR BI-RADS® Atlas, Breast Imaging Reporting and Data System (BI-RADS) breast composition category *d* have a 4- to 6-fold increased risk for breast cancer than those with ACR BI-RADS® breast composition category *a*.[17,18] However, this factor alone is generally not regarded as sufficient enough to place a woman in a high-risk category. Mathematical models vary in their ability to accurately incorporate risks associated with high-risk lesions, such as atypical lobular hyperplasia, atypical ductal hyperplasia, and lobular carcinoma in situ (LCIS). Many studies demonstrate that patients with a personal history of invasive breast cancer and/or ductal carcinoma in situ (DCIS) who are treated with breast-conserving surgery are at an increased risk to develop a second primary breast cancer. Most breast cancer risk assessment models are not applicable to these patients because they have already developed the disease; but they could be considered high risk, especially if they were diagnosed at a younger age, have a family history of breast cancer, and/or have other risk factors, such as mammographically dense breast tissue.

The Gail model

The Gail model was originally designed in 1989 and then modified in 1999.[19,20] The modified model is often called the National Cancer Institute–Gail model or the Breast Cancer Risk Assessment Tool (BCRAT). One of the primary differences in the newer version is that it includes only invasive cancers, whereas the original model included both invasive cancers and DCIS. It focuses primarily on nongenetic risk factors and includes limited information on family history. Validation data show that it performs best in the general population versus in patients who have a family history of the disease.[21]

The Gail model was developed based on data from the Breast Cancer Detection Demonstration Project (BCDDP), a breast cancer screening study that included 280,000 women aged 35 to 74 years, and from the National Cancer Institute's Surveillance, Epidemiology, and End Results Program. Specific risk factors were chosen, and a model of relative risks for various combinations of these factors was developed from the case-control data from the BCDDP.[19,20]

This model allows for inclusion of a woman's personal medical and reproductive history as well as a limited amount of family history information. Input factors include age, age at menarche, age at first live birth, number of first-degree female relatives with breast cancer, number of previous breast biopsies and results of those biopsies. Output from the model includes invasive breast cancer risk over a 5-year interval as well as a lifetime risk to 90 years of age. It is a readily available model via a user-friendly online interface at http://www.cancer.gov/bcrisktool/. The model was developed in the United States and is well validated for white women as well as those of African American, Asian, and Pacific Islander descent.[20,22–24] It needs further validation for Hispanic women and other ethnic subgroups. The Gail model is not accurate for women with the following:

- Personal history of breast cancer, LCIS, or DCIS
- Chest (mantle field) radiation treatment of lymphoma between 10 and 30 years of age

- Known mutation in a gene such as *BRCA1*, *BRCA2*, *TP53*, or *PTEN*

This model is only applicable to women aged 35 years and older. It only includes first-degree female relatives with breast cancer and does not factor in the age of onset, meaning that the effect of a sister with breast cancer diagnosed at 35 years of age is the same as that of a sister diagnosed at 90 years of age. It does not account for breast cancer in paternal relatives or a family history of male breast cancer. It may overestimate risk in patients with benign breast biopsies. Additionally, it is not recognized by the ACS as a model to identify candidates for breast MR imaging screening as an adjunct to mammography. The ACS does not count it as a model that is "largely dependent on family history."[2] The NCCN's guidelines endorse the Gail model specifically for identifying candidates for chemoprevention when the 5-year risk is 1.67% or greater.[4]

The Claus model
The Claus model is primarily accessible via its original publication,[25] which includes data on family history of female breast cancer, as well as a follow-up publication that also includes family history of ovarian cancer.[26] It was developed from the cancer and steroid hormone study, which was a population-based, case-control study involving 4730 patients aged 20 to 54 years with documented breast cancer matched with 4688 controls. The model assumes that breast cancer risk is transmitted as an autosomal-dominant trait, and its' risk estimates are based on the patients' relation to their affected relatives.[25] Output information from this model includes lifetime breast cancer risk to 79 years of age, including both invasive cancer and DCIS. It should not be used in patients who have tested positive for a highly penetrant gene mutation associated with breast cancer risk because it does not allow for inclusion of genetic test results and will, therefore, underestimate risk in those women.

This model allows for inclusion of the woman's age and a fairly comprehensive family history, including age of onset of cancer diagnoses in first- and second-degree relatives. Contrary to the Gail model, it includes family history on both the maternal and paternal side of the family; the data are presented in a series of tables that allow for various combinations of affected first- and second-degree relatives but no more than 2 total relatives affected. Certain combinations of relatives are not represented, such as an affected mother and a maternal grandmother; but it can be assumed that the magnitude of risk for this scenario is similar to that of an affected mother and a maternal aunt.[27]

Limitations include the fact this model does not include any hormonal or reproductive factors and it cannot account for male relatives with breast cancer. Furthermore, it has not been validated in the high-risk setting or in the general population, so some experts question its accuracy in these populations. It was based on a dataset of North American patients between 1980 and 1982, and the breast cancer risks of these women are lower than the current incidence of breast cancer in North America and most of Europe.[28,29] Thus, some experts suggest an upward adjustment of 3% to 4% for lifetime risk estimates less than 20% as calculated by this model. There are computerized versions of the Claus model available; but they often give lower risk figures than the published tables, perhaps because the tables make no adjustments for unaffected relatives.[30]

The Tyrer-Cuzick model
The Tyrer-Cuzick model integrates a wide variety of personal risk factors as well as an extensive family history of breast and ovarian cancer. There are 2 versions of this model, v6 or v7; both are available online. Output information includes risk for breast cancer over the next 10 years as well as lifetime risk for breast cancer, including both invasive cancer and DCIS. In this model, the term *lifetime* refers to patients' risk of breast cancer to 80 years of age in v6 and the risk to 85 years of age in v7. For this reason, v7 typically gives higher risk estimates than v6. The Tyrer-Cuzick model also calculates the probability of a *BRCA1/2* gene mutation.

This model incorporates age, height, weight, Jewish inheritance, age at menarche, menopausal status, age at first live birth, hormone replacement use, history of high-risk breast lesions (including atypia and LCIS), as well as extended paternal and maternal family history of both breast and ovarian cancer, including ages of onset. It also incorporates positive and negative *BRCA1/2* genetic test results. V7 allows for inclusion of male breast cancer in close relatives. It also asks for family size and unaffected relatives, which can affect the outcome of the risk assessment. The user interface allows for uncertainty, and any unknown factors can be left as a question mark; however, this will affect the accuracy of the outcome.

This model is based on a dataset from the International Breast Cancer Intervention Study in the United Kingdom that included Caucasian high-risk women only, so its applicability to the general population is uncertain but thought to be similar to that in the high-risk population.[21,31] V7 uses population-based breast cancer rates from the

Table 3
Commonly used breast cancer risk assessment models

Model	Family History of Breast Cancer	Hormonal, Reproductive, and Other Factors	Personal History of Breast Disease	Genetic Assumptions	Risks Calculated	Used to Identify Candidates for	Method of Administration
Gail/BCRAT[75,a]	First-degree female relative, no age of onset Includes affected relatives only	Age at menarche and first live birth	Breast biopsies, including ADH/ALH	No assumptions made	Lifetime to 90 y of age and 5 y, including invasive cancer only	Chemoprevention (based on 5-y risk of ≥1.67%)	Web based: http://www.cancer.gov/bcrisktool/
Claus[25]	First- and second-degree female relative, including age of onset Includes affected relatives only, specific combinations of up to 2 affected relatives	None	None	1 Autosomal dominant gene with age-dependent penetrance	Lifetime to 79 y, including invasive and DCIS	Breast MR imaging screening	Published tables Brisk Breast Cancer Risk Assessment mobile application
Tyrer-Cuzick, v6[76]	First-, second-, and third-degree female relatives, including age of onset and bilateral Includes information about family size and unaffected relatives	Age at menarche, first live birth, menopause; hormone replacement therapy use; body mass index	Breast biopsies, including ALH, ADH, LCIS	BRCA1/2 plus multiple genes of differing penetrance	Lifetime to 80 y and 10 y, including invasive and DCIS	Breast MR imaging screening (based on lifetime risk)	Software download: http://www.ems-trials.org/riskevaluator/

Model	Family history	Other factors	Breast biopsies	Genes	Risk estimate	Breast MR imaging screening	Software
Tyer-Cuzick, v7[77–79]	First-, second-, and third-degree female relatives, including age of onset and bilateral; also first-degree male relative with breast cancer. Includes information about family size and unaffected relatives	Age at menarche, first live birth, menopause; hormone replacement therapy use; body mass index	Breast biopsies, including ALH, ADH, LCIS	BRCA1/2 plus a multiple genes of differing penetrance	Lifetime to 85 y; 10 y, including invasive and DCIS	Breast MR imaging screening (based on lifetime risk)	Software download: http://www.ems-trials.org/riskevaluator/
BRCAPRO[34–36,77–79]	First-, second-, and third-degree female and male relatives, including age of onset and bilateral. Includes information on family size and unaffected relatives	None	None	BRCA1/2—Mendelian approach that assumes an autosomal dominant pattern of inheritance	Lifetime to 84 y, invasive cancer only	Breast MR imaging screening	CaGene software; full pedigree entry required: https://www4.utsouthwestern.edu/breasthealth/cagene/
BOADICEA[35,80,81]	First- and second-degree female and male relatives, including age of onset and bilateral. Includes information on family size and unaffected relatives	None	None	BRCA1/2 plus a polygenic component	Lifetime to 80 y, including invasive and DCIS	Breast MR imaging screening	Web-based; full pedigree entry required: http://ccge.medschl.cam.ac.uk/boadicea/

Abbreviations: ADH, atypical ductal hyperplasia; ALH, atypical lobular hyperplasia.
a Only applicable to patients older than 35 years without a history of LCIS.

United Kingdom from 2008, which are higher than those from 1994, which are used in v6. This difference is another reason why the lifetime risk estimates from v7 are typically higher than those from v6. This model does not adjust for non-Caucasian races; it may not perform well in women with atypical hyperplasia or LCIS, as it seems to overestimate risk in these cases.[32] In the clinical setting, it may underestimate risk in women with strong family histories and overestimate risk in women with less strong family histories.[33]

Other models

In addition to the Claus model and Tyrer-Cuzick model, the BRCAPRO and BOADICEA models are also endorsed by the ACS for identifying candidates for breast MR imaging screening as an adjunct to mammography. They both calculate lifetime breast cancer risk as well as the probability of a BRCA1/2 mutation. These models require input of a full pedigree and are, therefore, more cumbersome to use in the clinic. The BRCAPRO model is based on the likelihood of a BRCA1/2 mutation.[34–36] The BOADICEA model accounts for BRCA1/2 mutations as well as a polygenic factor that aims to address the idea that multiple genes exist that each have small effects on breast cancer risk but act multiplicatively when factored together. Like the Claus model, BRCAPRO and BOADICEA do not incorporate information about nonhereditary risk factors and will likely underestimate risk in these women. Additionally, the BRCAPRO model will underestimate risk in BRCA-negative, breast cancer–only families because it does not account for genes other than BRCA1/2 that can contribute to cancer risk.[21]

Future directions include models that incorporate additional risk factors to improve discriminatory power, which could be using a model that has already been developed and incorporating additional risk factors into it or developing a new model entirely. Tissue characteristics, such as mammographic density,[37–41] single-nucleotide polymorphisms,[42,43] and histologic features of biopsy tissue from women with benign breast disease, have been tested.[44] Additionally, efforts are underway to develop models that are more applicable to non-Caucasian populations, because many breast cancer risk assessment models are validated on white women only.[45]

Use of Models in Patients with Hereditary Breast Cancer Syndromes

For patients with a BRCA1/2 gene mutation, breast cancer risk can be calculated via models that incorporate information about these gene mutations, namely, Tyrer-Cuzick (both versions), BRCAPRO, and BOADICEA. Additionally, these models can also account for negative BRCA1/2 genetic testing in patients as well as BRCA1/2 test results in other relatives. The Claus and Gail models should not be used for patients who are BRCA1/2 positive or for patients who are a true negative, meaning a relative carries a BRCA1/2 mutation but the patient does not.

For patients with mutations in other high familial penetrance genes (see **Table 2**), risk assessment models should not be used, as they cannot account for mutations in TP53, PTEN, and so forth. Rather, risk estimates should be made based on data that are available in the literature and screening recommendations should be based on standard guidelines, such as NCCN.

For patients with mutations in genes with moderate familial penetrance, as well as those that are less well characterized, risk assessment models may still be helpful in understanding the patients' individual risk; but the estimates from the models should be interpreted along with the genetic test results. Many of these genes seem to vary in their penetrance depending on the strength of the family history; so, in these cases, risk assessment is more complicated. Genetic counselors or similar experts are highly recommended in these situations to provide accurate and comprehensive risk assessment based on the most recent literature as well as to ensure understanding and compliance on the part of the patients.

Clinical Application of Risk Assessment Models

Comprehensive and accurate breast cancer risk assessment requires a multifaceted approach. Thus, it is important to calculate patients' risk via multiple models but also to understand which models are not applicable to a specific patient or may be less likely to be accurate for them. **Table 4** shows examples of how a clinician might consider various risk assessment models in various situations. Each scenario assumes that hereditary breast cancer syndromes have been ruled out. The BRCAPRO model is not mentioned in **Table 4** because it has limited use in BRCA1/2-negative, breast cancer–only families. The BOADICEA model may be useful in certain situations as well; but given the required entry of a 3-generation pedigree, it is often not reasonable outside of a genetic counseling setting.

Some of these concepts can also be understood by examining the outputs of various

Table 4
Clinical application of various risk assessment models

If a Patient Has	Then the Following Models Might Not Be Applicable	Because	You Might Consider Instead Using
3 or more relatives with breast cancer	Claus	It only accounts for up to 2 relatives with breast cancer.	Tyrer-Cuzick v6 or v7
	Gail	It only accounts for first-degree relatives with breast cancer.	
A very strong family history of early onset breast cancer in multiple relatives	Tyrer-Cuzick	It can underestimate risk in patients with very strong family histories.	Claus
2 paternal female relatives with breast cancer (ie, aunt, grandmother)	Gail	It only accounts for first-degree relatives with breast cancer.	Claus Tyrer-Cuzick v6 or v7
A father or brother with breast cancer	Claus Gail Tyrer-Cuzick v6	They do not include male breast cancer.	Tyrer-Cuzick v7
Large family size with many unaffected relatives	Gail Claus	They do not include information about family size/unaffected relatives.	Tyrer-Cuzick v6 or v7
Aged <35 y	Gail	It is not for use in patients younger than 35 y.	Claus Tyrer-Cuzick v6 or v7
Personal history of LCIS	Gail	It is not for use in patients with LCIS.	Tyrer-Cuzick v6 or v7 (although it may overestimate risk in these patients)
	Claus	It does not incorporate nonhereditary factors.	
A history of radiation to the chest between 10–30 y (mantle cell radiation [ie, for treatment of lymphoma])	All of them	None of them incorporate this significant risk factor.	NCCN's guidelines for screening in this particular situation

risk assessment models for the following sample case:

A 50-year-old Caucasian woman presents for breast cancer risk assessment. She is not of Ashkenazi Jewish ancestry. She has never had a breast biopsy. She is premenopausal. She was 13 years of age at menarche, and her first live birth was at 28 years of age. The output of various risk assessment models will differ as shown in the **Table 5** based on the model used as well as with different family histories.

Comparing scenarios 1 and 2, the Gail model in unable to discriminate the differences in age of onset of the affected relatives because the Gail model does not incorporate the age at which relatives were diagnosed. The family histories are different between these two scenarios, with scenario 2 being more clinically significant because of the earlier age of breast cancer onset in the relatives. The Claus and Tyrer-Cuzick models are able to incorporate this difference, and the risks estimated for scenario 2 are higher than those for scenario 1.

Scenario 3 is also clinically significant because of 2 affected maternal relatives, one at a very early age. However, the Gail model does not incorporate the maternal aunt's diagnosis and, therefore, is underestimating risk. The Claus and Tyrer-Cuzick models are likely to be more

Table 5
Sample cases

Scenario	Family History of Breast Cancer	Gail	Claus	Tyrer-Cuzick v6	Tyrer-Cuzick v7	BRCAPRO
1	Mother @ 75 y Sister @ 60 y	27.7% to 90 y	9.8% to 79 y	22.9% to 80 y	30.7% to 85 y	10.7% to 84 y
2	Mother @ 55 y Sister @ 45 y	27.7% to 90 y	20.4% to 79 y	23.5% to 80 y	31.5% to 85 y	11.1% to 84 y
3	Mother @ 55 y Maternal aunt @ 35 y	16.8% to 90 y	22.2% to 79 y	22.4% to 80 y	29.9% to 85 y	11.4% to 84 y
4	Paternal aunt @ 35 y Paternal aunt @ 39 y Paternal grandmother @ 40 y	9.9% to 90 y	17% to 79 y (only account for the 2 paternal aunts)	23.6% to 80 y	29.8% to 85 y	14.8% to 84 y

accurate because they incorporate the aunt's diagnosis of early onset breast cancer.

Scenario 4 highlights the deficiencies of the Gail model with 3 affected paternal relatives at very young ages not included in the calculation. The Claus model is also likely underestimating risk because it can only account for up to 2 of these paternal relatives. Thus, for this scenario, the Tyrer-Cuzick model is probably most accurate for the patient.

Note that in all scenarios, the BRCAPRO risk estimates tend to be lower than the other models and do not adjust significantly with varying family histories because this model assumes no other hereditary influence to breast cancer risk, aside from the *BRCA1/2* genes. The BRCAPRO model will underestimate risk in breast cancer–only families.

Of note, scenarios 2 to 4 necessitate discussion of genetic testing, as per the NCCN's guidelines.[4] Thus, the risk calculations listed in **Table 5** for these scenarios would only apply if highly penetrant hereditary breast cancer syndromes had been ruled out. If any of these patients tested positive for a gene mutation, the risk assessment would be governed by the particular gene mutation that was identified.

Risk Assessment in the Breast Imaging Center

Given the importance of customized breast cancer screening plans, risk assessment should be on the forefront of all breast imaging centers. A visit to a breast imaging clinic may be the best time and place to triage patients into a risk category and can allow for improved clinical compliance.[82,83]

Software solutions are available to assess risk and can be integrated into the workflow of a busy breast center. Such programs can estimate breast cancer risk based on various models, for the purpose of identifying patients who are candidates for supplementary imaging screening as well as those who should consider chemoprevention. Additionally, some software programs can identify patients who should be referred for genetic counseling and testing based on clinical characteristics or the chance of a *BRCA1/2* mutation. These features rely on accurate collection and input of various personal and family history data from each patient, which should be elicited at each visit to the clinic as risk factors can change over time. A breast imaging clinic can synthesize this information, as well as mammographic breast density, to develop a personalized breast cancer screening algorithm (**Fig. 2**).

However, a disadvantage of relying on an imaging clinic to assess patients' breast cancer risk and their need for cancer genetic counseling/testing is that many women do not seek breast imaging services until they are in their 40s or perhaps even their 50s.[84,85] This strategy could miss an opportunity to identify a patient that may benefit from earlier screening, before 40 years of age. Approximately 2.7% of women between 20 and 29 years of age, 5.3% between 30 and 39 years of age, and 8.7% between 40 and 49 years of age report a family history of breast cancer, many of which included a relative diagnosed at a young age.[86] Breast cancer screening at earlier ages is recommended for those with specific hereditary breast cancer gene mutations as well as in patients with

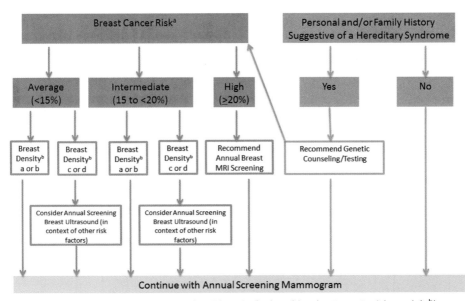

Fig. 2. Personalized Breast Cancer Screening Algorithm. [a]calculated by the Tyrer-Cuzick model. [b]breast composition is classified by the ACR BI-RADS® classification system.

a relative who was diagnosed with breast cancer before 50 years of age. In these situations, many guidelines recommend beginning screening 10 years before the earliest diagnosis in the relative. Although there is significant opportunity for patients to undergo accurate and comprehensive breast cancer risk assessment by their primary care or obstetrics/gynecology physician, studies show that this is not occurring consistently.[87] This finding underscores the importance of risk assessment as part of a woman's routine medical care. This risk assessment should begin in her early to mid 20s and be updated annually to capture any risk factors that may change over time.

HIGH-RISK SCREENING

Once breast cancer risk is determined, the next step is to consider how this information can be used. Guidelines and consensus statements are available to provide breast cancer screening recommendations. A practical way to look at imaging recommendations for high-risk screening is to group them into clinical categories (**Table 6**).

For patients with *BRCA1/2* mutations, beginning screening with annual breast MR imaging at 25 to 30 years of age and adding annual mammography at 30 years of age is widely accepted. The Society of Breast Imaging (SBI)/American College of Radiology (ACR) joint recommendations suggest annual mammography can begin at 25 years of age as well.[88] For patients who have not been tested themselves but have a first-degree relative with a *BRCA1/2*, *TP53* or *PTEN* mutation, annual

mammography and MR imaging are recommended by the ACS. All organizations listed have similar recommendations for patients with a history of mantle radiation, but recommendations vary by organization for patients at elevated risk due to a high-risk lesion. The recommended use for mammography is uniform for patients with a personal history of breast cancer, but the ACS' recommendation for MR imaging is less definitive at this time for this particular category of patients. The ACS is planning to update its guidelines for high-risk screening later this year.

When evaluating whether a patient is a candidate for breast MR imaging screening as an adjunct to mammography, the ACS supports using a variety of models that largely depend on family history, including BRCAPRO, Claus, and Tyrer-Cuzick. They acknowledge that these models are fundamentally different and predict varying outcomes. They have each been chosen purposefully to identify very different populations that are eligible for breast MR imaging screening. Therefore, even if only one of the ACS-endorsed models places patients at more than the 20% risk threshold, breast MR imaging screening should be considered. It is estimated that approximately 6% of women presenting for screening mammography will be high risk on at least one of the following models: Tyrer-Cuzick (v6), BRCAPRO, or Claus. The Tyrer-Cuzick model identified most of the eligible women (5.6%), and the other models identified a much smaller population. Only 0.2% of women were identified as *high risk/MR imaging candidates* on all 3 models.[31]

Table 6
Synthesis of practical risk categories and recommendations by organization

		Recommends Annual Mammography[a]			Recommends Annual MR Imaging		
		NCCN[86]	ACS[85]	SBI/ACR[31]	NCCN[86]	ACS[85]	SBI/ACR[31]
Genetic predisposition	BRCA1 or BRCA2 positive	≥30 y	≥30 y	≥25–30 y	≥25 y	≥25 y	≥25–30 y
	TP53 or PTEN positive	✗	✓	✗	✗	✓	✗
	5-y Gail model risk ≥1.7%	✓	✗	✗	✗	✗	✗
Family history	First-degree relative with BRCA1/2, TP53, or PTEN gene mutation and untested	✗	✓	✗	✗	✓	By 30 y
	Lifetime risk ≥20%[c]	✓	✓	≥25–30 y	✓	✓	≥25–30 y
Mantle radiation[d]	Between 10–30 y	✓	✓	8 y after radiation (not <25 y)	✓	✓	8 y after radiation
High-risk lesion	LCIS, ADH, or ALH	≥30 y	✗	Annually regardless of age	≥25 y	Not for or against	Consider based on high-risk lesion
Personal history	Any age	✓[b]	✓	Annually regardless of age	✗	Not for or against	Yes, at time of diagnosis
Dense breasts	ACR BI-RADS® breast composition category c or d[50]	✓	Yes but age to screen depends on risk assessment	Yes and consider supplemental screening with US	✗	Not for or against	✗

(✗) indicates the organization did not specify. (✓) indicates the exam is recommended by the organization.

Abbreviations: ACR, American College of Radiology; ADH, atypical ductal hyperplasia; ALH, atypical lobular hyperplasia; SBI, Society of Breast Imaging; US, ultrasound.

[a] NCCN considers the use of tomosynthesis when screening mammography is recommended.

[b] For DCIS, NCCN also indicates mammography at 6 to 12 months if after radiation and breast conservation.

[c] Lifetime risk based on models largely dependent on family history. Screening to begin 10 years before youngest family member but not less than 25 years of age.

[d] Typically therapeutic radiation to the chest.

Supplemental screening with whole-breast ultrasound in addition to mammography is something to be considered (based on the SBI/ACR's recommendations) for patients with ACR BI-RADS breast composition category *c* and *d*.[88]

The American Society of Breast Surgeons (ASBrS) recommends formal risk assessment for women aged 40 to 44 years. This conclusion was based on the ACS' guidelines, which state that average-risk women can wait until 45 years of to begin annual mammography screening but those who are at more than average risk should begin at 40 years of age.[84,89] Thus, the ASBrS recommends the use of a risk assessment tool in all women by 40 years of age to determine estimated lifetime risk for breast cancer as well as evaluation for the need for genetic counseling/testing when applicable. Women with a greater than 20% lifetime risk for breast cancer should begin screening at 40 years of age (or younger, if clinically indicated) with both annual mammography and breast MR imaging. Those at greater than 15% lifetime risk should begin annual screening mammography beginning at 40 years of age (or younger, if clinically indicated). A study found that, by following these guidelines, 50% of women between 40 and 44 years of age met the requirements for early mammography, 32% met the criteria for regular breast MR imaging screening, and 25% were eligible for genetic counseling/testing.[90]

Lastly, the USPSTF breast cancer screening recommendations in 2015 indicates that "women with a parent, sibling, or child with breast cancer are at higher risk for breast cancer and thus may benefit more than average-risk women from beginning screening in their 40s."[85] They also state that there is insufficient evidence for the addition of supplemental tools to a negative screening mammogram in women with dense breasts.[85]

SUMMARY

It is important to recognize that patients at high risk for breast cancer may benefit by following breast cancer screening paradigms that are more robust than those recommended for the average-risk population. Assessing individual cancer risk and using guidelines to determine if a patient is a candidate for genetic counseling and possibly genetic testing are essential components to comprehensive breast cancer screening.

REFERENCES

1. Saadatmand S, Bretveld R, Siesling S, et al. Influence of tumour stage at breast cancer detection on survival in modern times: population based study in 173,797 patients. BMJ 2015;351:h4901.
2. Saslow D, Boetes C, Burke W, et al. American Cancer Society guidelines for breast screening with MRI as an adjunct to mammography. CA Cancer J Clin 2007;57(2):75–89.
3. Berg WA, Zhang Z, Lehrer D, et al. Detection of breast cancer with addition of annual screening ultrasound or a single screening MRI to mammography in women with elevated breast cancer risk. JAMA 2012;307(13):1394–404.
4. National Comprehensive Cancer Network. Genetic/familial high-risk assessment: breast and ovarian (version 1.207). Available at: https://www.nccn.org/professionals/physician_gls/pdf/genetics_screening.pdf. Accessed September 20, 2016.
5. Moyer VA. Risk assessment, genetic counseling, and genetic testing for *BRCA*-related cancer in women: U.S. Preventive Services Task Force recommendation statement. Ann Intern Med 2014;160(4):271–81.
6. FORCE Web site. Available at: http://www.facingourrisk.org/understanding-brca-and-hboc/information/hereditary-cancer/hereditary-genetics/basics/signs-of-hereditary-breast-and-ovarian-cancer.php. Accessed September 20, 2016.
7. Frank TS, Deffenbaugh AM, Reid JE, et al. Clinical characteristics of individuals with germline mutations in *BRCA1* and *BRCA2*: analysis of 10,000 individuals. J Clin Oncol 2002;20:1480–90. Available at: https://www.myriadpro.com/hereditary-cancer-testing/hereditary-breast-and-ovarian-cancer-hboc-syndrome/prevalence-tables/.
8. Claus EB. Risk models used to counsel women for breast and ovarian cancer: a guide for clinicians. Fam Cancer 2001;1(3–4):197–206.
9. Plon SE, Cooper HP, Parks B, et al. Genetic testing and cancer risk management recommendations by physicians for at-risk relatives. Genet Med 2011;13(2):148–54.
10. Gilpin CA, Carson N, Hunter AG. A preliminary validation of a family history assessment form to select women at risk for breast or ovarian cancer for referral to a genetic center. Clin Genet 2000;58(4):299–308.
11. Evans DG, Eccles DM, Rahman N, et al. A new scoring system for the chances of identifying a *BRCA1/2* mutation outperforms existing models including BRCAPRO. J Med Genet 2004;41(6):474–80.
12. Bellcross CA, Lemke AA, Pape LS, et al. Evaluation of a breast/ovarian cancer genetics referral screening tool in a mammography population. Genet Med 2009;11(11):783–9.
13. Bellcross CA. Further development and evaluation of a breast/ovarian cancer genetics referral screening tool. Genet Med 2010;12(4):240.

14. Hoskins KF, Zwaagstra A, Ranz M. Validation of a tool for identifying women at high risk for hereditary breast cancer in population-based screening. Cancer 2006;107(8):1769–76.

15. Ashton-Prolla P, Giacomazzi J, Schmidt AV, et al. Development and validation of a simple questionnaire for the identification of hereditary breast cancer in primary care. BMC Cancer 2009;9:283.

16. Travis LB, Hill D, Dores GM, et al. Cumulative absolute breast cancer risk for young women treated for Hodgkin lymphoma. J Natl Cancer Inst 2005;97:1428–37.

17. American Cancer Society. Breast Cancer Facts & Figures 2015-2016. Atlanta: American Cancer Society, Inc; 2012.

18. Sickles EA, D'Orsi CJ, Bassett LW, et al. ACR BI-RADS® Mammography. In: ACR BI-RADS® Atlas, Breast Imaging Reporting and Data System. Reston (VA): American College of Radiology; 2013.

19. Gail MH, Brinton LA, Byar DP, et al. Projecting individualized probabilities of developing breast cancer for white females who are being examined annually. J Natl Cancer Inst 1989;81(24):1879–86.

20. Costantino JP, Gail MH, Pee D, et al. Validation studies for models projecting the risk of invasive and total breast cancer incidence. J Natl Cancer Inst 1999;91(18):1541–8.

21. Amir E, Evans DG, Shenton A, et al. Evaluation of breast cancer risk assessment packages in the family history evaluation and screening programme. J Med Genet 2003;40(11):807–14.

22. Spiegelman D, Colditz GA, Hunter D, et al. Validation of the Gail et al. model for predicting individual breast cancer risk. J Natl Cancer Inst 1994;86(8):600–7.

23. Bondy ML, Lustbader ED, Halabi S, et al. Validation of a breast cancer risk assessment model in women with a positive family history. J Natl Cancer Inst 1994;86(8):620–5.

24. Rockhill B, Spiegelman D, Byrne C, et al. Validation of the Gail et al. model of breast cancer risk prediction and implications of chemoprevention. J Natl Cancer Inst 2001;7(5):358–66.

25. Claus EB, Risch N, Thompson WD. Autosomal dominant inheritance of early onset breast cancer: implications for risk prediction. Cancer 1994;73(3):643–51.

26. Claus EB, Risch N, Thompson WD. The calculation of breast cancer risk for women with a first degree family history of ovarian cancer. Breast Cancer Res Treat 1993;28(2):115–20.

27. Amir E, Orit C, Freedman OC, et al. Assessing women at high risk of breast cancer: a review of risk assessment models. J Natl Cancer Inst 2010;102(10):680–91.

28. Jemal A, Siegel R, Ward E, et al. Cancer statistics, 2008. CA Cancer J Clin 2008;58(2):71–96.

29. Parkin DM, Bray F, Ferlay J, et al. Global cancer statistics, 2002. CA Cancer J Clin 2005;55(2):74–108.

30. Tischkowitz M, Wheeler D, France E, et al. A comparison of methods currently used in clinical practice to estimate familial breast cancer risks. Ann Oncol 2000;11(4):451–4.

31. Ozanne EM, Drohan B, Bosinoff P, et al. Which risk model to use? Clinical implications of the ACS MRI screening guidelines. Cancer Epidemiol Biomarkers Pred 2013;22(1):146–9.

32. Boughey JC, Hartmann LC, Anderson SS, et al. Evaluation of the Tyrer-Cuzick (International Breast Cancer Intervention Study) model for breast cancer risk predication in women with atypical hyperplasia. J Clin Oncol 2010;28(22):3591–6.

33. Rosner B, Colditz GA. Nurses' health study: log-incidence mathematical model of breast cancer incidence. J Natl Cancer Inst 1996;88:359–64.

34. Shannon KM, Lubratovish ML, Finkelstein DM, et al. Model-based predictions of BRCA1/2 mutation status in breast carcinoma patients treated at an academic medical center. Cancer 2002;94(2):305–13.

35. Berry DA, Iverson ES Jr, Gudbjartsson DF, et al. BRCAPRO validation, sensitivity of genetic testing of BRCA1/BRCA2, and prevalence of other breast cancer susceptibility genes. J Clin Oncol 2002;20(11):2701–12.

36. Enhus DM, Smith KC, Robinson L, et al. Pretest prediction of BRCA1 or BRCA2 mutation by risk counselors and the computer model BRCAPRO. J Natl Cancer Inst 2002;94(11):844–51.

37. Vachon CM, Pankratz VS, Scott CG, et al. The contributions of breast density and common genetic variation to breast cancer risk. J Natl Cancer Inst 2015;107(5) [pii:dju397].

38. Barlow WE, White E, Ballard-Barbash R, et al. Prospective breast cancer risk prediction model for women undergoing screening mammography. J Natl Cancer Inst 2006;98(17):1204–14.

39. Tice JA, Cummings SR, Smith-Bindman R, et al. Using clinical factors and mammographic breast density to estimate breast cancer risk: development and validation of a new predictive model. Ann Intern Med 2008;148(5):337–47.

40. Chen J, Pee D, Ayyagari R, et al. Projecting absolute invasive breast cancer risk in shite women with a model that includes mammographic density. J Natl Cancer Inst 2006;98(17):1215–26.

41. Brentnall AR, Harkness EF, Astley SM, et al. Mammographic density adds accuracy to both Tyrer-Cuzick and Gail breast cancer risk models in a prospective UK screening cohort. Breast Cancer Res 2015;17(1):147.

42. Mealiffe ME, Stokowski RP, Rhees BK, et al. Assessment of clinical validity of a breast cancer risk model combining genetic and clinical information. J Natl Cancer Inst 2010;102(21):1618–27.

43. Brentnall AR, Evans DG, Cuzick J. Distribution of breast cancer risk from SNPs and classical risk

factors in women of routine screening age in the UK. Br J Cancer 2014;110(3):827–8.

44. Pankratz VS, Degnim AC, Frank RD, et al. Model for individualized prediction of breast cancer risk after a benign breast biopsy. J Clin Oncol 2015;33(8):923–9.

45. Boggs DA, Rosenberg L, Adams-Campbell LL, et al. Prospective approach to breast cancer risk prediction in African American women: the black women's health study model. J Clin Oncol 2015;33(9):1038–44.

46. Ford D, Easton DF, Bishop DT, et al. Risks of cancer in BRCA1-mutation carriers. Breast Cancer Linkage Consortium. Lancet 1994;343(8899):692–5.

47. Antoniou A, Pharoah PD, Narod S, et al. Average risk of breast and ovarian cancer associated with BRCA1 or BRCA2 mutations detected in case series unselected for family history: a combined analysis of 22 studies. Am J Hum Genet 2003;72(5):1117–30.

48. Ford D, Easton DF, Stratton M, et al. Genetic heterogeneity and penetrance analysis of the BRCA1 and BRCA2 genes in breast cancer families. The Breast Cancer Linkage Consortium. Am J Hum Genet 1998; 62(3):676–89.

49. Chompret A, Brugières L, Ronsin M, et al. P53 germline mutations in childhood cancers and cancer risk for carrier individuals. Br J Cancer 2000;82(12): 1932–7.

50. Bougeard G, Renaux-Petel M, Flaman JM, et al. Revisiting Li-Fraumeni syndrome from TP53 mutation carriers. J Clin Oncol 2015;33(21):2345–52.

51. Tan MH, Mester JL, Ngeow J, et al. Lifetime cancer risks in individuals with germline PTEN mutations. Clin Cancer Res 2012;18(2):400–7.

52. Antoniou AC, Casadei S, Heikkinen T, et al. Breast-cancer risk in families with mutations in PALB2. N Engl J Med 2014;371(6):497–506.

53. van Lier MG, Wagner A, Mathus-Vliegen EM, et al. High cancer risk in Peutz-Jeghers syndrome: a systematic review and surveillance recommendations. Am J Gastroenterol 2010;105(6):1258–64 [author reply: 1265].

54. Pharoah PD, Guilford P, Caldas C, International Gastric Cancer Linkage Consortium. Incidence of gastric cancer and breast cancer in CDH1 (E-cadherin) mutation carriers from hereditary diffuse gastric cancer families. Gastroenterology 2001;121(6):1348–53.

55. Kaurah P, MacMillan A, Boyd N, et al. Founder and recurrent CDH1 mutations in families with hereditary diffuse gastric cancer. JAMA 2007;297(21):2360–72.

56. van der Post RS, Vogelaar IP, Carneiro F, et al. Hereditary diffuse gastric cancer: updated clinical guidelines with an emphasis on germline CDH1 mutation carriers. J Med Genet 2015;52(6):361–74.

57. Weischer M, Bojesen SE, Ellervik C, et al. CHEK2*1100delC genotyping for clinical assessment of breast cancer risk: meta-analyses of 26,000 patient cases and 27,000 controls. J Clin Oncol 2008;26(4):542–8.

58. Cybulski C, Wokołorczyk D, Jakubowska A, et al. Risk of breast cancer in women with a CHEK2 mutation with and without a family history of breast cancer. J Clin Oncol 2011;29(28):3747–52.

59. Ahmed M, Rahman N. ATM and breast cancer susceptibility. Oncogene 2006;25(43):5906–11.

60. Swift M, Morrell D, Massey RB, et al. Incidence of cancer in 161 families affected by ataxia-telangiectasia. N Engl J Med 1991;325(26):1831–6.

61. Thompson D, Duedal S, Kirner J, et al. Cancer risks and mortality in heterozygous ATM mutation carriers. J Natl Cancer Inst 2005;97(11):813–22.

62. Zhang B, Beeghly-Fadiel A, Long J, et al. Genetic variants associated with breast-cancer risk: comprehensive research synopsis, meta-analysis, and epidemiological evidence. Lancet Oncol 2011; 12(5):477–88.

63. Steffen J, Nowakowska D, Niwińska A, et al. Germline mutations 657del5 of the NBS1 gene contribute significantly to the incidence of breast cancer in Central Poland. Int J Cancer 2006; 119(2):472–5.

64. Seminog OO, Goldacre MJ. Risk of benign tumours of nervous system, and of malignant neoplasm, in people with neurofibromatosis: population-based record-linkage study. Br J Cancer 2013;108(1):193–8.

65. Madanikia SA, Bergner A, Ye X, et al. Increased risk of breast cancer in women with NF1. Am J Med Genet A 2012;158A(12):3056–60.

66. Rafnar T, Gudbjartsson DF, Sulem P, et al. Mutations in BRIP1 confer high risk of ovarian cancer. Nat Genet 2011;43(11):1104–7.

67. Seal S, Thompson D, Renwick A, et al. Truncating mutations in the Fanconi anemia J gene BRIP1 are low-penetrance breast cancer susceptibility alleles. Nat Genet 2006;38(11):1239–41.

68. Easton DF, Lesueur F, Decker B, et al. No evidence that protein truncating variants in BRIP1 are associated with breast cancer risk: implications for gene panel testing. J Med Genet 2016; 53(5):298–309.

69. Le Calvez-Kelm F, Oliver J, Damiola F, et al. RAD51 and breast cancer susceptibility: no evidence for rare variant association in the Breast Cancer Family Registry study. PLoS One 2012;7(12):e52374.

70. Coulet F, Fajac A, Colas C, et al. Germline RAD51C mutations in ovarian cancer susceptibility. Clin Genet 2013;83(4):332–6.

71. Loveday C, Turnbull C, Ramsay E, et al. Germline mutations in RAD51D confer susceptibility to ovarian cancer. Nat Genet 2011;43(9):879–82.

72. Vogt S, Jones N, Christian D, et al. Expanded extracolonic tumor spectrum in MUTYH-associated polyposis. Gastroenterology 2009;137(6):1976–85.e1-10.

73. Rennert G, Lejbkowicz F, Cohen I, et al. MutYH mutation carriers have increased breast cancer risk. Cancer 2012;118(8):1989–93.

74. Damiola F, Pertesi M, Oliver J, et al. Rare key functional domain missense substitutions in MRE11A, RAD50, and NBN contribute to breast cancer susceptibility: results from a Breast Cancer Family Registry case-control mutation-screening study. Breast Cancer Res 2014;16(3):R58.

75. Heikkinen K, Rapakko K, Karppinen SM, et al. RAD50 and NBS1 are breast cancer susceptibility genes associated with genomic instability. Carcinogenesis 2006;27(8):1593–9.

76. Madigan MP, Ziegler RG, Benichou J, et al. Proportion of breast cancer cases in the United States explained by well-established risk factors. J Natl Cancer Inst 1995;87(22):1681–5.

77. Tyrer J, Duffy SW, Cuzick J. A breast cancer prediction model incorporating familial and personal risk factors. Stat Med 2004;23(7):1111–30.

78. Berry DA, Parmigiani G, Sanchez J, et al. Probability of carrying a mutation of breast-ovarian cancer gene BRCA1 based on family history. J Natl Cancer Inst 1997;89:227–38.

79. Parmigiani G, Berry D, Aguilar O. Determining carrier probabilities for breast cancer-susceptibility genes BRCA1 and BRCA2. Am J Hum Genet 1998;62:145–58.

80. Antoniou AC, Pharoah PD, McMullan G, et al. A comprehensive model for familial breast cancer incorporating BRCA1, BRCA2 and other genes. Br J Cancer 2002;86:76–83.

81. Antoniou AC, Pharoah PP, Smith P, et al. The BOADICEA model of genetic susceptibility to breast and ovarian cancer. Br J Cancer 2004;91:1580–90.

82. Brinton JT, Barke LD, Freivogel ME, et al. Breast cancer risk assessment in 64,659 women at a single high-volume mammography clinic. Acad Radiol 2012;19(1):95–9.

83. Brinton JT, Barke LD, Freivogel ME, et al. Informing women and their physicians about recommendations for adjunct breast MRI Screening: a cohort study. Health Commun 2017;3:1–7.

84. Oeffinger KC, Fontham ET, Etzioni R, et al. Breast cancer screening for women at average risk: 2015 guideline update from the American Cancer Society. JAMA 2015;314(15):1599–614.

85. Siu AL, On behalf of the U.S. Preventative Services Task Force. Screening for breast cancer: U.S. Preventative Services Task Force recommendation statement. Ann Intern Med 2016;164(4):279–96.

86. Ramsey SD, Yoon P, Moonesinghe R, et al. Population-based study of the prevalence of family history of cancer: implications for cancer screening and prevention. Genet Med 2006;8:571–5.

87. Murff HJ, Greevy RA, Syngal S. The comprehensiveness of family cancer history assessments in primary care. Community Genet 2007;10:174–80.

88. Lee CH, Dershaw DD, Kopans D, et al. Breast cancer screening with imaging: recommendations from the Society of Breast Imaging and the ACR on the use of mammography, breast MRI, breast ultrasound, and other technologies for the detection of clinically occult breast cancer. J Am Coll Radiol 2010;7(1):18–27.

89. Available at: https://www.breastsurgeons.org/new_layout/about/statements/PDF_Statements/Screening_Mammography.pdf. Accessed September 5, 2016.

90. Plichta JK, Coopey SB, Griffin ME, et al. Application of the 2015 ACS and ASBS Screening Mammography Guidelines: Risk Assessment is Critical for Women Ages 40-44. Presented at ASBS Annual Meeting, Massachusetts General Hospital. Boston, 2016. Available at: https://www.breastsurgeons.org/docs2016/press/PLICHTA-Risk_based_screening-slides.pdf.

Breast Tomosynthesis
Clinical Evidence

Steven Poplack, MD

KEYWORDS

• Digital breast tomosynthesis • Diagnostic evaluation • Trial outcomes

KEY POINTS

• The data on the efficacy and effectiveness that has accumulated in the last 20 years is consistent and compelling.
• Most published outcomes suggest that screening with DBT improves cancer detection and reduces false positive recalls.
• Diagnostic imaging with DBT of non-calcified findings has equivalent or superior performance compared to digital mammography.

INTRODUCTION

In January 2016, the United States Preventive Services Task Force updated their breast cancer screening recommendations and classified digital breast tomosynthesis (DBT), concluding that "the current evidence is insufficient to assess the benefits and harms of digital breast tomosynthesis (DBT) as a primary screening method for breast cancer."[1] This was primarily based on the absence of randomized controlled trials of DBT. In sharp contrast to this conclusion, nearly 20 years of scientific and service data have accumulated that clearly confirm the efficacy of the DBT technology and strongly suggest its effectiveness in both screening and diagnostic applications. Beginning in 1997 with the first scientific publication on DBT[2] and continuing with the ongoing results reporting of a wide variety of clinical trials, the data supporting the use of DBT are both consistent and compelling. This article catalogs the scientific and clinical evidence of DBT, highlighting some of the most important studies that have been reported to date.

EARLY OBSERVATIONAL STUDIES: 1997 TO 2008

Modern DBT was first introduced into the peer reviewed literature in 1997 by Niklason and colleagues[2] in a proof of principle experiment conducted at the Massachusetts General Hospital (MGH) using a prototype modification of the senographe DMR (GE Medical Systems, Milwaukee, WI). Three radiologists with mammography expertise rated lesion and margin visibility and diagnostic confidence of DBT images (at the slice of interest) and film mammography (FM) images of 6 abnormalities contained within 4 mastectomy specimens. Images were viewed side by side on a high luminance view box. The abnormalities included subtle findings (irregular mass, calcifications, round mass), a discrete round mass, architectural distortion, and an obvious 3 cm mass. DBT was superior to FM in the evaluation of all of the subtle abnormalities and the area of architectural distortion. Only the obvious mass had comparable ratings. The investigators concluded that DBT is "capable of producing high-quality breast images that may contain information that is currently not visible with conventional imaging" and that the value of DBT was most evident in the setting of radiographically dense tissue.

After a 10 year hiatus, Poplack and colleagues,[3] described the first in vivo DBT experience in a consecutive series of clinical subjects. The study was intended to evaluate the efficacy of DBT in the setting of diagnostic imaging. Ninety-eight women with 99 abnormalities recalled from digital

Breast Imaging Section, Mallinckrodt Institute of Radiology, Washington University School of Medicine, 510 South Kingshighway Boulevard, St. Louis, MO 63110, USA
E-mail address: poplack@wustl.edu

Radiol Clin N Am 55 (2017) 475–492
http://dx.doi.org/10.1016/j.rcl.2016.12.010
0033-8389/17/© 2017 Elsevier Inc. All rights reserved.

mammography (DM) screening were enrolled. Current practice at that time included screening with DM and diagnostic work up with FM; therefore, subjects underwent FM diagnostic evaluation per usual clinical protocol. DBT full-field images were obtained with a prototype unit, Genesis (Hologic Inc), and matched to the FM diagnostic views, Lorad MIV (Hologic Inc, Danbury, CT), in up to 3 projections. One mm DBT slices were viewed on a prototype workstation. One radiologist specializing in breast imaging subjectively compared the diagnostic image quality of DBT with FM based on lesion conspicuity and feature analysis. At a separate session, the radiologist reviewed the DM screening examination with the additional DBT images to determine recall status, providing a reason for no recall.

The results for both diagnostic and screening DBT applications were remarkable. For the diagnostic imaging comparison, DBT was superior to FM in 37 out of 99 (37%), equivalent in 51 out of 99 (52%), and inferior in 11 out of 99 (11%) of the cases based on subjective image quality. Eight of the 11 (73%) inferior ratings involved calcifications. The adjunctive use of DBT for screening led to a 40% (37/92) reduction in false positive (FP) recalls. The study provided insight into the nature of DBT recall reduction. Most, 71% (32/45), came under the heading of no abnormality seen and were thought to reflect superimposition of normal fibroglandular tissues. The remainder of the recalls, 27% (12/45), reflected definitive lesion characterization (7/12) and detection of multiple benign masses (5/12).

A third important pilot observational study evaluated the cancer detection potential of DBT. In this study, Andersson and colleagues[4] assessed the conspicuity of subtle breast malignancy defined as questionably visible or occult on DM. DBT was performed on a modified DM unit, Mammomat Novation (Siemens Medical, Erlangen, Germany). Two experienced breast radiologists compared single-view (1v) DBT with 1v DM and 2-view (2v) DM on a prototype workstation and rendered a nonblinded consensus opinion. The DBT projection was selected to correspond with the DM view in which the cancer was judged to be least well seen, and defaulted to the mediolateral oblique (MLO) projection when the cancer was occult on DM. The readers rated each case by modality on a 4-point visibility scale, reported final Breast Imaging Reporting and Data System (BIRADS), overall breast density, breast density within 1 cm of the cancer, and mammographic finding type.

There were 40 breast cancers in 36 women, with an average subject age of 59 years and median tumor size of 11 mm. Almost all, 39 out of 40 (98%) were invasive cancer with only a single case of pure ductal carcinoma in situ (DCIS). Both invasive lobular carcinoma, 10 out of 39 (26%), and tubular carcinoma, 3 out of 39 (8%), were over-represented relative to a typical invasive cancer distribution. Two-thirds (24/36) of breasts had dense composition (heterogeneously dense or extremely dense). Cancer was significantly ($P<.01$) more visible with DBT than with either 1v DM or 2v DM. Visibility was rated higher with 1v DBT than 2v DM in 11 out of 40 (28%) cancers. BIRADS assessment was upgraded by DBT in 11 subjects compared with 2v DM. The investigators concluded that 1v DBT was better than DM in visualizing and classifying mammographically subtle cancer.

Summary

- Early studies showed a decrease in recall with DBT, primarily because of the ability to discount superimposed tissue.
- Increase in cancer conspicuity was appreciated with DBT when the malignancies were either mammographically subtle or occult.
- Calcifications were not as well characterized on DBT, possibly due to long exposure times.

READER STUDIES: 2008 TO 2012

Over the course of the next 5 years, 16 small to intermediate-scale DBT reader studies were published in the English language in peer reviewed journals from the United States and Europe.[5–20] For the most part, these studies consisted of small-scale rating trials that evaluated the efficacy of DBT in different clinical settings (ie, screening or diagnostic breast imaging) or in the assessment of distinct mammographic finding types (eg, calcifications or masses). Studies ranged from 30 to 376 subjects and involved up to 20 mammography readers with varying levels of mammography expertise, although none of the readers had a high-volume experience with DBT due to its novelty. Highlights from some of those studies are noted here.

SCREENING STUDIES: 2008 TO 2012

Under the leadership of David Gur, researchers from the University of Pittsburgh Medical Center (UPMC) published 2 pilot performance studies using a common image data set of 125 unilateral examinations enriched with 35 cancers. Eight breast radiologist specialists compared DM alone with the combination of DM and 2v DBT. In the first study,[6] the readers also evaluated DBT source images and 2v DBT only. DM was acquired using the Selenia (Hologic Inc) and DBT with the Genesis (Hologic Inc). Unilateral examinations were viewed on a prototype workstation that recorded lesion localization, screening BIRADS, likelihood of malignancy, and time to interpretation. The first study reported a statistically significant 30% decrease in FP recalls ($P<.0001$) when comparing DM only with combined DM/DBT, and a 10% nonsignificant recall reduction ($P = .09$) comparing DM with DBT. The investigators concluded that the "Use of digital breast tomosynthesis for breast imaging may result in a substantial decrease in recall rate." The second study assessed DBT screening performance using receiver operator characteristic (ROC) curve analysis.[13] ROCs were generated for cancer cases and for all (benign and malignant) cases. For cancer cases, there was an overall higher performance level for each of the 8 breast radiologist readers, with a mean improvement of 16% (range of 5%–34%) with the use of combined DM/DBT. On average, 6 additional cancers were identified (from a pool of 35) at the expense of 8 additional FP findings in 125 examinations. The increase in FP ratings occurred in combination with correctly detected cancer cases (ie, true positives) and did not occur in the setting of noncancer cases. In cases that were truly negative, there were fewer FP for combined DM/DBT than DM only. Gur and colleagues[13] concluded that adjunctive DBT improved observer performance.

At about the same time, Gennaro and colleagues[7] conducted a clinical performance study of 2v DM versus MLO 1v DBT in 200 women with at least 1 abnormality detected by DM or ultrasound (US). The contralateral breast comprised the normal cases. DM was acquired using the Senographe 2000D (GE Healthcare), whereas DBT was performed on a prototype DBT unit (GE Healthcare). After exclusions, the study group consisted of 376 breasts with 63 cancers, 177 benign lesions, and 136 normal cases. DBT was viewed as both 1 mm slices and 10 mm slab reconstructions. Six radiologists rated lesion conspicuity and assessed final BIRADS on combined DM and DBT image sets over multiple reader sessions with a 1-week to 4-week interval between sessions. ROC curves were generated by reader and in aggregate. The overall area under the curve (AUC) for 1v DBT (0.851) was no different than the AUC of 2v DM (0.836), $P = .645$. However, 4 readers had slightly greater AUC for 1v DBT and 2 readers had slightly greater AUC for 2v DM. The mean sensitivity for DBT was 69.8% and for DM was 74.3%. The mean specificity was 88.9% and 84.8% for DBT and DM, respectively. The overall mean conspicuity of 1v DBT was higher or equal to 2v DM in 79% of all abnormalities, 81% of cancers, and 79% of benign abnormalities. The investigators commented that the better lesion conspicuity afforded by DBT did not lead to improved assessment and concluded that 1v (MLO) DBT was not inferior to 2v DM.

Svahn and colleagues[10] compared DM with 1v (MLO) DBT and added a third arm combining MLO DBT with craniocaudal (CC) DM in an enriched image set analysis of 25 cancer cases and 25 noncancer cases. Cancer cases were restricted to women with subtle DM screen detected and symptomatic women with suspicious US findings. DM was acquired using the Mammomat Novation (Siemens Medical) and DBT performed with a DBT prototype modification of the Mammomat Novation (Siemens Medical). Five expert readers assessed suspicious findings with a final BIRADS score. Combined CC DM/ (MLO) DBT (AUC = 0.833) performed better than 1v (MLO) DBT (AUC = 0.81), which in turn performed better than 2v DM (AUC = 0.76). Only the comparison of DM/DBT with DM attained statistical significance; however, the investigators noted that the biggest step in performance occurred from DM to 1v DBT.

Using similar methodology, Svahn and colleagues[16] reported observer performance results from a larger cohort of subjects restricting the comparison to 1v DBT versus DM. The unilateral breasts of 185 women comprised the study cohort, consisting of 95 cancers in 89 breasts and 96 breasts that were normal or benign. Breast density of the malignant breasts was classified as predominantly fat in 9 out of 89 (10%), scattered in 26 out of 89 (29%), heterogeneously dense in 50 out of 89 (56%), and extremely dense in 4 out of 89 (5%). DBT that was 1v significantly outperformed DM for all 5 readers in 2 separate ROC analyses. DBT had a significantly higher sensitivity than DM (90% vs 79%). On average, 10 additional cancers were detected by DBT, although the FP fraction was not significantly different. The cancer detection benefit was seen in invasive cancer rather than DCIS, whereas DCIS was detected more frequently by DM. The investigators concluded that MLO DBT was more accurate than 2v DM but cautioned readers that this result required confirmation in larger population-based trials.

Wallis and colleagues[19] also compared 2v DM with 1v DBT but also compared 2v DBT and used a DBT system that had not previously been reported. The study group included symptomatic women and women recalled for an abnormal DM screen, including 64 women with malignant (40) or benign (24) pathologic findings and 66 normal women. Predominantly fatty breasts were excluded. The predominant finding type was mass in 30 out of 64 (47%), calcifications in 23 out of 64 (36%), architectural distortion or asymmetry in 7 out of 64 (11%), and DM occult findings in 4 out of 64 (6%). DM was acquired with MicroDose D40 (Sectrea Mamea, Solna, Sweden) or Senographe Essential (GE Medical Systems). DBT was performed with a modification of the MicroDose DM system (Sectra Mamea). This system reconstructed images of 3 mm slice thickness. The 2 groups of 10 readers were high-volume readers (mean 12,350 examinations per year) with variable (2.5–25 years) mammography experience. One group compared 2v DM to 2v DBT and the other group compared 2v DM with 1v DBT, rating the probability of malignancy (POM) and recall decision.

Overall, 2v DBT performed significantly better than 2v DM (AUC 0.851 vs 0.772, $P = .21$), which applied to both masses and calcifications. No difference was seen comparing 1v DBT with 2v DM. When readers were aggregated by years of experience (ie, <10 years vs ≥10 years) only less experienced readers had significantly better performance with 2v DBT than 2v DM ($P = .03$ vs $P = .25$) Experience had no effect on the 1v DBT comparison. Recall rates decreased by 11% for 2v DBT and 9.5% for 1v DBT. Wallis and colleagues[19] concluded that 2v DBT performed better than 1v DM only in readers with fewer than 10 years of mammography experience.

Summary
- Multiple (4) different DBT manufacturers report generally consistent results.
- DBT that is 2v (alone or in combination with DM) is more accurate than 2v DM.
- DBT that is 1v is not inferior to 2v DM.

DIAGNOSTIC STUDIES 2008 TO 2012
Noncalcified Abnormalities

Although the main thrust of investigation involved screening applications, trials estimating the diagnostic utility of DBT were also conducted at this time. Three small-scale studies compared DBT with spot compression views in the diagnostic evaluation of noncalcified abnormalities.[11,15,17]

Hakim and colleagues[11] reported the results of a subject rating study of 25 women with noncalcified abnormalities comparing screening DM and spot DM diagnostic views with screening DM and 2v DBT. Four readers subjectively rated diagnostic utility and assessed final BIRADS and the need for US. DBT was subjectively preferred to spot DM in 50% and was equivalent in 30% of cases. Approximately two-thirds of benign cases were rated as BIRADS 1, 2, or 3; and 92% of cancer cases were rated as BIRADS 4 or 5. Of the 2 false-negative DBT reads, the mass was deemed suspect based on change from

prior examinations, which were not available to study readers. If DBT had been used clinically, 12% of cases would not have required US. The investigators suggested that DBT may have an important future role in the diagnostic evaluation of some noncalcified abnormalities.

Subsequently, in October 2011, separate groups in Europe and the United States published results of a comparison of DBT with mammographic focal compression views in the diagnostic evaluation of noncalcified abnormalities.[15,17] Tagliafico and colleagues[15] evaluated 52 consecutive women who underwent both DBT and digital focal compression views in 2 projections using the Selenia Dimensions (Hologic Inc) by 2 readers who were blinded to clinical outcome. Nine of 52 (17%) noncalcified findings were malignant. The modalities had equivalent diagnostic performance with an AUC of 1 (DBT) and 0.96 (DM compression), $P = .43$, although subjective lesion conspicuity was significantly higher with DBT (mean 4.1) than DM (mean 2.9), $P<.001$.

Nearly simultaneously, researchers from the University of Michigan reported results comparing DBT with mammographic spot compression views (MSVs), including DM and FM focal compression and focal magnification, of 67 noncalcified masses recommended for biopsy, of which 30 out of 67 (45%) were malignant.[17] DBT was acquired with a prototype of a combined DBT and a whole-breast US system (GE Global Research, Niskayuna, NY). Four blinded readers evaluated 93 matched image sets for mass conspicuity and POM. On average for all 4 readers, there were no significant differences in accuracy, AUC-DBT equal to 0.91 and AUC-MSV equal to 0.90, $P = .60$. Based on recommendation for biopsy, the use of DBT would have resulted in the diagnosis of 7 additional cancers and 5 additional benign biopsies, or 1.8 true positive assessments for every 1.3 FP assessments per reader.

Calcifications

The results of early DBT reader trials of calcifications were less consistent than those assessing noncalcified abnormalities. Two small-scale reader studies on DBT were published in 2011 from the UPMC and from the MGH. Spangler and colleagues[12] at UPMC reported a multireader, enriched case study that compared 2v DM with 2v DBT using Selenia (Hologic Inc) and a Hologic prototype DBT system. Five readers reviewed 100 image sets consisting of 20 cancers, 40 biopsy-proven benign abnormalities, and 40 negative examinations in a crossed modality, blinded study design. Readers provided both screening and final BIRADS. Detection was based on all cases and characterization based only on the subset of cases detected by both modalities. Kopans and colleagues[14] at MGH reported a subjective comparison of MLO DBT versus 2v DM of 119 cases of DM-detected calcifications. DM was performed with Selenia (Hologic Inc) and Senographe 2000D (GE Health Care) units and DBT was acquired with a General Electric prototype DBT system. Two unblinded readers with 5 to 35 years of mammography experience evaluated the 2v DM and MLO DBT views on a 5-point clarity scale.

The results of these 2 studies differ slightly. In the UPMC study, there was no significant difference in the AUC based on the final BIRADS; however, detection sensitivity and specificity were worse with DBT than DM. Based on final BIRADS, with BIRADS 3 considered positive, DBT had a higher false-negative rate of 12% (9/74) versus 4% (3/37), and a lower FP rate 77% (93/121) versus 85% (105/123) compared with DM. Based on screening BIRADS, sensitivity was DM equal to 84% and DBT equal to 75%, and specificity was DM equal to 71% and DBT equal to 64%. Four cancers were not detected by DM, whereas 14 cancers were occult on DBT. The investigators concluded that DM was more sensitive for the detection of calcifications than DBT but that diagnostic performance of previously detected calcifications was comparable. The MGH study did not evaluate detection because all abnormalities were identified at the outset. On average, DBT was judged superior in 42%, equivalent in 50%, and worse in only 8% of the abnormalities. There was a high degree of interobserver agreement, κ equal to 0.96. The investigators concluded that calcifications can be demonstrated with 1v (MLO) DBT with superior or equivalent image clarity compared with 2v DM.

Summary
- DBT evaluates noncalcified abnormalities with equal accuracy and greater conspicuity than focal compression or magnification DM views.
- DBT shows mixed results for calcifications: detection may be inferior to DM but after detection DBT has similar accuracy compared with standard DM views.

LARGER READER TRIALS 2012 TO 2015

Before 2012, DBT trials were limited to single institutions and involved relatively few subjects. The interval from 2012 through 2015 marked a period of transition in the nature and scope of DBT-related trials that were reported. This period is bookended by 2 large multireader trials conducted in the United

Kingdom[21–23] and includes 3 important industry-sponsored enriched reader trials.[24–27] These 5 trials helped establish and validate the efficacy of the DBT technology.

Early in 2012, Michelle and colleagues[21] published the results of a single-institution trial of 738 women recalled for abnormal FM. Participants underwent 2v combined DM/DBT with Selenia Dimensions (Hologic Inc). Five readers evaluated standard CC and MLO images from each modality sequentially, progressing from FM to DM to DBT. Images were scored for lesion type, lesion size, and POM. Of the 759 lesions, 555 out of 759 (73%) were normal or benign, and 204 out of 759 (27%) were malignant, including 147 out of 204 (72%) invasive breast cancers and 57 out of 204 (28%) cases of DCIS. Accuracy significantly improved with each adjunctive modality: AUC FM equal to 0.788, AUC FM + DM equal to 0.895 (P = .0001), and AUC FM + DM + DBT equal to 0.967 (P = .0001). The addition of DBT increased the confidence of a malignant diagnosis and resulted in better classification of normal and benign findings. When analyzed by finding type, there was a significant improvement in the evaluation of noncalcified abnormalities but no benefit in the evaluation of calcifications only.

In January 2013, the results of the industry-sponsored DBT premarket approval (PMA) trials appeared in the peer reviewed literature[24] and on the federal investigational Web site, clinicaltrials.gov.[24,26,27] The methodology of the PMA trials was similar for the 3 industry sponsors. Each study garnered cases from multiple institutions that formed the basis of enriched data sets subsequently interpreted by multiple blinded readers. Accuracy was judged by the AUC at ROC analysis (**Fig. 1**) and the effect on recall rate or FP recalls of the competing screening technologies (ie, 2v DM versus the vendor-specific DBT screening platform).

The Hologic combined DM/DBT single compression platform, was the first system to be investigated and approved by the Food and Drug Administration (FDA) for commercial use in 2011. Results from the Hologic-sponsored multi-institutional multireader trial were published in 2 peer reviewed journals.[24,25] This trial accrued 1192 subjects from 5 institutions from July 2006 through May 2007 yielding 997 eligible DM/DBT image data sets and consisting of normal (ie, nonrecalled) screening examinations, positive (ie, recalled) screens with variable outcomes, and DM/DBT examinations from women presenting for biopsy of a suspicious abnormality. All cancer cases were included and noncancer cases were selected randomly. Two reader trials ensued that differed

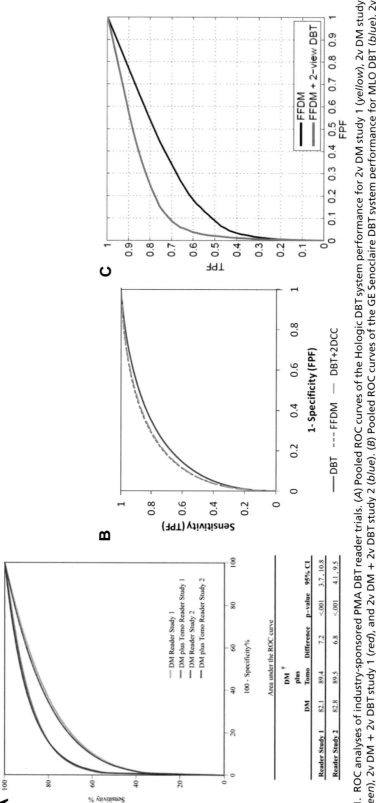

Fig. 1. ROC analyses of industry-sponsored PMA DBT reader trials. (A) Pooled ROC curves of the Hologic DBT system performance for 2v DM reader trials. (A) Pooled ROC curves of the Hologic DBT system performance for 2v DM study 1 (yellow), 2v DM study 2 (green), 2v DM + 2v DBT study 1 (red), and 2v DM + 2v DBT study 2 (blue). (B) Pooled ROC curves of the GE Senoclaire DBT system performance for MLO DBT (blue), 2v DM (red dashed), and MLO DBT/CC DM (green). (C) Pooled ROC curves of the Siemens Mammomat Inspiration DBT System for 2v DM (black) and 2v DM/2v DBT (red). (From [A] Rafferty EA, Park JM, Philpotts LE, et al. Assessing radiologist performance using combined digital mammography and breast tomosynthesis compared with digital mammography alone: results of a multicenter, multireader trial. Radiology 2013;266:104–13, with permission; [B] Senoclaire. PMA P130020: FDA Summary of Safety and Effectiveness Data. Available at: http://www.accessdata.fda.gov/cdrh_docs/pdf13/P130020B.pdf. Accessed August 12, 2015; and [C] Digital Breast Tomosynthesis. Mammomat Inspiration with Tomosynthesis Option. PMA P140011: FDA Summary of Safety and Effectiveness Data. Available at: http://www.accessdata.fda.gov/cdrh_docs/pdf14/P140011B.pdf. Accessed August 12, 2015.)

in reader number, lesion localization, and reader training. In study 1, 12 readers interpreted 312 image sets consisting of 264 noncancer cases and 48 cancer cases. In study 2, 15 readers interpreted 310 image sets consisting of 259 noncancer cases and 51 cancer cases. None of the readers in either study had prior experience with DBT interpretation but underwent formal training and review of 150 combined DM/DBT cases. The training of the 2 reader groups differed in that additional examples of malignant lobulated masses with circumscribed margins were included for reader group 2. Each reader group scored the DM examination first, then the DBT examination. Cases assessed as category 0 were also given a final BIRADS assessment. In study 2, readers also listed the location of the abnormality and scored an additional intermediate step of the 1v (MLO) DBT examination before assessing 2v DBT.

The results of studies 1 and 2 were very similar, demonstrating an overall improvement in accuracy with the addition of 2v DBT. The AUC increased significantly by approximately 7% in both studies, $P<.001$. Accuracy depended on finding type. The AUC improved significantly by 9% to 10% for noncalcified abnormalities, $P<.001$, but only slightly by 1% to 4% for calcifications, $P = .7 – .8$. When MLO DBT was added to DM there was an intermediate improvement in overall accuracy, an increase in AUC of 3.6%, $P = .009$. Sensitivity improved by 11% in study 1 and by 16% in study 2. The enhanced sensitivity of DM/DBT primarily reflected invasive cancer detection. Specificity increased in study 1 by 5% but decreased in study 2 by 2%. The differences between modalities in sensitivity and specificity were not statistically significant. Both the positive predictive values (PPVs) and negative predictive values of DM/DBT were greater than the DM alone. In both studies, the mean FP recall rate significantly improved, $P<.001$. All 27 readers experienced a reduction in FP recalls ranging from 6% to 67%, with $P<.001$ in 25 out of 27 readers. Similar to the ROC analysis, there was an intermediate benefit in FP recall rate with the addition of 1v DBT. The mean FP recall rate of DM equaled 44%, for DM/1v DBT equaled 27% and for DM/2v DBT equaled 24%. The addition of 1v or 2v DBT was significantly better than DM alone, $P<.001$ and DM/2v DBT was significantly better than DM/1v DBT, $P<.001$.

The design and results from the multi-institutional multireader PMA trial sponsored by General Electric are available solely on the federal clinical trials Web site.[26] The data from this trial were garnered from 5 sites in the United States and one site in Canada. It involved 753 subjects accrued from June 2007 through March 2010, yielding 444 image sets enriched with 67 cancers, 56 recalls, and 321 normal examinations. Imaging was acquired with a GE full-field digital mammography (FFDM) system and a DBT prototype modification of the GE Senographe DS FFDM system. The modalities compared were 2v DM versus 1v MLO DBT versus combined MLO DBT/CC DM. Seven Mammography Quality Standards Act (MQSA)-certified radiologists received 8 hours of hands-on training of approximately 100 DBT cases. Image sets were randomized into 2 groups and divided into 3 modality-specific sessions and reviewed by the 7 readers in a crossover design with a 1-month interval (memory wash) between reading sessions. Readers provided a screening BIRADS score, a final BIRADS, and POM on a 7-point scale, as well as identified abnormalities by finding type, location, and maximum lesion size.

The results of this trial validated the combination of 1v MLO DBT and 1v CC DM as comparable with standard 2v DM but did not support screening with 1v MLO DBT only. At ROC analysis, the combination of MLO DBT/CC DM proved noninferior to 2v DM, whereas 1v MLO DBT was inferior based on the noninferiority criterion of a less than 5% difference of the lower limit of the 97.5% confidence interval for the AUC. The AUC was highest for 2v DM at 0.853, intermediate for MLO DBT/CC DM at 0.842, and lowest for 1v MLO DBT at 0.820. The AUC difference between DM and DM/DBT was -0.011 (97.5% CI -0.047–0.028), whereas the AUC difference for 1v MLO DBT was -0.0331 (97.5% CI -0.073–0.002). Other endpoints included sensitivity, specificity, and recall rate. The combined MLO DBT/CC DM approaches were slightly less sensitive and more specific than 2 v DM. The sensitivity of 2v DM was 0.83 (95% CI 0.77–0.90) versus 0.79 (95% CI 0.72–0.85) for MLO DBT/CC DM, whereas the specificity was 0.67 (95% CI 0.64–0.70) versus 0.74 (95% CI 0.71–0.77), respectively. Recall rate was lower for MLO DBT/CC DM at 34% (95% CI 0.31, 0.37) compared with 2v DM at 41% (95% CI 0.37, 0.44).

Similar to the Hologic DBT approach, the Siemens-sponsored multicenter, enriched multi-reader trial was intended to prove superiority of combined 2v DBT/2v DM when compared with 2v DM.[27] The study involved 7 institutions that enrolled 698 subjects from May 2011 through September 2013, yielding an enriched image data set of 300 cases, including 50 cancers, 85 screening recalls, and 165 normal examinations. Subject images were acquired from women undergoing screening and diagnostic mammography with the Siemens commercially available DM systems and a prototype version of the Mammomat

Inspiration DBT system. Twenty-two MQSA-qualified radiologists with a minimum of 5 years of mammography experience and representing a broad spectrum of clinical breast practice underwent pretrial DBT training that included supervised review of 65 DM/DBT cases and a subsequent test of 70 DM/DBT image sets. Readers sequentially reviewed bilateral 2v DM, DM plus MLO DBT, and then DM plus 2v DBT. Readers provided a screening BIRADS (ie, assessment categories 0, 1, 2). For all BIRADS 0 examinations, the finding type and slice location was identified and final BIRADS and POM scores were issued. The primary outcome measure was an ROC analysis based on POM scores of 490 breasts (53 cancer, 90 benign, 437 normal) with secondary outcomes of sensitivity, specificity, and noncancer recall rate. A separate analysis of DM/MLO DBT was not reported.

Both the primary and secondary outcome measures confirmed the superiority of the combined DM/DBT examination to DM alone. The addition of 2v DBT increased the mean (for all readers) AUC by 10.1%, $P<.0001$ (95% CI 6.3%–13.9%). The mean FP recall rate decreased significantly from 43.8% to 35.5% with adjunctive DBT. Based on final BIRADS analysis, sensitivity increased and specificity was unchanged regardless of whether a probably benign assessment was considered positive or negative. Subset ROC analyses based on mammographic breast composition and finding type were also performed. There was little difference in the benefit provided by adjunctive DBT based on dichotomous breast density (ie, dense vs nondense). The AUC for dense breasts increased by 11.7% (DM = 0.734, DM/DBT = 0.851) and by 8.3% for nondense breasts (DM = 0.787, DM/DBT = 0.870). In contrast, there was a substantial difference in the improvement in the evaluation of masses compared with calcifications. With the addition of 2v DBT, the AUC for calcifications increased by 4.5% (DM = 0.744, DM/DBT = 0.790), whereas it increased by 10.9% (DM = 0.782, DM/DBT = 0.891) for masses.

Summary of PMA trials
- PMA trials validated the use of DBT for breast cancer screening.
- Hologic and Siemens use adjunctive DBT screening platforms (ie, 2v DM + 2v DBT).
- General Electric uses a hybrid DBT screening platform (ie, CC DM + MLO DBT).
- ROC analyses (shown in **Fig. 1**)
  ○ 2v DM + 2v DBT outperforms 2v DM
  ○ CC DM + MLO DBT equals 2v DM.

More recently, a large multi-institutional multireader trial was conducted in the United Kingdom with the aim of performing statistically valid subset analyses and addressing some of the limitations of earlier reader trials.[22,23] The TOMosynthesis with digital MammographY (TOMMY) trial from the United Kingdom was powered to allow for subset analysis and was conducted by multiple institutions and readers to minimize single-center and individual reader biases. This trial included a synthesized mammogram (SM) which is a digital mammogram that is generated from the tomosynthesis data set and allows for elimination of the digital mammogram. A dataset of 7060 examinations was retrospectively evaluated by 26 readers from 6 sites from the National Health Services Breast Cancer Screening Program. This set included combined DM/DBT/SM examinations from 6020 out of 7060 (85%) women 47 or more years old recalled for an abnormal DM screen and 1040 out of 7060 (15%) high-risk women ages 40 to 49 years presenting for screening. DM/DBT examinations of both breasts were acquired with the same compression using the Selenia Dimensions (Hologic Inc) commercial DBT unit. Synthesized images were created from the DBT dataset using C-View 2011 software (Hologic Inc). None of the women had previously had DBT. On average, the 26 readers had 10 years of screening mammography experience and underwent a 1-day DBT training course consisting of 80 cases. Weekly reading sets were randomly assigned with a mix of normal, benign, and cancer cases. Readers interpreted DM, DM/DBT, and SM/DBT for any given case, blinded to outcome and without comparison mammography. Recall status, lesion location, and a 5-point suspicion score was recorded and slice locations were noted for DBT examinations. For DM/DBT examinations, readers also compared DM with DBT, rating lesion visibility, lesion extent, lesion discrimination, and overall opinion.

Although the thrust of the trial was subset evaluation, overall results were also provided. There were 6828 examinations comparing bilateral 2v DM to 2v DM/DBT, including 5691 noncancer and 1137 cancer cases. Cancer was detected by both modalities in 921 out of 1137 (81%) and by neither of the modalities in 50 out of 1137 (4%). DM/DBT detected cancer in 95 out of 1137 (8%) and DM alone detected cancer in 71 out of 1137 (6%). There was a 34% increase in cancer detection with the adjunctive use of DBT and a statistically significant 56% reduction in FP recalls. The AUC was significantly better ($P<.001$) for both DBT arms than the DM alone arm with AUC (DM) equal to 0.84, AUC (DM/DBT) equal to 0.89, AUC(SM/DBT) equal to 0.88. Sensitivity was not significantly different between modalities overall: DM equal to 87%, DM/DBT equal to 89%, and

SM/DBT equal to 88%. Specificity was significantly (P<.001) better for adjunctive DBT: DM equal to 57%, DM/DBT equal to 70%, and SM/DBT equal to 72%.

In subset analysis combination DM/DBT outperformed DM alone in multiple areas. The AUC of DM/DBT for greater than 50% dense composition was significantly better than DM (DM = 0.83 vs DM/DBT = 0.87, P<.001). This was driven by improvement in specificity. DM/DBT was significantly better than DM in several subgroups. Sensitivity of DM/DBT was higher than DM in women ages 50 to 59 years equal to 91% versus 87% (P = .01) and breast density greater than 50% equal to 93% versus 86% (P = .03), Invasive cancer size 11 to 20 mm equal to 93% versus 86% (P<.001), grade 2 invasive cancer histology equal to 91% versus 87% (P = .01), finding types of mass equal to 92% versus 89% (P = .04), and architectural distortion or asymmetry 82% versus 71%. Sensitivity was not improved for calcifications. Also of note, DM/DBT was not more sensitive in the detection of larger invasive cancers (ie, tumor >20 mm). The investigators acknowledged that DBT cancer detection may have been underestimated because nearly all of the cancers were from the screening recall group (ie, initially detected by DM). Comparative results for specificity were more striking. Specificity was significantly better for DM/DBT than DM alone both overall and for all subsets. Gilbert and colleagues[23] concluded that DM/DBT had its greatest potential benefit for younger women and women with dense breast composition but also suggested that it was of value for all screening eligible women in light of its potential for FP recall reduction and specificity improvement.

Summary of larger nonindustry-sponsored United Kingdom trials
- Superior accuracy of combined 2v DM/DBT than 2v DM alone.
- Improved accuracy driven by a reduction in FP recalls.
- Subset analyses demonstrate improved sensitivity of DBT for (1) noncalcified abnormalities, (2) younger women, (3) dense breast composition, and (4) smaller invasive tumor size.

POPULATION-BASED TRIALS

Perhaps the most important scientific trials of DBT that have been published are 3 prospective population-based studies conducted in Europe. These 3 trials are particularly noteworthy because of the rigor of the scientific methodology used. They involve 2 of the 3 currently FDA-approved tomosynthesis units. Although they reflect a European screening mammography practice perspective, the consistency of the results (Table 1) suggests that study outcomes are more widely applicable to a variety of screening mammography practice settings.

The Oslo Tomosynthesis Screening Trial (OTST) has been variably reported in 3 publications.[28–30] The first of 2 nearly simultaneous publications reported the interim results of 2v DM compared with combined 2v DM and 2v DBT in the Norwegian Breast Cancer Screening Program based in Oslo, Norway.[28] The second publication reported the effect of double-reading on both DM and DM/DBT arms of the trial.[29] The most recent publication[30] investigated the impact of synthetically reconstructed planar images versus conventional DM in conjunction with DBT over 2 different synthetic reconstruction software versions.

In the primary publication, Skaane and colleagues[28] reported results from the first half of data collection of the OTST. This interim report was planned to verify that study results were within European quality assurance guidelines and to allow for design adjustments to meet statistical goals. In accordance with the Oslo arm of the Norwegian Breast Cancer Screening Program, 29,652 women ages 50 to 69 years who were on a biennial screening schedule were invited for screening mammography. Based on technical staff availability alone, 12,631 women underwent screening mammography with combined 2v DM/DBT using Selenia Dimensions (Hologic Inc). Ten women were excluded based on nonbreast malignancy and interval cancer development. Examinations were interpreted at the breast imaging center of the Ullevaal University Hospital by 8 readers with 2 to 31 years of screening mammography experience in mode-balanced sessions, including 4 modes (ie, DM alone, DM + CAD, DM + DBT, SM + DBT). Results of the comparison of DM versus DM + DBT were reported.

Both of the performance outcomes (ie, FP recall rate and cancer detection rate [CDR]) improved with the addition of DBT. The FP rate of DM was 6.1% (771/12,621) and decreased to 5.3% (670/12,621) for DM/DBT. After adjustment for reader-specific performance levels, this reflected a statistically significant 15% decrease in FP recall rate of 0.85 (P<.001; 98.5% CI 0.76–0.96). There was an even larger effect on cancer detection. With the addition of DBT, the CDR increased 31% from 6.1 to 8.0 per 1000 women. This translated to a 27% increase in reader-adjusted cancer detection or 1.27 (P = .001; 98.5% CI 1.06–1.53). Importantly, the increase in cancer detection reflected an increase in invasive cancer detection by 25

Table 1
Outcomes of European population based screening trials of digital breast tomosynthesis

Trial Name	Design	Population, Accrual Period, Subject Age	Number of Examinations and Readers	Vendor or Examination Type and #Views	Results: FP Recalls	Results Cancer Detection Rate per 1000
Oslo Tomosynthesis Screening Trial[28]	Prospective, reader, single-institution, invitation	Screening unspecified Nov. 2010–Dec. 2011 50–69	12,631 examinations 8 readers, single-read	Selenia Dimensions, Hologic Inc 2v DM vs 2v DM/2v DBT	↓ 13%, 6.1% (DM) vs 5.3% (DM/DBT) Adjusted: ↓ 15%, 0.85 (0.76, 0.96), $P<.001$.	↑ 31%, 6.1 (DM) vs 8.0 (DM/DBT) Adjusted: ↑ 27%, 1.27 (1.06, 1.53), $P = .001$
Screening with Tomosynthesis OR Standard Mammography (STORM)[31]	Prospective, reader, 2 institutions, invitation	75%–80% incidence, 20%–25% prevalence Aug. 2011–June 2012 48–71 y Median 58	7292 women (examinations) 8 readers, independent double-read	Selenia Dimension, Hologic Inc 2v DM vs 2v DM/2v DBT	↓ 17% 4.5% (DM) vs 3.5% (DM/DBT) $P<.0001$	↑ 53%, 5.3 (DM) vs 8.1 (DM/DBT) $P<.0001$
Malmo Breast Tomosynthesis Screening Trial[32]	Prospective, reader, single-institution, invitation	80% incidence, 20% prevalence Jan. 2010–Dec. 2012 40–74 Mean 56	7500 women 6 readers, independent double-read	Mammomat Inspiration, Siemens MLO DBT vs 2v DM, vs MLO DBT/CC DM	↑ 43%, 2.0% (DM) vs 2.8% (DBT) $P<.0001$	↑ 43%, 6.3 (DM) vs 8.9 (DBT) $P<.05$
Total	—	Range 40–74	27,423 women	—	Range 2.8%–5.3%	Range 8.0–8.9

over DM alone rather than 1 less DCIS detection than DM alone. Of the 25 additional invasive cancers detected by DM/DBT, 40% (10/25) were grade 2 or grade 3. The only cautionary outcome for DM/DBT was the time for image interpretation, which approximately doubled from 45 seconds (DM) to 91 seconds (DM/DBT), $P<.001$.

The second European population-based trial was conducted in Italy and was also published in 2013. Similar to the Oslo trial, the Screening with Tomosynthesis OR standard Mammography (STORM) trial also compared combined DM/DBT with DM and reported a similar reduction in FP recalls with simultaneous increase in cancer detection.[31] Participating subjects were asymptomatic women ages 48 or more years attending screening in the Trento and Verona (Italy) screening programs from August 2011 to June 2012. Historically, approximately 75% to 80% of the subjects attending these screening programs had incidence screening. Participants underwent a combined 2v DM/DBT screening examination with Selenia Dimensions (Hologic Inc). Each examination was read independently by 2 of 8 study radiologists with 3 to 13 years of mammography experience and basic training in DBT. The DM examination was interpreted initially and the combined DM/DBT was read later that day.

Study outcome measures included CDR and FP recall rate. Overall, 59 cancers were detected in 57 women. Approximately two-thirds (39/59) were detected by both modalities. DM/DBT detected an additional 20 cancers, whereas DM alone detected no additional cancers. Eighty-five percent (17/20) of cancers detected only by DM/DBT were invasive. The CDR was 5.3 per 1000 examinations (95% CI 3.8–7.3) for DM only and 8.1 per 1000 examinations (95% CI 6.2–10.4) for DM/DBT. This reflected a 51% increase in CDR of 2.7 cancers per 1000 screening examinations ($P<.0001$). Overall, there was a 5.5% FP recall rate (395/7235). Of the 395 women recalled who did not have cancer, both DM and DM/DBT recalled 181, DM alone recalled 141 and DM/DBT recalled 73. The difference in FP recalls based on modality was statistically significant, $P<.0001$. If positivity was based only on the results of DM/DBT, the investigators estimated a 17.2% (68/395) reduction in FP recall rate (95% CI 13.6–21.3). A subset analysis based on age (<60 vs ≥60 years) and breast density (fat-scattered vs heterogeneously extremely dense) showed no differences between subgroups in the beneficial effect of DM/DBT on CDR and FP recall rate, although the number of women with dense breasts only accounted for 17.4% (1215/7292) of the study population.

The most recently reported European population-based screening trial of DBT occurred in Malmo,

Sweden.[32] Although similar in design to the OTST and STORM, it used different DBT technology and reported slightly different results compared with its predecessors. The Malmo Breast Tomosynthesis Screening Trial (MBTST) compared 1v DBT with reduced compression (DBT*) versus 2v DM versus a combination of 1v MLO DBT* and 1v CC, using the Mammomat Inspiration (Siemens AG) DBT and DM technology. The investigators reported interim results on CDR, recall rate, and PPV of the initial 7500 participants from the planned accrual of 15,000 subjects. A random sample of women undergoing screening either yearly (ages 40–55 years) or biennially (ages 56–74 years) were invited to participate from January 2010 to December 2012. The average participant age was 56 years (range 40–76). Consenting subjects underwent 2v DM followed by 1v MLO DBT with approximately 50% reduced compression based on compressive force. The method for reduced compression is described in greater detail in an earlier publication.[33] Full breast compression occurred in approximately 10% of participants. Six readers with a mean of 26 years of mammography experience (range 8–41 years) participated in blinded double-reading of 2 independent arms and scored each examination in stepwise fashion based on a 5-point POM scale. In the DM arm, the reader first interpreted the 2v DM, then compared with the prior DM. In the DBT arm, the reader initially interpreted the MLO DBT view, then added the CC DM view, then compared the examination with prior DM examinations. All positive screening interpretations underwent arbitration. Unlike other studies, lobular carcinoma in situ (LCIS) was considered a cancer outcome in addition to invasive cancer and DCIS.

The beneficial outcomes of DBT in the MBTST are similar to the preceding 2 trials. Like the OTST and STORM, cancer detection increased significantly by 43% from 6.3 out of 1000 (2v DM) to 8.9 out of 1000 (MLO DBT), $P<.0001$. DM detected a single DBT occult DCIS, whereas DBT detected 21 DM occult malignancies, including 16 invasive cancers, 2 microinvasive cancers, 3 DCIS, and 1 LCIS. The addition of the CC DM view did not result in additional cancer detection. DBT detected DM occult cancers in all density categories. Of the 17 macroinvasive cancers detected by DBT alone, 10 were grade 2 or 3, and 2 had lymph node metastases. Although there were no statistical differences in cancer characteristics between DBT only and cancers detected with both modalities, the DM occult cancers tended to have a more favorable prognosis and occurred in younger women.

Unlike the other 2 trials, the FP recall rate of MLO DBT was significantly greater than the FP recall rate of 2v DM, $P<.0001$; although the benchmark FP recall rate was actually lower for 1v DBT than in either the OTST or STORM. DBT that was 1v falsely recalled 212 out of 7432 subjects (2.9%), whereas 2v DM falsely recalled 150 out of 7432 subjects (2.0%). FP recalls include subjects recalled for clinical symptoms in both arms. The investigators state that the increased conspicuity of benign lesions and islands of fibroglandular tissue likely contributed to the increase in recall rate. In a subsequent analysis, Lang and colleagues[34] reported that the increase in FPs was largely due to increased detection of stellate distortions and that DBT was better at characterizing round lesions with a resulting decrease in the recall of fibroadenomas and cysts. Over the course of the study, the investigators noted a reduction in FP DBT recalls, which stabilized at a rate of 1.5% and may be attributed to a learning curve. Interestingly, the PPV from screening mammography (PPV[1]) or likelihood of cancer from a positive screen was 24% for both MLO DBT (67/282) and 2v DM (47/197). The investigators conclude that 1v DBT may be a feasible approach to breast cancer screening with gains in cancer detection, acceptable FP rates, and advantages of reduced compression and decreased radiation dose and interpretation time.

Summary of European population-based screening trials of DBT (Table 1)

- DBT leads to increased cancer detection.
  - DBT detects approximately 2 to 3 additional cancers per 1000 women than DM.
  - Increased DBT cancer detection primarily involves invasive cancer not DCIS.
- DBT results in favorable recall rates.
  - DBT FP recall rate ranges from 2.8% to 5.3%.
  - Two of 3 trials show approximate 15% decrease in FP recall rate with DBT.

CLINICAL OUTCOMES OF DIGITAL BREAST TOMOSYNTHESIS SCREENING: 2013 TO 2016

To date, there have been no prospective population-based scientific trials of DBT in the United States. However, important clinical outcomes related to DM/DBT screening in substantial numbers of women have been described. These service reports describe differences in performance measures between screening modalities (DM and DM/DBT) in women attending facilities that did or did not offer DBT screening and within a facility before and after the implementation of DBT screening.[35–37]

Haas and colleagues[35] reported outcomes of 13,158 women presenting for screening mammography to 4 facilities with variable DBT screening resources between October 2011 and September 2012. Six thousand and one hundred women had combined DM/DBT images (Dimensions, Hologic Inc) and 7058 women had DM images (Selenia, Hologic Inc). Women with breast size exceeding the large image receptor size and with breast prostheses were excluded. Examinations were interpreted by 8 dedicated breast imagers with 2 to 23 years of mammography experience. Differences in recall rates and cancer detection rates were assessed and multivariate regression analysis was used to identify confounders.

There was a statistically significant 30% reduction in recall rate and a nonstatistical trend for increased cancer detection with the combination DM/DBT. The recall rate of DM alone was 12% (95% CI 11.3%–12.8%) and decreased to 8.4% (95% CI 7.7%–9.1%) with DM/DBT, $P<.01$. The benefit in recall rate remained statistically significant for women with scattered, heterogeneous, and extremely dense breasts ($P<.01$) and in women younger than 40, 40 to 49, and 50 to 59 ($P<.01$), and in women 60 to 69 years old ($P = .01$). After controlling for age, breast density, and breast cancer risk, the adjusted odds of recall for DM/DBT versus DM alone was 0.62 (95% CI 0.55–0.70) or 38% lower likelihood of recall with DM/DBT screening. CDR increased insignificantly by 9.5% from 5.2 per 1000 women to 5.7 per 1000 women.

In 2014, Friedewald and colleagues[36] published the largest service experience with combined DM/DBT screening involving 13 geographically diverse, academic, and nonacademic centers in the United States, and 139 specialist and nonspecialist radiologists. This study reported audit results on 454,850 screening examinations with DM (n = 281,187) and DM/DBT (n = 173,663). It compared DM screening 1 year before DBT implementation (time period 1) with DM/DBT screening in the same facilities after DBT implementation (time period 2), which varied at each site until a cut-off date of December 31, 2012. Two sites converted completely to DM/DBT screening, whereas 11 out of 13 sites converted partially, offering both DM and DM/DBT screening in the second time period. All facilities used Selenia Dimensions (Hologic Inc) DBT systems. Outcome measures reflected typical practice audit performance measures, including recall rate, biopsy rate per 1000 women, PPV[1], PPV with biopsy performed (PPV[3]), CDR per 1000 women, and whether the cancers were invasive or in situ.

The results of this study showed significant improvements in recall rate, PPVs, and invasive cancer detection, with a slight increase in biopsy rate. The average age of women undergoing DM was 57.0 years and those having DM/DBT was 56.2 years. There was a 16% statistically significant decrease in recall rate from 10.7% (DM) to 9.1% (DM/DBT), $P<.001$. Most, or 85% (11/13), sites showed a reduction in recall rate, whereas 2 out of 13 facilities showed an increase. The PPV[1] increased from 4.3% (DM) to 6.4% (DM/DBT), $P<.001$, a relative increase of 49%, and the PPV[3] went from 24.2% (DM) to 29.2% (DM/DBT), $P<.001$. Overall, cancer detection increased by 1.2 cancers per 1000 women, DM equal to 4.2 versus DM/DBT equal to 5.4, $P<.001$. Invasive cancer detection increased relatively by 41% from 2.9 (DM) to 4.1 (DM/DBT), $P<.001$, whereas DCIS detection remained stable at 1.4 for both modalities. The number of women who underwent biopsy following a positive screen increased by 1.2 per 1000 women, DM equal to 18.1 versus DM/DBT equal to 19.3, $P = .004$. The investigators concluded that adjunctive DBT provided benefits in both recall rate reduction and cancer detection.

Although compelling, the results from the 2 trials previously discussed primarily describe the outcomes of DBT in the prevalence screening round. Performance measures related to incidence screening with DBT are largely unknown. In a recent study from University of Pennsylvania, McDonald and colleagues[37] compared outcome measures from a 1-year interval before DBT implementation with 3 successive years of screening with combined DM/DBT at both a population level and at the individual woman level.

At the population level, outcome measures from DM screening preceding DM/DBT implementation was compared with 3 successive years of DM/DBT screening after implementation. At the University of Pennsylvania, DM screening was completely converted to combined DM/DBT (Selenia Dimensions, Hologic Inc) screening in September 2011. The year preceding the transition (ie, September 1, 2010–August 30, 2011) served as the DM alone reference (ie, year 0) and the 3 subsequent years (October 1, 2011–September 30, 2014) constituted years 1, 2, and 3 of combined DM/DBT screening. Overall, there were 44,468 screening examinations in 23,958 women with a mean age of 56.8 years. There were 10,728 examinations occurring in the reference DM (year 0), 11,007 examinations in DM/DBT (year 1), 11,157 examinations in DM/DBT (year 2), and 11,576 examinations in DM/DBT (year 3). The yearly population cohorts were not identical but shared similar subject characteristics. There was a slight increase in women undergoing mammography without comparison examinations after DBT implementation. BIRADS assessments of 0, 4, and 5 were considered test positive and BIRADS assessments of 1, 2, and 3 were test negative. The index recall rate for DM was 10.4%, decreasing to 8.8% in DM/DBT (year 1), 9.0% DM/DBT (year 2), and 9.2% DM/DBT (year 3). Despite a slight increase from years 1 to 3, this reduction maintained significance for all DM/DBT years 1 to 3, $P<.0001$, $P = .005$, $P = .0025$, respectively. PPV[1] also improved each year from DM (year 0) of 4.4% to DM/DBT (year 1) equal to 6.2%, DM/DBT (year 2) equal to 6.5%, and DM/DBT (year 3) equal to 6.7% but was only significant for DM/DBT years 2 and 3. PPV with biopsy recommendation (PPV[2]) and PPV[3] showed nonsignificant increases. CDR also improved from DM (year 0) equal to 4.6 per 1000 women, to 5.5 DM/DBT (year 1), 5.8 DM/DBT (year 2), and 6.1 DM/DBT (year 3) but the increase was not statistically significant. The increase in invasive cancer detection predominated over DCIS. The interval cancer rate decreased from 0.7 to 0.5 per 100 women ($P = .603$) from DM (year 0) to the DM/DBT year 1.

The investigators also reported an individual level analysis of the cohort of unique women undergoing DM/DBT screening. There were 12,079 unique women with 1 DM/DBT screen, 6293 with 2 DM/DBT screens, and 3023 with 3 DM/DBT screens within the study period. The recall rate of the DBT prevalence examination was 13% (no priors) and 11.1% (DM prior), decreasing to 7.8% ($P<.0001$) and 5.9% ($P<.0001$) for women with 2 and 3 DM/DBT screens, respectively. CDR was highest at 11.2 per 1000 women on the first DM/DBT screen. Although it decreased to 6.2 and 7.3 in women with 2 and 3 DM/DBT screens, it remained considerably higher than the index CDR of DM at 4.6, which included both prevalence and incidence screens. The PPV[1] of the first DM/DBT examination was 8.6 (no priors) and 11.7 (with DM priors), dipping slightly with the 2 DM/DBT screens to 7.9% and increasing to 12.4% with 3 DM/DBT screens. Similar to CDR, the PPV[1] was much higher than the PPV[1] of 4.4% for DM only.

In summary, this study suggests an ongoing benefit of DM/DBT screening at both the population and individual levels. At the population level, DM/DBT screening seems to maintain reduction in recall rate and improvements in PPV and CDR, especially invasive cancer detection. Some of these outcomes do not meet statistical significance but that is probably due to the relatively small numbers of cancers in the study. The woman level outcomes are equally remarkable. The data indicate an expected higher recall rate with prevalence screening followed by a marked reduction with successive DM/DBT screens. There seems to be a dip in cancer detection and PPV[1] at screen 2 and partial rebound in screen 3. Although the number of women with 3 DM/DBT screens in the 3 year interval reported here is too low to draw definitive conclusions, it suggests very high-quality metrics for annual DM/DBT screening; for example, recall rates less than 6%, PPV[1] over 12%, and CDR greater than 7 per 1000 women.

CLINICAL PERFORMANCE

Over the past 5 years there have been several important single-institution reports on issues that focus on the clinical practice of DBT. These publications provide guidance on several issues that are unique to DBT. They help inform clinical practice in areas ranging from implementation to clinical management.

INTERPRETATION TIME

One of the important practical issues related to DBT implementation is the time required to interpret DBT examinations. Screening with FM and DM involves CC and MLO views generating 2 images for each breast. In contrast, the 3 current FDA-approved vendors reconstruct the set number of low-dose images into 1 mm slices, generating between 20 and 100 images per DBT view depending on breast thickness.

Although several DBT studies have reported DBT interpretation time, only a few studies were specifically designed to address this logistical issue.[8,38,39] Bernard and colleagues[38] prospectively evaluated the effect of DBT screening on both technologist examination acquisition time and radiologist examination interpretation time using the Selenia Dimensions (Hologic Inc) combined DM/DBT system. The examination acquisition time from the start of first view initial positioning to the release of last view compression was measured in 40 women, 20 with DM and 20 with DM/DBT by 7 mammography technologists. Three experienced breast radiologists interpreted an enriched image set of 10 cancer and 90 noncancer cases in separate DM and DM/DBT reading modes. On average, the image acquisition of DM/DBT was 26% longer than DM only: DM equal to 193 seconds versus DM/DBT equal to 243 seconds, $P<.01$. Average examination interpretation time increased by 44 seconds or 135% from DM to DM/DBT: DM equal to 33 seconds versus DM/DBT equal to 77 seconds, $P<.01$.

Dang and colleagues[39] also compared interpretation times of DM versus DM/DBT with a study design intended to mimic clinical practice. Ten radiologists with 1.5 to 21 years of mammography experience and a minimum of 17 months of DBT experience prospectively interpreted DM or DM/DBT screening examinations in uninterrupted 60 minute sessions from July 2012 to January 2013. Each radiologist read a minimum of 5 sessions per modality. Sessions were interpreted in usual clinical practice, including the use of prior comparison examinations and computer-aided detection software. Average interpretation time increased by 0.9 minutes (or 47%) from DM equal to 1.9 minutes to DM/DBT equal to 2.8 minutes, $P<.0001$. On average, approximately 10 fewer DM/DBT studies were interpreted per hour: DM equal to 34.0 versus DM/DBT equal to 23.8. Increasing breast imaging experience correlated with decreasing additional DBT interpretation time.

Summary
- Screening mammography examination interpretation time increases by 50% to greater than 100% with the addition of DBT.

DIAGNOSTIC EVALUATION OF SCREENING DIGITAL BREAST TOMOSYNTHESIS RECALLS

Although lengthier DBT interpretation times may decrease practice efficiency, the effect of DBT screening on the efficiency of diagnostic breast imaging may somewhat mitigate this problem. In an early study of the diagnostic potential of screening DBT, Brandt and colleagues[40] reported that standard DBT views were considered adequate for mammographic evaluation in 99% (156/158) for 2 of 3 readers and in 93% (147/158) for the third reader. In contrast, an average of 3 additional diagnostic DM views were needed to evaluate DM screening recalls.

In a recent study, Lourenco and colleagues[41] compared screening outcomes and described the downstream effect on diagnostic breast imaging in 2 screening cohorts before and after DM/DBT implementation. A total of 25,948 screening examinations consisting of 2v DM only (n = 12,577, March 2011 through February 2012) using Senographe Essential, Senographe DS, or Senographe 2000D (GE Healthcare), and combined DM/DBT (n = 12,921, March 2012 through February 2013) using Selenia Dimensions (Hologic Inc) were accrued. The recall rate decreased by 31%, from 9.3% to 6.4%, $P<.00001$ with the use of DM/DBT. DM screening recalled a greater proportion of asymmetries and focal asymmetries, whereas DM/DBT recalled a greater proportion of masses, calcifications, and architectural distortion, $P<.00001$. There were no statistically significant differences in PPV[3] or CDR between screening modalities.

The use of diagnostic modalities depended significantly on the nature of the screening examination. Additional diagnostic mammographic views, 40.2% versus 28.4%, $P<.0001$ and additional diagnostic mammography and US 57.2% versus 43.3%, $P<.0001$, were used more frequently with DM screening than with DM/DBT screening. In contrast, the use of US only was more common for DM/DBT screening than DM screening, 2.6% versus 28.3%, $P<.0001$. The investigators suggested that screening DBT may take the place of additional mammography in diagnostic evaluation.

DIAGNOSTIC DIGITAL BREAST TOMOSYNTHESIS

As previously noted, several early diagnostic reader studies suggested comparable or superior performance of DBT than DM in the evaluation of noncalcified abnormalities.[11,15,17] Larger reader trials that evaluated performance by finding type showed similar results.[22,23,25,27]

With this hypothesis in mind, Morel and colleagues[42] from Kings College Hospital (London, UK) compared DBT with DM spot magnification views in a diagnostic breast imaging population. Three hundred and forty-one women either recalled from DM screening or presenting for diagnostic evaluation of a clinical concern underwent diagnostic imaging with either coned compression magnification mammography (CCMM) or DBT (Selenia Dimensions, Hologic Inc) in a single projection. One of 7 breast imaging specialists with 6 to 24 months of DBT experience evaluated the 2v DM plus CCMM or 2 v DM plus 1v DBT separated by a 2 week interval. Each radiologist identified the finding type and rated the POM. There were 354 lesions, including 279 soft tissue abnormalities and 75 calcifications. Twenty-nine percent (103/354) were malignant, 23% (82/354) were benign, and 58% (169/354) were normal. The adjunctive use of DBT outperformed CCMM for all lesions: AUC DBT equal to 0.93 versus AUC CCMM 0.87, $P = .0014$; and for soft tissue lesions: AUC DBT 0.97 versus AUC CCMM equal to 0.90, $P = .005$. There was no difference in the AUC for calcifications. There were 3 FN interpretations in the CCMM group and none in the DBT group. The sensitivity and specificity was higher for DBT (99% and 64%, respectively) than CCMM (95% and 54%, respectively). There was a decrease in low POM DBT assessments, possibly due to an increased confidence level. The investigators concluded that DM was more accurate than CCMM in the diagnostic evaluation of mammographic abnormalities. At the Kings College Hospital, this led to a change in clinical protocol to evaluate noncalcified findings with 2v DBT rather than CCMM.

MANAGEMENT OF ARCHITECTURAL DISTORTION

Because of its unique ability to detect subtle architectural distortion, the management of distortion that is only visible with DBT is problematic. In addition to malignant causes, architectural distortion may arise in benign entities, most notably from surgical scarring and complex sclerosing lesions,[34] leading to FP results and diminishing the accuracy of DBT. In an attempt to provide guidance for clinical management, 2 studies have described clinical experiences with architectural distortion that is seen primarily or only on DBT.

From a pool of 9982 screening DM/DBT examinations, 3 breast radiologists evaluated 51 cases recalled for architectural distortion without associated scar marker, mass, or calcification.[43] At consensus review, approximately half, 25 out of 51 (49%), were considered not genuine architectural distortion and were excluded, highlighting the inconsistency in the interpretation of this finding. Of the remaining 26, the majority, 19 of 26 (73%), were only visible on DBT, 15 out of 19 on 2vs, and 4 out of 19 on 1v only. Image-guided biopsy and/or surgical excision occurred in 14 out of 26 (54%) and resulted in 7 cancers, PPV[3] equal to 50% (7/14), including 5 invasive carcinomas and 2 DCIS; 1 associated with atypical papillary lesion and 1 associated with a complex sclerosing lesion. All invasive cancers were visible with US. Follow-up of 2 probably benign assessments and 6 negative assessments was limited. The investigators concluded that DBT detects architectural distortion better than DM, especially in dense breast composition, leading to increased cancer detection. They also suggested that architectural distortion that was not visible with US was likely due to a complex sclerosing lesion rather than malignancy.

Subsequent studies were conducted by Freer and colleagues[44] and Houssami and Skaane.[45] The former reported the outcomes of 36 cases of DBT detected architectural distortion not visible with mammography or US that underwent DBT-guided wire localized surgical excision. The mean size of the architectural distortion was 7.9 mm. In addition to diagnostic mammography and US, 31% (11/36) had breast MR imaging. Two had MR imaging correlates that did not provide an adequate target for MR imaging–guided biopsy and 9 had no MR imaging correlate. Almost all, 97% (35/36), of localized excisions were successful. One case was relocalized at 6 weeks due to imaging pathologic findings discordance and upgraded to invasive cancer. There were 17 cancers, including 13 invasive cancers and 4 cases of DCIS, with a PPV[3] equal to 47% (17/36). Of note, 45% (5/11) of the cases that were imaged with MR imaging were malignant. The mean size of invasive cancer was 7.5 mm (range 5–12 mm). The remaining 53% (19/36) were benign, including 5 high-risk lesions (ie, atypical ductal hyperplasia, atypical lobular hyperplasia, and LCIS), 14 complex sclerosing lesions, 3 cases of sclerosing adenosis, and 1 prior percutaneous biopsy site. The investigators concluded that sonographically occult DBT-detected architectural distortion required tissue sampling and that DBT-guided wire localization was feasible and accurate.

Summary of diagnostic DBT
- DBT evaluation of noncalcified abnormalities is superior to DM evaluation with spot magnification.
- DBT detects architectural distortion better than DM, which leads to increased cancer detection.
- Architectural distortion that is only visible on DBT has a substantial likelihood of malignancy.

SUMMARY

Over the last 20 years, we have witnessed a rapid evolution in the clinical investigation of DBT. Beginning with proof of principle pilot observational studies and culminating in prospective population-based screening trials and outcome reporting from clinical practice. The amount and intensity of DBT research conducted over this period is impressive.

Published outcomes strongly suggest simultaneous improvements in cancer detection and FP recalls to varying degrees with DBT screening. Furthermore, the cancer detection benefit primarily involves detection of invasive cancer rather than DCIS, which is important given current concerns for potential overdiagnosis and overtreatment. The data also indicate equivalent or improved performance in diagnostic imaging with DBT, particularly of noncalcified findings.

REFERENCES

1. Siu AL, U.S. Preventive Services Task Force. Screening for breast cancer: U.S. Preventive Services Task Force recommendation statement. Ann Intern Med 2016;164(4):279–96.
2. Niklason LT, Christian BT, Niklason LE, et al. Digital tomosynthesis in breast imaging. Radiology 1997; 205:399–406.
3. Poplack SP, Tosteson ED, Kogel CA, et al. Digital breast tomosynthesis: initial experience in 98 women with abnormal digital screening mammography. AJR Am J Roentgenol 2007;189:616–23.
4. Andersson I, Ikeda DM, Zackrisson S, et al. Breast Tomosynthesis and digital mammography: a comparison of breast cancer visibility and BIRADS classification in a population of cancers with subtle mammographic findings. Eur Radiol 2008; 18:2817–25.
5. Good WF, Abrams GS, Catullo VJ, et al. Digital breast tomosynthesis: a pilot observer study. AJR Am J Roentgenol 2008;190:865–9.
6. Gur D, Abrams GS, Chough DM, et al. Digital breast tomosynthesis: observer performance study. AJR Am J Roentgenol 2009;193:586–91.
7. Gennaro G, Toledano A, di Maggio C, et al. Digital breast tomosynthesis vs digital mammography: a clinical performance study. Eur Radiol 2010;20: 1545–53.
8. Zuley ML, Bandos AI, Abrams GS, et al. Time to diagnosis and performance levels during repeat interpretations of digital breast tomosynthesis. Acad Radiol 2010;17:450–5.
9. Fornvik D, Zachrisson S, Ljungberg O, et al. Breast tomosynthesis: accuracy of tumor measurement compared with digital mammography and ultrasonography. Acta Radiol 2010;51:240–7.
10. Svahn T, Andersson I, Chakraborty D, et al. The diagnostic accuracy of dual-view digital mammography, single-view breast tomosynthesis and a dual-view combination of breast tomosynthesis and digital mammography in a free-response observer performance study. Radiat Prot Dosimetry 2010; 139:113–7.
11. Hakim CM, Chough DM, Ganott MA. Digital breast tomosynthesis in the diagnostic environment: a subjective side-by-side review. AJR Am J Roentgenol 2010;195:172–6.
12. Spangler ML, Zuley ML, Sumkin JH, et al. Detection and classification of calcifications on DBT and DM: a comparison. AJR Am J Roentgenol 2011;196:320–4.
13. Gur D, Bandos AI, Rockette HE, et al. Localized detection and classification of abnormalities on FFDM and tomosynthesis examinations rated under an FROC paradigm. AJR Am J Roentgenol 2011; 196:737–41.
14. Kopans D, Gavenonis S, Halpern E, et al. Calcifications in the breast and DBT. Breast J 2011;17:638–44.
15. Tagliafico A, Astengo D, Cavagnetto F, et al. One to one comparison between digital spot compression view and DBT. Eur Radiol 2012;22:539–44.

16. Svahn TM, Chakraborty DP, Ikeda D, et al. Breast tomo-synthesis and digital mammography: a comparison of diagnostic accuracy. Br J Radiol 2012;85:1074–82.

17. Noroozian M, Hadjiiski L, Rahnama-Moghadam S, et al. DBT is comparable to mammographic spot views for mass characterization. Radiology 2012;262:61–8.

18. Gur D, Zuley ML, Anell MI, et al. Dose reduction in DBT screening using synthetically reconstructed projection images: an observer performance study. Acad Radiol 2012;19:166–71.

19. Wallis MG, Moa E, Sanca F, et al. Two-view and single-view tomosynthesis vs. FFDM. Radiology 2012;262:788–96.

20. Skaane P, Gullien R, Bjornadal H, et al. DBT: initial experience in a clinical setting. Acta Radiol 2012; 53:524–9.

21. Michelle MJ, Iqbal A, Wasan RK, et al. A comparison of the accuracy of film-screen mammography, FFDM, and DBT. Clin Radiol 2012;67:976–81.

22. Gilbert FJ, Tucker L, Gillan MGC, et al. The TOMMY trial: a comparison of TOMosynthesis with digital MammographY in the UK NHS Breast Screening Programme – a multicentre retrospective reading study comparing the diagnostic performance of dig-ital breast tomosynthesis and digital mammography with digital mammography alone. Health Technol Assess 2015;19(4):i–xxv.

23. Gilbert FJ, Tucker L, Gillan MGC, et al. Accuracy of digital breast tomosynthesis for depicting breast cancer subgroups in a UK retrospective reading study. Radiology 2015;277:697–706.

24. Rafferty EA, Park JM, Philpotts LE, et al. Assessing radiologist performance using combined digital mammography and breast tomosynthesis compared with digital mammography alone: results of a multi-center, multireader trial. Radiology 2013;266:104–13.

25. Rafferty EA, Park JM, Philpotts LE, et al. Diagnostic ac-curacy and recall rates for digital mammography and digital mammography combined with one-view and two-view tomosynthesis: results of an enriched reader study. AJR Am J Roentgenol 2014;202:273–81.

26. Digital Breast Tomosynthesis. Senoclaire. PMA P130020: FDA Summary of Safety and Effectiveness Data. Available at: http://www.accessdata.fda.gov/cdrh_docs/pdf13/P130020B.pdf. Accessed August 12, 2015.

27. Digital Breast Tomosynthesis. Mammomat Inspira-tion with Tomosynthesis Option. PMA P140011: FDA Summary of Safety and Effectiveness Data. Avail-able at: http://www.accessdata.fda.gov/cdrh_docs/pdf14/P140011B.pdf. Accessed August 12, 2015.

28. Skaane P, Bandos AI, Gullien R, et al. Comparison of digital mammography alone and digital mammog-raphy plus tomosynthesis in a population-based screening program. Radiology 2013;267:47–56.

29. Skaane P, Bandos AI, Eben EB, et al. Prospective trial comparing full-field digital mammography (FFDM) versus combined FFDM and tomosynthesis in a population-based screening programme using independent double reading with arbitration. Eur Ra-diol 2013;23:2061–71.

30. Skaane P, Bandos AI, Eben EB, et al. Two-view dig-ital breast tomosynthesis screening with syntheti-cally reconstructed projection images. Radiology 2014;271:655–63.

31. Ciatto S, Houssami N, Bernardi D, et al. Integration of 3D digital mammography with tomosynthesis for population breast-cancer screening (STORM): a prospective comparison study. Lancet Oncol 2013; 14:583–9.

32. Lang K, Andersson I, Rosso A, et al. Performance of one-view breast tomosynthesis as a stand-alone breast cancer screening modality: results from the Malmo Breast Tomosynthesis Screening Trial. Eur Radiol 2016;26:184–90.

33. Fornvik D, Andersson I, Svahn T, et al. The effect of reduced breast compression in breast tomosynthe-sis: human observer study using clinical cases. Ra-diat Prot Dosimetry 2010;139:118–23.

34. Lang K, Nergarden M, Andersson I, et al. False pos-itives in breast cancer screening with one-view breast tomosynthesis: An analysis of findings lead-ing to recall, work-up and biopsy rates in the Malmo Breast Tomosynthesis Screening Trial. Eur Radiol 2016;26(11):3899–907.

35. Haas BM, Kalra V, Geisel J, et al. Comparison of to-mosynthesis plus digital mammography and digital mammography alone for breast cancer screening. Radiology 2013;269:694–700.

36. Friedewald SM, Rafferty EA, Rose SL, et al. Breast cancer screening using tomosynthesis in combina-tion with digital mammography. JAMA 2014;311: 2499–507.

37. McDonald ES, Oustimov A, Weinstein SP, et al. Effectiveness of digital breast tomosynthesis compared with digital mammography: outcomes analysis from 3 years of breast cancer screening. JAMA Oncol 2016;2:737–43.

38. Bernard D, Ciatto S, Pellegrini M, et al. Application of breast tomosynthesis in screening: incremental ef-fect on mammography acquisition and reading time. Br J Radiol 2012;85:1174–8.

39. Dang PA, Freer PE, Humphrey KL, et al. Addition of tomosynthesis to conventional digital mammog-raphy: effect on image interpretation time of screening examinations. Radiology 2014;270:49–56.

40. Brandt DR, Craig DA, Hoskins TL, et al. Can digital breast tomosynthesis replace conventional diag-nostic mammography views for screening recalls without calcifications? A comparison study in a simulated clinical setting. AJR Am J Roentgenol 2013;200:291–8.

41. Lourenco AP, Barry-Brooks M, Baird GL, et al. Changes in recall type and patient treatment

following implementation of screening digital breast tomosynthesis. Radiology 2014;274:337–42.

42. Morel JC, Iqbal A, Wasan C, et al. The accuracy of digital breast tomosynthesis compared with coned compression magnification mammography in the assessment of abnormalities found on mammography. Clin Radiol 2014;69:1112–6.

43. Partyka L, Lourenco AP, Mainiero MB. Detection of mammographically occult architectural distortion on digital breast tomosynthesis screening: initial clinical experience. AJR Am J Roentgenol 2014;203:216–22.

44. Freer PE, Niell B, Rafferty EA. Preoperative tomosynthesis-guided needle localization of mammographically and sonographically occult breast lesions. Radiology 2015;275:377–83.

45. Houssami N, Skaane P. Overview of the evidence on digital breast tomosynthesis in breast cancer detection. Breast 2013;22:101–8.

Breast Tomosynthesis
Practical Considerations

Sarah M. Friedewald, MD

KEYWORDS

- Digital breast tomosynthesis • Screening mammography • Hanging protocols • Magnification views
- Diagnostic mammography • Skin calcifications

KEY POINTS

- DBT simultaneously decreases false-positive examinations and increases cancer detection.
- Practical approaches to interpretation of DBT enables accurate reading and increases speed.
- Ways to decrease recall requires appreciation of benign findings at the time of screening.
- Implementation of DBT may be stepwise because of financial constraints. Therefore, institutions may have different approaches to successful DBT integration into practice.

▶ Video content accompanies this article at http://www.radiologic.theclinics.com/.

INTRODUCTION

Benefits of screening mammography have been proven with seven randomized controlled trials demonstrating a significant decrease in mortality when women are screened. Additionally, screening mammography is a low-cost imaging modality that is easily accessible to patients in many parts of the world.[1]

However, traditional digital mammography (DM) is limited in sensitivity, particularly in women with dense breasts. The Breast Cancer Surveillance Consortium published data on the sensitivity of DM in 365,426 women aged 40 to 74 years. The highest sensitivity of DM for the detection of breast cancer was found in women who have almost entirely fatty breasts, ranging from 81.2% to 92.7%, and the lowest sensitivity was reported in women with extremely dense breasts, ranging from 57.1% to 71.3%.[2]

DM has also undergone harsh criticism for the perceived risks associated with screening yearly. The United States Preventive Services Task Force (USPSTF) in 2009 published guidelines for breast cancer screening in women in the United States that differed from recommendations from medical societies, such as the American College of Radiology and the American Congress of Obstetricians and Gynecologists. Specifically, the USPSTF stated women should be offered screened biennially beginning at age 50 rather than annually at age 40.[3] These guidelines were updated in 2016 with similar recommendations.[4]

The USPSTF cited that the "harms" associated with screening, such as false-positive findings and unnecessary biopsies, burdens patients with a significant amount of anxiety and unnecessary biopsies. Other critics of mammography are concerned about the false-positives contributing to the rising cost of health care.

In 2015, the American Cancer Society emphasized the risks with screening, but stated that the "contentious nature of debates surrounding breast cancer screening" were concerning and that "a more productive discussion would be focused on how to improve the performance of screening mammography."[5]

Many published studies have shown that digital breast tomosynthesis (DBT) improves on these limitations, namely the decreased sensitivity and high false positives when screening with traditional DM. DBT has therefore been rapidly implemented

Department of Radiology, Lynn Sage Comprehensive Breast Center, Prentice Women's Hospital, Feinberg School of Medicine, Northwestern University, 250 East Superior Street, Room 4-2304, Chicago, IL 60611, USA
E-mail address: sarah.friedewald@nm.org

Radiol Clin N Am 55 (2017) 493–502
http://dx.doi.org/10.1016/j.rcl.2016.12.004
0033-8389/17/© 2017 Elsevier Inc. All rights reserved.

into clinical practice since the United States Food and Drug Administration (FDA) approval in 2011 and at a significantly increased rate relative to DM from analog mammography. Review of the practical considerations of DBT is highlighted in this article.

SCREENING WITH TOMOSYNTHESIS

There are three sets of data obtained when screening patients with DM in combination with DBT (**Fig. 1**, Videos 1 and 2). The projection images represent the raw data and consist of multiple low-dose images acquired at varying angles across the breast. A set number of projection images are obtained, which are determined by the manufacturer, regardless of breast thickness. These projection images are then reconstructed into thin slices and are the data set interpreted by the radiologist. The number of reconstructed slices depends on the compression thickness of the breast. Therefore, the thicker the breast, the more images to interpret. Most manufactures of DBT systems set the slice thickness at 1 mm as a default; however, this can be adjusted. For example, if the breast compresses to 6 cm, there are 60 images to review in that single projection. Although decreasing the

number of images by increasing the slice thickness is helpful in appreciating the relationship of calcifications in a group, the advantages of removing superimposed tissue is decreased. Therefore, one must consider this trade off when setting a standard protocol for interpretation.

The last data set includes the traditional DM images, which are useful for calcification evaluation and comparison with prior films. Asymmetries are also better appreciated with the DM images and therefore are necessary to review for optimal interpretation.

Image Interpretation

As with any type of imaging study, it is critical to have a systematic approach for interpretation of images. This becomes particularly important with tomosynthesis because of the large number of images that are generated for review. As proven with DM interpretation, optimal screening environments, such as reading in dark rooms with little to no interruptions, can contribute to improved performance. Additionally, batch reading where successive screening examinations are interpreted without the patient waiting has been shown to be superior to "on-line screening" interpretation,

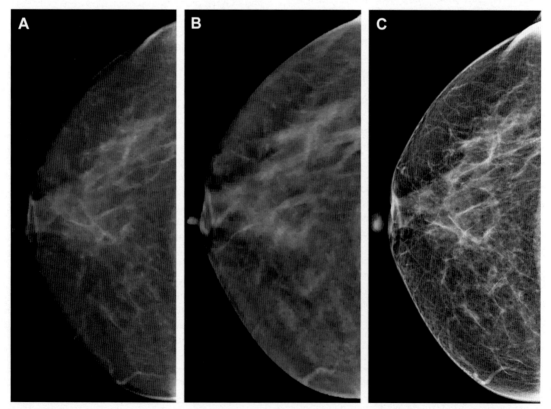

Fig. 1. Images acquired in a combination DM and DBT examination. (*A*) Projection images (video) (*B*) Reconstructed images (video) (*C*) DM obtained under the same compression, co-registered with the DBT images.

where results are given to the patient immediately after intepretation.[6] Additionally, toggling between current examinations and prior examinations on the same screen may decrease perception errors. This is compared with a "trend" hanging protocol where the current examination is on one end of the monitor and the prior examinations (same view) successively get older as one moves toward the other end of the monitor. When placing images side by side in the trend hanging protocol, differences in breast lesions may not be as well perceived because of the change in eye gaze, resulting in "change blindness" or inability to detect differences between two objects.[7] This is particularly applicable in breast imaging where differences in breast tissue patterns may indicate pathology. In addition to accuracy, interpretation speed may also be improved with toggling. One study has shown that toggling between current and prior DM films decreases interpretation time by 6 seconds. There was also a trend toward improved accuracy by 5%, although this pilot study was too small to show a statistical difference.[8] Because of the large data sets in DBT, toggling between DM and DBT has the potential to improve interpretation time and accuracy.

The method chosen to interpret the data sets must be consistent to improve efficiency and decrease errors. One approach to image interpretation is as follows: interpret the DM images first and make an assessment before evaluating the DBT images. If no abnormality is detected, then review the DBT images and make an assessment.

Scrolling through the reconstructed DBT images is challenging because of the tendency for distraction as different portions of the breast come in and out of focus. This is particularly true if multiple abnormalities are present in the breast. The risk of missing a lesion is heightened if the breast is large. One approach to managing the volume of data is to review one portion of the image while scrolling, rather than reviewing the entire image and then moving on to the next image slice. For example, focusing on the lower half of the image (either medial on the craniocaudal view or inferior on the mediolateral oblique view) and then scrolling through the entire data set allows for complete evaluation of that portion of the breast. Then moving one's focus to the upper half of the image (lateral on the craniocaudal view and superior on the mediolateral oblique view) and scrolling through the data set completes the interpretation. If the breast is large, then compartmentalizing the breast into smaller portions is appropriate. This approach minimizes the potential to miss lesions (**Fig. 2**).

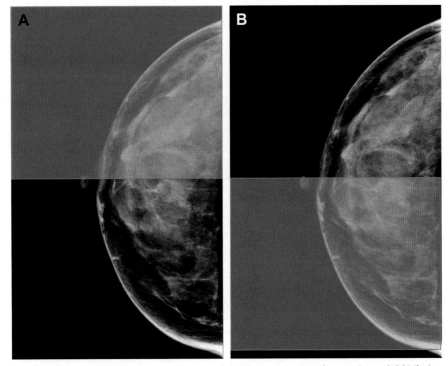

Fig. 2. One method to interpret reconstructed images. (*A*) When reviewing the craniocaudal (CC) view, keep eyes focused on the lower half of the image (medial breast) and scroll through the entire set of images. (*B*) Then, move eyes to the upper half of the image (lateral breast) and scroll through the entire set of images again.

The cine speed at which the reader interprets the reconstructed images can also be varied. Some find that distortions are better perceived when scrolling through the images at higher cine speeds. This requires back and forth scrolling many times to ensure all portions of the breast are reviewed. Others prefer slower speeds and therefore have fewer passes through the breast.

BENEFITS OF DIGITAL BREAST TOMOSYNTHESIS
Increase in Cancer Detection

Detection of abnormalities in mammography is often limited by superimposed tissue. Tomosynthesis has been shown, in nearly all published studies, to increase invasive cancer detection.[9] This is primarily caused by the ability to effectively "remove" superimposed tissue that obscures lesions while the reader scrolls through the reconstructed images. Architectural distortion of normal breast structures and masses are particularly well visualized on tomosynthesis (**Fig. 3**). Ductal carcinoma in situ has not contributed to the increase in cancer detection, largely because ductal carcinoma in situ typically presents mammographically as grouped calcifications. The distribution of the calcifications is better appreciated on DM and therefore the DBT images are noncontributory.

Decrease in Recall
Asymmetries
The developing asymmetry can either represent normal asymmetric breast tissue caused by summation artifact or has the potential to be malignant. Because of the high positive predictive value for malignancy of developing asymmetries detected at screening found in one study (12.8%), this finding must be recalled with DM.[10] However, the ability to decipher normal superimposed tissue from true lesions allows for reduction in recall when DBT is added to DM. The appearance of normal overlapping structures, such as crossing vessels and normal Cooper's ligaments, is appreciated on each slice, decreasing the need to recall the patient for additional views in some cases (**Fig. 4**).

Skin lesions
Another advantage of screening with DBT is with the ability to detect indeterminate calcifications on DM that are located within the skin. Skin

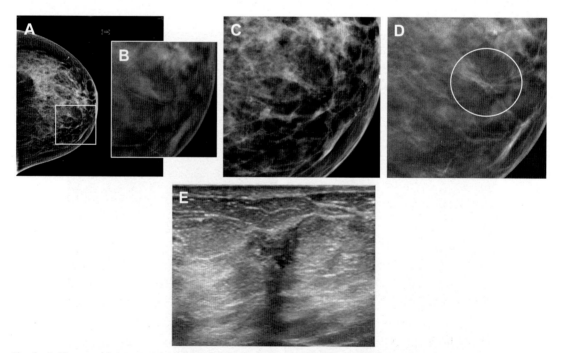

Fig. 3. A 45-year-old woman who presented for a combination DBT and DM screening mammogram. (*A*) DM CC view of the left breast is negative with particular attention to the medial region (*white box*). (*B*) The same area with DBT reconstructed slices (video). A spiculated mass appears in and out of focus. (*C*) DM image compared with (*D*) DBT reconstructed slice showing a spiculated mass seen only on the DBT image (*circle*). (*E*) Ultrasound evaluation of the inner left breast shows an irregular hypoechoic mass that was biopsied and proven to be invasive ductal carcinoma.

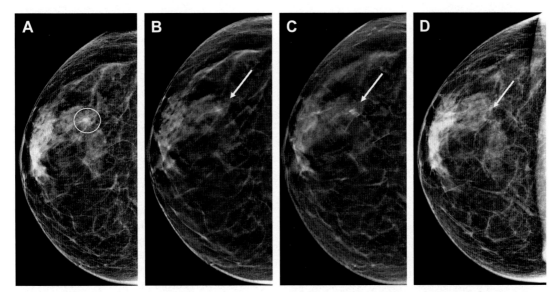

Fig. 4. Example of superimposed tissue that mimics an asymmetry on DM. (*A*) DM image demonstrating an asymmetry in the outer right breast on the CC view that needs to be recalled without the DBT images (*circle*). (*B, C*) Single reconstructed slices that show the asymmetry representing normal crossing breast structures (*arrow*). (*D*) Repeat CC view shows that the asymmetry does not persist on the DM image (*arrow*).

calcifications are typically dismissed if they display the classic lucent centers. However, some skin calcifications appear heterogeneous and therefore are not diagnostic at the time of screening. Assuming that skin is approximately 3 mm thick, with DBT, identification of the calcifications on

the first or last three reconstructed slices proves that the calcifications are within the skin and therefore do not need to be called back for additional diagnostic imaging (**Fig. 5**).

However, the reverse is not true; not all skin calcifications are located within the first or last three

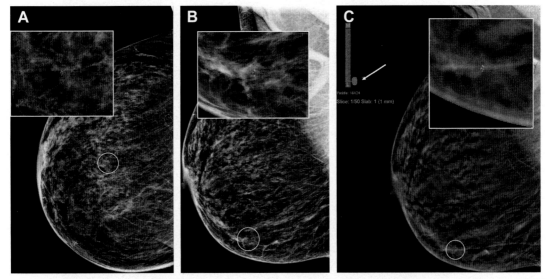

Fig. 5. Skin calcifications that appear indeterminate on DM images but are clearly within the skin on DBT. (*A*) CC view showing indeterminate calcifications in the right breast (*circle*) digitally magnified in the box. (*B*) Mediolateral oblique view in the same patient with the indeterminate calcifications in the lower right breast (*circle*) digitally magnified in the box. (*C*) The calcifications located in the lower breast (*circle*) and digitally magnified (*box*) are in focus on the first slice (*arrow*), and therefore are definitively within the skin.

slices. Reasons for alternative locations of skin calcifications include the following:

1. Skin calcifications may be located in skin that is not touching the detector or the compression paddle.
2. The scroll bar measures the maximum compressed thickness, usually in the posterior breast, and remains a fixed thickness regardless of the paddle flex. Flexing of the compression paddle anteriorly because of decreased breast thickness near the nipple causes the skin to be located deeper into the scroll bar.
3. In several systems, extra reconstructed slices are added to the compression paddle side of the stack so that inaccuracies of compression measurement (specifically underestimation of compression thickness) does not exclude portions of the breast from display. Therefore, in cases where the compression measurement is accurate, the calcifications may appear deeper into the stack, as extra slices are added after the true end of tissue.

If the calcifications are within the skin touching the detector plate, they project in the first three slices and do not have to be recalled. If the calcifications are in the last three slices of the stack, the same holds true. However, if the skin calcifications are located deeper in the stack, they remain indeterminate and must be recalled to verify their location.

Nipple

Sometimes the nipple appears to represent a mass or asymmetry on DM but is in reality not positioned properly in profile. This is proven with tomosynthesis and can potentially eliminate the need to recall the patient. In these cases, the nipple is typically touching the detector and can be seen as a mass on the first three slices (**Fig. 6**).

Vessel turns

Serpiginous vessels can create the appearance of a mass on DM. However, with DBT, the vessel is followed and the turn distinguished from a mass. This ability to differentiate between a normal vessel and a mass contributes to the decrease in false-positive recalls (**Fig. 7**).

LEARNING CURVE

The addition of DBT to DM adds data at the time of screening. Although this added information is ultimately helpful to the reader, it takes time to be confident that some abnormalities do not need to be recalled. In fact, early after DBT implementation, recall rates may initially increase. This is not exclusively caused by the increased detection of abnormalities on the prevalent DBT screen, but is

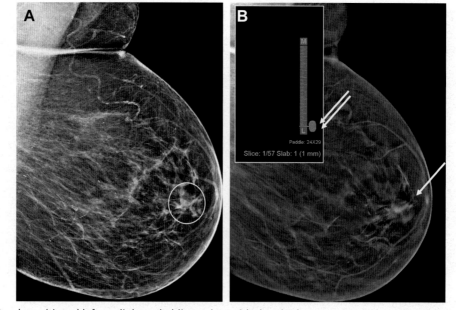

Fig. 6. Poorly positioned left mediolateral oblique view with the nipple appearing as a mass on the DM images. (*A*) DM left mediolateral oblique view with an asymmetry in the anterior breast (*circle*). (*B*) Reconstructed DBT slice showing the mass (*arrow*) is on the first slice (*double arrow*) proving that the nipple is touching the detector.

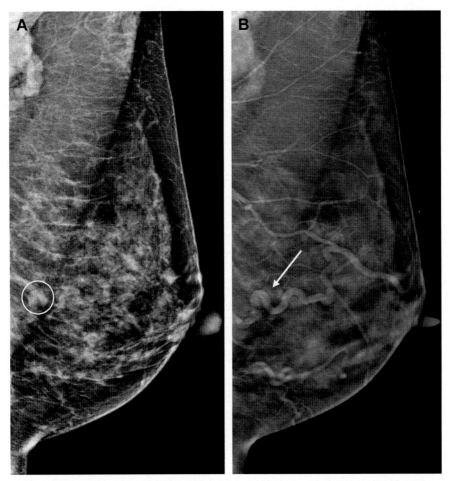

Fig. 7. Vessel turn appearing as an asymmetry on DM. (*A*) Indeterminate asymmetry on DM in the posterior right breast (*circle*). (*B*) DBT reconstructed slice showing that the asymmetry represents a vessel turn (*arrow*).

also caused by inexperience whereby the radiologist continues to call back normal superimposed tissue unnecessarily. One way to gain confidence in decreasing recall of asymmetries is to call back the patient as you would if you were reading DM alone. Beginning with a low pretest probability that these abnormalities represent a malignancy, confirmation with diagnostic imaging and ultrasound is particularly helpful. After reading enough cases, one becomes more familiar with the appearance of superimposed structures and therefore can confidently dismiss an asymmetry on DM when appropriate.

Repeated exposure to DBT contributes to decreased recall rates as evidenced by a study by McDonald and coworkers,[11] who showed that with the first round of screening with DBT, the recall rates were 130 of 1000 women screened (compared with a baseline of 104 of 1000 with DM alone) but decreased after the second round of screening with DBT to 78 of 1000 recalled/

screened, and finally a recall rate of 59 of 1000 women screened was achieved after the third round of DBT screening.

DIAGNOSTIC MAMMOGRAPHY WITH DIGITAL BREAST TOMOSYNTHESIS

The standard paradigm for diagnostic mammographic work-up after an abnormality is detected on a screening examination is not mandatory when screening patients with tomosynthesis.[12] When a clear mass is identified with DBT, the borders are more accurately appreciated and distinguished from background tissue. For example, if a distinct abnormality is detected and margins are well appreciated, the likelihood that diagnostic mammography will aid in the work-up is reduced. Therefore, skipping diagnostic mammography and going straight to ultrasound is more efficient and decreases unnecessary radiation to that patient. This is not appropriate when there are subtle findings, incomplete visualization of lesion margins, or with microcalcifications.

Tomosynthesis and Magnification Views

To obtain magnification views in DM, the breast is placed on a platform with a large air gap between the breast and the detector. The x-ray beams are perpendicular to the breast and are captured on the detector. However, with DBT, the x-ray tube moves at an angle across the breast. With the largest angles, the x-ray beam overshoots the detector. Because of this technical limitation, magnification cannot be achieved with DBT and therefore, traditional DM diagnostic evaluation of indeterminate calcifications with magnification is still required (**Fig. 8**).

IMPLEMENTATION
Hybrid Implementation

The capital expenditure required to purchase mammography equipment can be difficult to obtain. Therefore, not all institutions have the capability to convert all mammography machines overnight with DBT units. This has been historically demonstrated with the slow conversion of analog machines to DM in the United States. At 5 years after DM FDA approval (January 28, 2000) the number of DM units that were accredited was 874, representing only 6.4% of the market. However, the adoption of DBT is at a significantly faster pace, likely because of the clear advantages of tomosynthesis described previously, namely increase in cancer detection

and decrease in recall rate. At 5 years after FDA approval of DBT on February 11, 2011, a total of 3362 units were accredited representing 20.8% of the market.[13,14]

However, the transition from DM to DBT is complicated because there are many more images to interpret and the time it takes to read a screening examination is two to three times as long as DM.[15] Allocation of physician effort must therefore be considered. With the reduction in recall after screening with DBT, the volume of diagnostic imaging should decrease concomitantly. Physician time can then be shifted to screening (**Table 1**).

Because our institution adopted DBT soon after FDA approval, and we had only one DBT-capable machine, we could only offer the technology to a fraction of our patients. Additionally, there were only a few other institutions with the technology and no standard implementation protocol had been established. Therefore, our approach to incorporating DBT into our practice was cautious. We chose to begin imaging patients in the diagnostic setting that have longer appointment times than screening. This extended time enabled the physicians to become accustomed to the new images and reading times and allowed the technologists to become familiar with the technology.

Eventually, as funds became available, we were able to acquire additional units. We then transitioned from using DBT in the diagnostic setting to the screening environment because we could guarantee that all patients would be screened

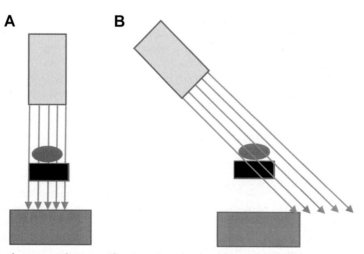

Fig. 8. Comparison of exposure for magnification views between DM and DBT. Light blue box represents X-ray tube, gray oval represents breast. Black box represents the magnification stand. Blue box represents detector. Arrows represent X-ray beam. (*A*) Schematic representing DM exposure for a CC magnification view. The X-ray beam hits the detector. (*B*) Schematic representing proposed DBT exposure for CC magnification view. Many of the X-rays miss the detector because of the angle of the X-ray tube.

Table 1
FDA-accredited units 5 years after DM was approved (June 1, 2005) and 5 years after DBT was approved (June 1, 2016)

	FDA Accredited Units as of June 1, 2005			FDA Accredited Units as of June 1, 2016		
	Facilities	Units	%	Facilities	Units	%
Total	8911	13,621	100	8740	16,155	100
Analog	—	12,747	93.6	—	285	1.8
FFDM	—	874	6.4	—	12,508	77.4
DBT	—	0	0	—	3,362	20.8

with DBT, maximizing the number of patients exposed to the new technology.

Other institutions have chosen to implement DBT differently. For example, at Baylor College of Medicine, they chose to begin screening patients with DBT and not perform routine diagnostic imaging with DBT. Their focus was to maximize the advantages of the benefits of DBT by increasing cancer detection and reducing the unnecessary recalls. However, after 24 months of screening with tomosynthesis, they moved to a hybrid model based on room availability and specific scenarios that needed DBT (asymmetries and architectural distortion).[16]

SUMMARY

DBT has been rapidly adopted in the United States as an improved mammography screening tool and it is anticipated that DBT will continue to be installed as facilities update their equipment. The main advantages of the technology are to improve cancer detection while decreasing false positive recalls thereby improving on the limitations of DM. Appreciating normal findings at the time of screening contributes toward this end and is dependent on the reader's experience. The pathway to successful incorporation of DBT into clinical practice may differ at each facility. However, optimal interpretation of images is paramount to achieving best performance with this technology.

SUPPLEMENTARY DATA

Supplementary data related to this article can be found online at http://dx.doi.org/10.1016/j.rcl.2016.12.004.

REFERENCES

1. Hendrick RE, Helvie MA. Mammography screening: a new estimate of number needed to screen to prevent one breast cancer death. Am J Roentgenol 2012;198(3):723–8.

2. Kerlikowske K, Zhu W, Tosteson AN, et al. Identifying women with dense breasts at high risk for interval cancer: a cohort study. Ann Intern Med 2015; 162(10):673–81.

3. U.S. Preventive Services Task Force. Screening for breast cancer: U.S. Preventive Services Task Force recommendation statement. Ann Intern Med 2009; 151:716–26.

4. Siu AL, on behalf of the U.S. Preventive Services Task Force. Screening for breast cancer: U.S. Preventive Services Task Force recommendation statement. Ann Intern Med 2016;164:279–96.

5. Oeffinger KC, Fontham ET, Etzioni R, et al. Breast cancer screening for women at average risk: 2015 guideline update from the American Cancer Society. JAMA 2015;314:1599–614.

6. Burnside ES, Park JM, Fine JP, et al. The use of batch reading to improve the performance of screening mammography. Am J Roentgenol 2005; 185(3):790–6.

7. Simonsa DJ, Rensink RA. Change blindness: past, present, and future. Trends Cogn Sci 2005;9(1): 16–20.

8. Drew T, Aizenman AM, Thompson MB, et al. Image toggling saves time in mammography. J Med Imaging 2016;3(1):011003.

9. Friedewald SM, Rafferty EA, Rose SL, et al. Breast cancer screening using tomosynthesis in combination with digital mammography. JAMA 2014; 311(24):2499–507.

10. Leung JWT, Sickles EA. Developing asymmetry identified on mammography: correlation with imaging outcome and pathologic findings. Am J Roentgenol 2007;188:667–75.

11. McDonald ES, Oustimov A, Weinstein SP, et al. Effectiveness of digital breast tomosynthesis compared with digital mammography: outcomes analysis from 3 years of breast cancer screening. JAMA Oncol 2016;2(6):737–43.

12. Noroozian M, Hadjiiski L, Rahnama-Moghadam S, et al. Digital breast tomosynthesis is comparable

to mammographic spot views for mass characterization. Radiology 2012 Jan;262(1): 61–8.

13. U.S. Food and Drug Administration. MQSA national statistics. 2016. Available at: http://www.fda.gov/ Radiation-EmittingProducts/MammographyQuality StandardsActandProgram/FacilityScorecard/ucm 113858.htm. Accessed August 13, 2016.

14. U.S. Food and Drug Administration. Digital accreditation. 2016. Available at: http://www.fda.gov/Radiation-EmittingProducts/MammographyQualityStandards ActandProgram/FacilityCertificationandInspection/ ucm114148.htm. Accessed August 13, 2016.

15. Dang PA, Freer PE, Humphrey KL, et al. Addition of tomosynthesis to conventional digital mammography: effect on image interpretation time of screening examinations. Radiology 2014;270(1): 49–56.

16. Ebuoma LO, Roark AA, Sedgwick EL. Practical considerations for integrating digital breast tomosynthesis into clinical practice. J Am Coll Radiol 2015; 12(9):944–6.

Synthesized Digital Mammography Imaging

Phoebe E. Freer, MD*, Nicole Winkler, MD

KEYWORDS

- Digital breast tomosynthesis • Synthesized mammography • Breast cancer screening
- Digital mammography

KEY POINTS

- Early studies suggest that synthesized mammography (SM) may be used appropriately to replace acquired full-field digital mammography (FFDM) when using digital breast tomosynthesis (DBT) for screening.
- Replacing FFDM with SM when using DBT screening decreases the radiation dose by approximately one-half, making DBT more widely available clinically.
- Inherent differences in image quality and lesion visibility exist and the clinical radiologist should be aware of these differences if switching to SM technology.

Video content accompanies this article at http://www.radiologic.theclinics.com/.

INTRODUCTION

Digital breast tomosynthesis (DBT) has been adopted rapidly in academic and private practices for both screening and diagnostic imaging for breast cancer since its approval by the US Food and Drug Administration (FDA) in 2011.[1] The technology has been used to screen more than 8 million women since 2011, and more than 2400 systems are installed across all 50 states.[2] The use of DBT in screening has been demonstrated to drastically reduce the recall rate saving women from additional testing and anxiety involved with a false-positive mammogram.[3–5] Simultaneously, DBT screening has been found to increase the cancer detection rate, especially for invasive cancer, compared with standard mammography.[3,5] Additionally, because dense breast notification legislation has become more widespread across the country, early studies suggest that DBT may have some of its greatest incremental benefit over the 2-dimensional standard mammogram in women with heterogeneously dense breasts. Therefore, DBT screening as a primary breast cancer screening modality may be even more appealing because it could satisfy some state requirements for supplemental screening for dense breasts.[6,7] Synthesized digital mammography refers to 2-dimensional mammography that is computer generated from the DBT dataset and allows for the benefits of DBT without the increased dose over traditional mammography.

IMAGING PROTOCOLS

For screening purposes, the FDA initially approved the use of DBT in conjunction with standard 2-dimensional full-field digital mammograms

Disclosure Statement: The authors have nothing to disclose.
Department of Radiology and Imaging Sciences, University of Utah Hospital and Huntsman Cancer Institute, 30 North 1900 East, Salt Lake City, UT 84132, USA
* Corresponding author. Department of Radiology, University Medical Center, 30 North 1900 East, Salt Lake City, UT 84132.
E-mail address: phoebe.freer@hsc.utah.edu

Radiol Clin N Am 55 (2017) 503–512
http://dx.doi.org/10.1016/j.rcl.2016.12.005

(FFDMs), as opposed to using the DBT alone.[8–10] The standard full-field mammogram depiction of the breast allows for[1] easier assessment of breast density,[2] assessment of symmetry from breast to breast[3] compared with prior 2-dimensional mammograms, and[4] may help in the detection and assessment of distribution of calcifications.[11] Therefore, many users of DBT obtain both a DBT and standard 2-dimensional FFDM at the time of imaging. Some approved manufacturers allow for DBT and FFDM to be obtained sequentially in a single compression, with both studies registered to one another in an acquisition time that takes a matter of seconds. Other manufacturers have different acquisition methods resulting in obtaining a standard FFDM craniocaudal mammogram with a DBT mediolateral oblique image as a standard screening protocol.[10] Alternatively, other users may obtain FFDM and DBT for each view under different compressions.[12]

The current imaging protocol of obtaining DBT with FFDM exposes the patient to virtually double the radiation dose of mammography alone,[13,14] although it still falls below the FDA limit for screening mammography of 3 mGy. However, it is important to realize that the total radiation dose from a combination FFDM + DBT examination is comparable to the radiation of dose from an FFDM examination alone in the early days of digital mammography, as seen in the DMIST (Digital Mammographic Imaging Screening Trial) trial.[14] Efforts to decrease the dose have been underway to more closely approximate the average glandular dose of a single modern FFDM examination.

Therefore, much interest—and research—has focused on constructing a synthesized mammogram (SM) from the DBT dataset that mimics the acquired FFDM mammogram without the need to obtain a separate exposure. Different vendors are at different states of readiness with their SM technology for clinical use. However, one manufacturer currently has FDA approval[15] (**Fig 1**, Video 1).

SYNTHESIZED MAMMOGRAM TECHNIQUE

The only SM that is currently approved by the FDA for clinical use (C-View, Hologic, Inc, Bedford, MA) is a mathematical reconstruction of the acquired tomosynthesis slices. The reconstruction to create the SM is essentially a weighted summation and filtering technique from each of the DBT projection slices to construct an image by using a technique similar to a maximum intensity projection. An SM may be obtained in any view in which the DBT is acquired, including spot compression. The processing algorithm conserves the contrast of linear and point structures on each tomosynthesis slice. The reconstruction protocol applies a proprietary technique that enhances architectural distortion and spiculations as well as calcifications and other high-contrast features.

IMAGING FINDINGS

At present, only a single vendor has gained FDA approval of SM technology for clinical use.[15] In their vendor-supported study that was presented to the FDA to gain approval, the investigators designed a reader study with an enriched data set of 293 total cases (selected from a set of 2299 possible cases), 77 of which were cancers, and 216 were noncancer cases.[16] Fifteen board-certified radiologists who were MQSA qualified (Mammography Quality Standards Act of 1992) with various levels of clinical experience were trained to use the workstation and served as readers. The primary endpoint of the study design was noninferiority of the area under the curve (AUC) for SM + DBT compared with standard mammography alone (FFDM). The study used a probability of malignancy scale with readers interpreting each case separately both as the SM + DBT or the FFDM cases, with each modality separated by a month between session sets. Overall, the study was successful in demonstrating noninferiority of SM + DBT to FFDM and demonstrated a 14% decrease in the recall rate of noncancer cases in the dataset when switching from FFDM to SM + DBT (from 46.3% to 32.3% in this enriched dataset that had a high percentage of abnormal or previously recalled cases, and therefore a much higher expected rate of recalls than standard practice). Additionally, the overall sensitivity with SM improved slightly, by 0.6% (from 86.2% for FFDM to 86.8% for SM + DBT), and overall specificity improved, by 10% (from 64.8% for FFDM to 74.8% for SM + DBT). The positive likelihood ratio was significantly greater (improved positive predictive value) when reading SM + DBT than FFDM alone. The negative likelihood ratio was decreased when reading SM + DBT (improved negative predictive value), although this trend was not significant.[16]

SYNTHESIZED MAMMOGRAPHY IN CLINICAL USE

Studies of early prototypes of SM technology lacked initial promise and suggested that SM technology may be suboptimal for clinical use.[17] One of the first reader studies evaluating a prototype of SM found that the average sensitivity for SM + DBT was decreased at 0.772 compared

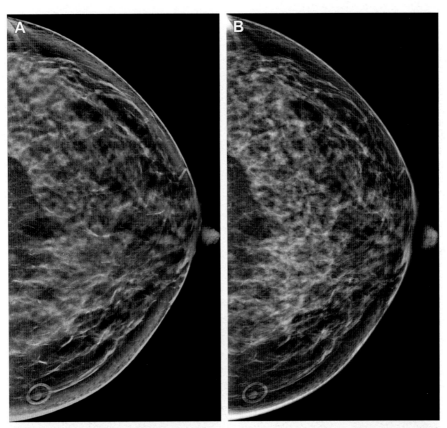

Fig. 1. Normal synthesized mammogram obtained in combination mode. (*A*) Normal synthesized left craniocaudal (CC) mammogram. The corresponding normal full-field digital mammogram left CC is shown in (*B*).

with the average sensitivity for FFDM + DBT of 0.826. Moreover, in this reader study using an early prototype of SM technology, 16 clusters of microcalcifications (out of a study set of 114 mammograms), were missed by 100% of the 10 radiologist readers when reading the SM + DBT mode.[17]

However, since then, clinical studies using later prototypes of SM technology similar to the model that gained approval by the FDA have demonstrated far more promise, suggesting that SM may be of sufficient quality to use clinically as a replacement for FFDM.[18,19] Zuley and colleagues[18] performed a retrospective reader study using 8 MQSA-qualified radiologists of various experience (3–24 years), reading 123 examinations selected from a set of 1184 cases collected during clinical practice as part of a research protocol. Each examination was interpreted using either FFDM + DBT or SM + DBT, with each mode separated by at least 2 months. Interestingly, this study was also designed to first directly compare the initial interpretation of the SM alone (without the DBT) with the FFDM alone (without the DBT), and subsequently gave the reader the DBT data for each

mode, allowing the more relevant comparison of SM + DBT to FFDM + DBT. The study also used the accuracy of the probability of malignancy ratings to generate AUC curves. They found that the AUC for SM + DBT was 0.916 and AUC for FFDM + DBT 0.939 (95% confidence interval [CI], -0.011 to 0.057; $P = .19$). Interestingly, 100% of the individual readers performed slightly better with FFDM + DBT compared with SM + DBT, but not to a statistically significant amount when taken as an aggregate group. The authors also noted that for the cases that had a subsequent biopsy-proven cancer, there was a substantive shift toward the reader giving a higher Breast Imaging Reporting and Data Systems (BIRADS; toward BIRADS 4C and BIRADS 5) when using SM versus FFDM. This shift may be owing to the SM reconstruction algorithm, which overemphasizes spiculated lines. However, there was no significant difference, because the total number of biopsy-proven malignant cases that were given a BIRADS 3 or higher by the reader did not differ. This study also showed more promise at recognizing calcifications than the study by Gur and associates,[17] which used an earlier prototype. There was 88% sensitivity using

FFDM + DBT versus 86% using SM + DBT for 9 cases that were malignant but were visible as microcalcifications only. The authors summarize that the SM technology is likely of sufficient quality to be used clinically to replace FFDM. A limitation of the study is that it included a majority of cases that had been imaged with an older research prototype of DBT using 11 slices for the acquisition, instead of the 15 that are used in the clinically available model. Thus, it is probable that many of the dataset cases were using an SM that was noisier than would be if the DBT to create the SM had been acquired with the current technology. Additionally, newer versions of processing software of SM technology have become clinically available since the study from Zuley and colleagues,[18] and therefore the same results may not directly apply.

A robust prospective vendor-sponsored study of SM technology in the clinical realm performed by Per Skaane and colleagues[19] in Norway demonstrated similar results. The investigators included 24,901 cases that were interpreted independently as either FFDM + DBT or as SM + DBT. This study assessed both an earlier version of the software for reconstruction of SMs, and a later, more advanced version. For the period involving the later software version, 12, 270 women were included. There was no difference in the false-positive rates between the standard FFDM + DBT technology and the SM + DBT technology (4.6% vs 4.5%, respectively; ratio, 0.99; 95% CI, 0.88–1.11; P = .85). Similarly, there was no difference in the cancer detection rate when switching from FFDM + DBT to SM + DBT (7.8

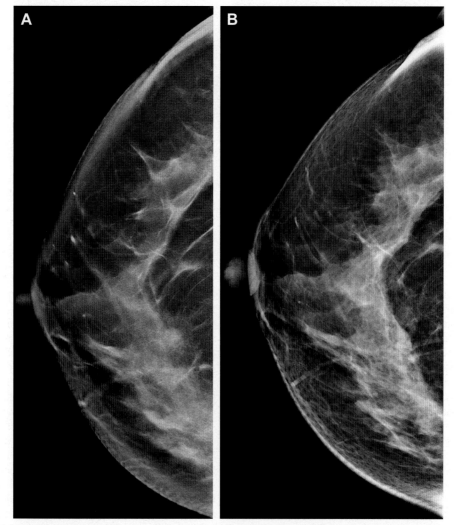

Fig. 2. Right breast motion. (A) is a synthesized right craniocaudal mammogram that shows motion blur. Compare this image with the full-field digital mammogram acquisition (B), which shows no motion.

in 1000 for FFDM + DBT and 7.7 in 1000 for SM + DBT; ratio = 0.98; 95% CI, 0.74–1.30; *P* = .89). However, the cancers that were detected using each modality were not the same cancers: that is, there were 14 cancers that were detected only by the FFDM + DBT readers and a different 12 cancers that were detected only by the SM + DBT readers. Per the authors, there is no difference in the size, grade, radiologic signs of cancer, or underlying breast density in these discordant examinations. It was seen, however, that the positive predictive value (%) of recalls increased for the SM + DBT compared with the FFDM + DBT. The authors conclude based on their study that the SM technology is likely ready

for clinical use to replace standard FFDM when using DBT, to decreasing the radiation dose by 45%.

Even more recently, the results of the STORM-2 (Screening with Tomosynthesis or Mammography-II) trial were published, again confirming that SM technology, in conjunction with DBT, may produce similar results for breast cancer screening as FFDM + DBT.[20] The large Italian trial included 9677 screening cases that were sequentially double read, first as FFDM, and then followed by either FFDM + DBT or SM + DBT. The cancer detection rate for SM + DBT was similar to, and in fact, slightly higher, than FFDM + DBT (8.8 in 1000 [95% CI, 7.0–10.8] vs 8.5 in 1000 [95% CI, 6.7–10.5], respectively), with both DBT reading

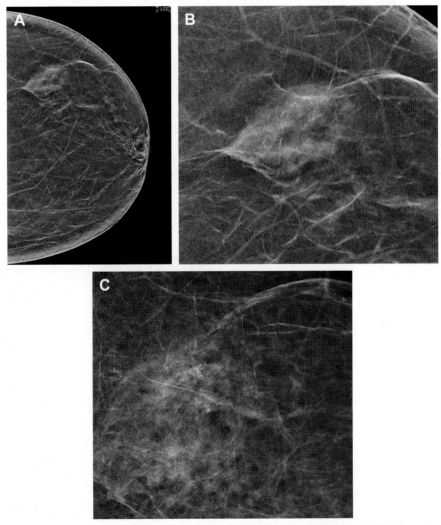

Fig. 3. Amorphous calcifications not visible on synthesized mammogram. (*A*) Synthesized left breast craniocaudal view that seems to be normal. No calcifications are visible on digital zoom image (*B*), prompting the radiologist to recall the patient for a magnification view (*C*). The mediolateral oblique synthesized projection (not shown) also did not show these calcifications. Stereotactic biopsy was recommended revealing atypical ductal hyperplasia.

modes having a significantly higher cancer detection rate than FFDM alone (6.3 in 1000; 95% CI, 4.8–8.1; P<.0001). Note that the cancer detection rate in Europe is quite a bit higher than expected in most US breast screening practices, owing to the biennial screening regimen. Additionally, the STORM-2 trial is also one of the only published studies to show an increased recall rate when switching from FFDM to DBT. However, this is likely secondary to the inherently low recall rate in this study itself (3.42%; 95% CI, 3.07–3.80) for FFDM, which is typical of European practice. Additionally, unlike other studies, the STORM-2 trial did not use a sequential double-reading design and did not use arbitration for recalled cases, both of which would increase the false-positive rate. Interestingly, the recall rate for the SM + DBT (4.45%; 95% CI, 4.05–4.89) was higher than the recall rate for FFDM + DBT (3.97%; 95% CI, 3.59–4.38), demonstrating inherent differences between the FFDM image and the SM image. Additionally, this suggests that there may be a learning curve associated with interpreting SM images.

It should be noted that most studies that have evaluated the use of SM have compared the use of SM + DBT with the use of FFDM or FFDM + DBT, rather than comparing the use of SM alone, with the use of FFDM. Because the SM is generated from a DBT image, the SM cannot be obtained without acquiring a DBT; therefore, the comparison of SM + DBT with other screening mammographic techniques is the clinically relevant question. However, because DBT takes longer to interpret than mammography,[21] Zuley and colleagues[18] investigated the use of the SM alone versus FFDM alone. Interestingly, when analyzing the AUC, SM was found to be essentially no different than the FFDM (AUC for SM was 0.894 vs 0.889 for FFDM; 95% CI, 0.062–0.054; P = .86). However, it was noted that 5 of the 8 readers performed somewhat *better* with SM than FFDM, but that the differences were small and therefore the mean AUCs were not significantly different.

DIFFERENCES BETWEEN FULL-FIELD DIGITAL MAMMOGRAPHY AND SYNTHESIZED MAMMOGRAPHY

In multiple studies, the latest iterations of clinically available SM technology have been demonstrated to be of acceptable quality for clinical use; and, when used with the DBT images obtained to make the SM, have been shown to have improved cancer detection rates. Moreover, most studies have demonstrated improved recall rates compared with FFDM. However, in these studies, it is clear that some cancers detected by

FFDM + DBT may not be as well-depicted on the SM + DBT, whereas other cancers are better depicted on the SM image compared with the FFDM.[19] In a study using phantoms, Nelson and colleagues[22] explored what accounts for some of the differences in quality, detection, and noise between FFDM and SM. They acquired phantom images with FFDM + DBT as well as with SM + DBT. Both sets of images were reviewed by radiologists, as well as by an automated software program. In their study, there was improved visualization of medium and large microcalcifications with SM; however, there was poorer resolution for small microcalcifications. Additionally, there was overall decreased resolution with SM. Specifically, SM had a significantly poorer depiction of fibers and specks. In fact, when using the American College of Radiology mammography accreditation phantom and scoring criteria, FFDM was rated consistently better quality than SM, with up to 70% of SM failing to meet the minimum American College of Radiology requirements for film screen mammography. Their conclusion is that SM may depict high-contrast objects, as well as medium and large microcalcifications better than FFDM, but overall SM has lower resolution and more noise. Additionally, for imaging findings that are small or are low contrast and have a similar appearance to background noise, SM fares the worst. This conclusion makes sense when considering that SM is reconstructed from a low-dose, lower resolution projection images of tomosynthesis and,

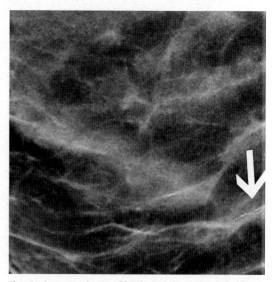

Fig. 4. Overemphasis of high-density pixels mimicking linear calcifications on synthesized view (*white arrow*). It is a right mediolateral oblique synthesized screening mammogram showing linear high-density foci in the posterior breast mimicking calcifications.

thus, is inherently of lower resolution than FFDM. Despite the lower resolution of SM, the reader studies support clinical use of SM, which are interpreted with DBT. The benefit of radiation dose reduction outweighs the small risk of missing low-density findings while maintaining equivalent cancer detection compared with FFDM + DBT.

PEARLS, PITFALLS, AND VARIANTS

- SM may be obtained in combination mode where FFDM is acquired along with tomosynthesis and noncombination mode where only tomosynthesis is acquired and 2-dimensional mammogram is synthesized from the tomosynthesis dataset. The former allows you to obtain cases with both FFDM and SM to familiarize yourself with SM (see **Fig. 1**, Video 1).
- The use of SM without FFDM reduces dose by approximately one-half and reduces acquisition time by approximately 30% compared with combination FFDM + DBT.[14,19]
- Motion can be more difficult to detect on SM compared with FFDM. The projection images are useful to assess for the presence of motion (**Fig. 2**, Videos 2 and 3).
- SM images should always be interpreted along with DBT images (**Fig. 3**, Video 4).
- The reconstruction algorithm for SM is designed to emphasize calcifications. Pixels that meet a certain density threshold may be overemphasized on SM creating the appearance of calcifications when, in fact, there are none (**Fig. 4**, Video 5).
- Architectural distortion is often enhanced on SM, which may aid in the detection of malignancy, but as a consequence may also increase detection of benign complex sclerosing lesions and radial scars (**Fig. 5**, Video 6).

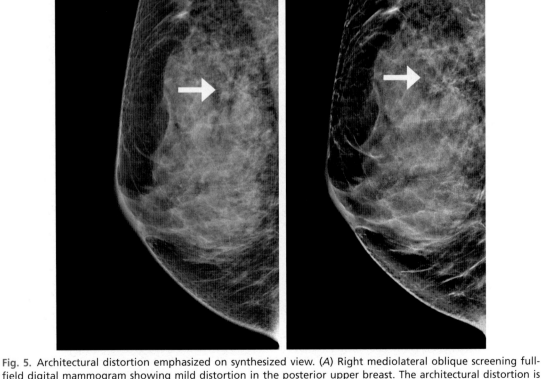

Fig. 5. Architectural distortion emphasized on synthesized view. (*A*) Right mediolateral oblique screening full-field digital mammogram showing mild distortion in the posterior upper breast. The architectural distortion is more emphasized on the synthesized view (*B*) (*white arrows*).

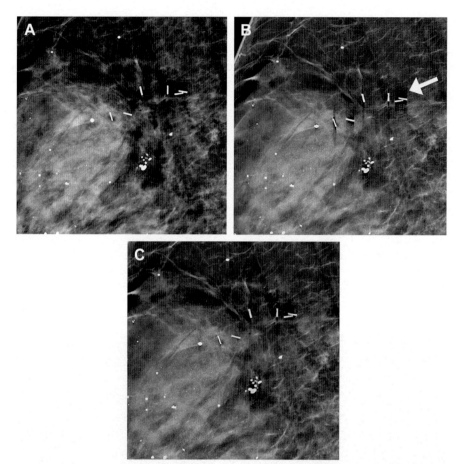

Fig. 6. Slinky artifact and postprocessing artifact reduction. (*A*) Digital zoom full-field digital mammogram (FFDM) mediolateral oblique image of a prior lumpectomy site showing multiple surgical clips and dystrophic calcifications. The concomitantly acquired FFDM (*B*) shows multiple repeating black lines above and below the clips and calcifications called the "slinky" artifact (*white arrow*). The synthesized mammogram was reprocessed from the tomosynthesis dataset with metal reduction software showing reduced artifact (*C*).

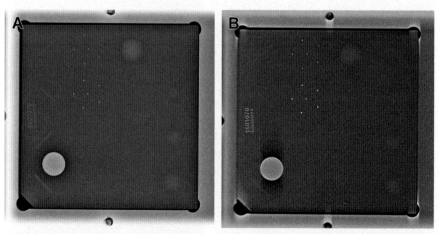

Fig. 7. A full-field digital mammogram (FFDM) phantom versus synthesized mammography (SM) phantom. Both phantoms were obtained in the same acquisition using FFDM + DBT + SM. (*A*) The FFDM of the phantom, which shows 5 masses, 5 fibers, and 4 groups of specks. (*B*) The SM of the phantom which shows 4 masses, 4 fibers, and 3 groups of specks. Note that the higher contrast material (higher density mass and specks) is more conspicuous on SM than on FFDM, but the lower contrast material is not visible on SM.

- Surgical clips, biopsy markers, and metallic skin markers result in a "slinky" artifact that may obscure subtle findings. Nonmetallic scar markers are helpful to reduce artifact. Postprocessing can also be used to reduce metal artifact if offered by the manufacturer (Fig. 6).
- Some findings, such as high-contrast masses or spiculations, may be better visualized on SM relative to FFDM, whereas other findings such as low-contrast masses and microcalcifications are less conspicuous on SM relative to FFDM (Fig. 7).

WHAT THE REFERRING PHYSICIAN NEEDS TO KNOW

- Dose reduction is the main benefit of SM, but only if FFDM is not also obtained. SM allows patients to be screened with DBT, gaining the benefits of tomosynthesis, with a minimal dose difference relative to FFDM.
- SM viewed with tomosynthesis acquisition is likely adequate for interpretation in clinical practice without the addition of FFDM.

SUMMARY

The recent development of SM allows for the advantages of DBT, namely, an inherent reduced recall rate and improved cancer detection rate, at nearly the same radiation dose as FFDM. However, its adoption in clinical practice is new and, as such, should be used with caution. The inherent differences between SM and FFDM may account for differences in detection of findings. Specifically, the SM images are of lower resolution and increased noise compared with FFDM, and small microcalcifications, or low-contrast small objects equivalent to fibers on phantoms, may be less well-visualized on SM compared with FFDM. Additionally, because SM is generated from the DBT dataset, it is designed for use in conjunction with DBT rather than as a stand-alone image. One should not be lulled into thinking that review of the DBT reconstructed images can be eliminated.

SUPPLEMENTARY DATA

Supplementary data related to this article can be found online at http://dx.doi.org/10.1016/j.rcl.2016.12.005.

REFERENCES

1. United States Food and Drug Administration. Selenia Dimensions 3D system – P08003. 2013. Available at: http://www.fda.gov/MedicalDevices/ProductsandMedical Procedures/DeviceApprovalsandClearances/Recently-ApprovedDevices/ucm246400.htm. Accessed July 24, 2016.
2. Available at: http://mygenius3d.com/pro/difference/; Hologic, Inc, Bedford (MA). Accessed July 13, 2016.
3. Friedewald SM, Rafferty EA, Rose SL, et al. Breast cancer screening using tomosynthesis in combination with digital mammography. JAMA 2014; 311(24):2499–507.
4. Rose S, Tidwell A, Bujnock L, et al. Implementation of breast tomosynthesis in a routine screening practice: an observational study. AJR Am J Roentgenol 2013;200(6):1401–8.
5. Skaane P, Bandos AI, Gullien R, et al. Comparison of digital mammography alone and digital mammography plus tomosynthesis in a population-based screening program. Radiology 2013;267(1):47–56.
6. Freer PE, Slanetz PJ, Haas JS, et al. Breast cancer screening in the era of density notification legislation: summary of 2014 Massachusetts experience and suggestion of an evidence-based management algorithm by multi-disciplinary expert panel. Breast Cancer Res Treat 2015;153(2):455–64.
7. Rafferty EA, Durand MA, Conant EF, et al. Breast cancer screening using tomosynthesis and digital mammography in dense and nondense breasts. JAMA 2016;315(16):1784–6.
8. US Food and Drug Administration, Department of Health and Human Services. Letter re: Selenia Dimensions 3D System. Available at: http://www.accessdata.fda.gov/cdrh_docs/pdf8/p080003a.pdf. Accessed July 13, 2016.
9. US Food and Drug Administration, Department of Health and Human Services. Letter re: SenoClaire. Available at: http://www.accessdata.fda.gov/cdrh_docs/pdf13/P130020a.pdf. Accessed July 13, 2016.
10. US Food and Drug Administration, Department of Health and Human Services. Letter re: MAMMOMAT Inspiration with tomosynthesis option. Available at: http://www.accessdata.fda.gov/cdrh_docs/pdf14/P140011a.pdf. Accessed July 13, 2016.
11. Spangler ML, Zuley ML, Sumkin JH, et al. Detection and classification of calcifications on digital breast tomosynthesis and 2D digital mammography: a comparison. AJR Am J Roentgenol 2011;196(2):320–4.
12. American College of Radiology and Society of Breast Imaging. Position Statement: ACR and SBI guidance on DBT "off label" use. Available at: http://www.acr.org/About-Us/Media-Center/Position-Statements/Position-Statements-Folder/20150109-ACR-and-SBI-Guidance-on-DBT-Off-Label-Use. Accessed July 23, 2016.
13. Svahn TM, Houssami N, Sechopoulos I, et al. Review of radiation dose estimates in digital breast tomosynthesis relative to those in two-view full-field digital mammography. Breast 2015;24(2):93–9.

14. Feng SS, Sechopoulos I. Clinical digital breast tomo-synthesis system: dosimetric characterization. Radiology 2012;263(1):35–42.

15. US Food and Drug Administration, Department of Health and Human Services. Letter re: Selenia Dimensions 3D system. Available at: http://www.accessdata.fda.gov/cdrh_docs/pdf8/p080003s001a.pdf. Accessed July 14, 2016.

16. US Food and Drug Administration. US Food and Drug Administration (FDA) Review: Radiology Advisory Panel Meeting: Hologic Selenia Dimensions 3D System with C-View Software Module. Available at: http://www.fda.gov/downloads/AdvisoryCommittees/CommitteesMeetingMaterials/MedicalDevices/MedicalDevicesAdvisoryCommittee/RadiologicalDevicesPanel/UCM325901.pdf. Accessed July 10, 2016.

17. Gur D, Zuley ML, Anelloa MI, et al. Dose reduction in digital breast tomosynthesis (DBT) screening using synthetically reconstructed projection images: an observer performance study. Acad Radiol 2012; 19(2):166–71.

18. Zuley ML, Guo B, Catullo VJ, et al. Comparison of two-dimensional synthesized mammograms versus original digital mammograms alone and in combination with tomosynthesis images. Radiology 2014; 271(3):664–71.

19. Skaane P, Bandos A, Eben E, et al. Two-view digital breast tomosynthesis screening with synthetically reconstructed projection images: comparison with digital breast tomosynthesis with full-field digital mammographic images. Radiology 2014;271(3): 655–63.

20. Bernardi D, Macaskill P, Pellegrini M, et al. Breast cancer screening with tomosynthesis (3D mammography) with acquired or synthetic 2D mammography compared with 2D mammography alone (STORM-2): a population-based prospective study. Lancet Oncol 2016;17(8):1105–13.

21. Dang PA, Freer PE, Humphrey KL, et al. Addition of tomosynthesis to conventional digital mammography: effect on image interpretation time of screening examinations. Radiology 2014;270(1): 49–56.

22. Nelson JS, Wells JR, Baker JA, et al. How does c-view image quality compare with conventional 2D FFDM? Med Phys 2016;43(5):2538.

Breast Density Legislation and Clinical Evidence

Regina J. Hooley, MD

KEYWORDS

• Ultrasound • Screening • Density • Legislation • Breast • Cancer • Risk

KEY POINTS

- Breast density legislation is increasing in popularity, and more than half of the United States have enacted such laws since 2009.
- Dense breast tissue is common and is associated with decreased mammographic sensitivity, as well as increased breast cancer risk.
- Supplemental screening with ultrasound, tomosynthesis, and MRI are complimentary to mammography, although each modality is associated with its own limitations.

INTRODUCTION

Connecticut passed the first breast density awareness notification law in 2009, and now over half of the United States has also followed. Although radiologists have been aware of the significance of breast density and its impact on the sensitivity of mammography for decades, most primary care physicians and women undergoing screening mammography were previously unaware of differences in breast density along with its relationship to breast cancer risk and mammographic accuracy. Breast density is now a hot topic and is fueled primarily by the successful grassroots efforts of patient advocates behind breast density inform legislation.

Women are diagnosed with dense breast tissue based on the amount of fibroglandular tissue relative to fatty tissue present on mammography. Women with dense breast tissue may opt for supplemental screening, usually with ultrasound or MRI. Radiologists are on the forefront of the breast density platform, since they are responsible for diagnosing women with dense breast tissue and, increasingly, offering women—either by choice or by law—a discussion over the implications of having dense breast tissue and the options regarding supplemental screening. Therefore, radiologists must be knowledgeable of the current evidence related to optimal breast density determination, its effect on mammography and breast cancer risk, and the associated risks and benefits of different supplemental screening tests.

BREAST DENSITY LEGISLATION
The Origins of Breast Density Legislation

In 2004, Nancy Cappello self-palpated a breast lump only 6 weeks after having a normal mammogram. Ultrasound subsequently revealed a 2.5 cm suspicious breast mass, and she was ultimately diagnosed with stage IIIC breast cancer metastatic to 13 axillary lymph nodes.[1] Cappello was surprised by her diagnosis of late-stage cancer, particularly since she faithfully had annual mammography. Moreover, she was bewildered when multiple doctors were unsurprised by her diagnosis, because, they explained, she had dense breast tissue as was clearly and consistently described on all of her mammogram reports.

Disclosure Statement: Research Grant: Philips; Consultant: Fuji Film, Siemens, Hologic.
Department of Radiology and Biomedical Imaging, Yale University School of Medicine, 333 Cedar Street, PO Box 208042, New Haven, CT 06520, USA
E-mail address: regina.hooley@yale.edu

Radiol Clin N Am 55 (2017) 513–526
http://dx.doi.org/10.1016/j.rcl.2016.12.006

Cappello searched lay publications but found no information about dense breast tissue. Having a PhD in psychology, Cappello then easily searched the scientific and medical literature, discovering that not only is dense breast tissue common,[2,3] but also represents a risk factor for breast cancer[5,6] and is the strongest predictor of the failure of mammography screening.[7-9] She also found multiple studies showing that supplemental screening ultrasound performed in the addition to mammography could find early stage mammographically occult invasive cancers.[10-15]

Overwhelmed by this information, Cappello decided to take action. At first she believed that providing access to screening breast ultrasound would allow more women to choose supplemental screening. A former chief of special education in Connecticut, she successfully helped craft legislation to mandate insurance coverage for screening whole breast ultrasound (SWBUS), which easily passed state legislation in 2005. She spread her message during speaking engagements throughout Connecticut, but soon discovered that the initial legislation was unsuccessful, because many women were still not given the option to choose SWBUS; additionally, most doctors remained dismissive about the importance of dense breasts. As a result, Cappello worked with her state senators to craft new legislation designed to provide standardized communication to women regarding the findings of dense breast tissue on their mammography reports. The initial legislation failed in 2007, as only a single community radiologist testified in its favor, and multiple radiologists, including members of the Connecticut Radiology Society, testified against it. In response, Cappello founded AreYouDense.org, which is also linked to a nonprofit organization. The website provided a path to efficient widespread community outreach and support.

In a second attempt, CT 09-41 "An Act Requiring Communication of Mammographic Density Information to Patients," was introduced in 2009. By then the multi-institutional results of the ACRIN 6666 were published, showing that SWBUS could detect an additional 4.2 cancers per 1000 women screened in women with dense breasts, elevated risk, and a negative mammogram.[16] Fueled with this new scientific evidence and more community support, the billed easily passed. Despite initial opposition, the Connecticut Radiology Society supported the bill in the closing hours to help influence the verbiage of the final legislation. On May 20, 2009, Governor Jodi Rell, herself diagnosed with breast cancer a few years earlier while in office, signed the landmark legislation that went on to spark a nationwide breast density inform grassroots effort.

Texas, New York, Virginia, and California soon followed Connecticut's lead, enacting similar breast density inform legislation by early 2013. Despite the success of the initial breast density inform laws, there were numerous early opponents including the American College of Obstetricians and Gynecologists (ACOG), Planned Parenthood, insurance companies, and many state radiology societies. Opponents cited concerns about the lack of strong scientific evidence proving mortality reduction related to providing patients breast density information and supplemental screening. There were also concerns about increased patient anxiety, false-positive results, and increased health care costs generated by additional diagnostic testing.

The Current Status of Breast Density Legislation

There are 27 states with mandatory breast density inform laws in effect, as of this writing. These laws require patients receive some level of information about their breast density present on their mammogram. However, breast density reporting is variable by state, and although some state laws are similar, there is no nationwide standard.[17] For example, the Connecticut law specifically states that supplemental screening with ultrasound or MRI could be beneficial, while the California and Pennsylvania laws do not specifically mention the option of supplemental screening. Three states have also passed breast density inform related bills suggesting, but not mandating, that patients be informed of their breast density (**Table 1**).

Five states have insurance mandates for screening ultrasound, but only 3 states with insurance mandates also have active breast density laws. New Jersey law mandates insurance coverage for SWBUS in women with a normal mammogram and extremely dense breasts only, while Connecticut requires insurance coverage for all women with dense breasts subject to an individual's deductible, plus a maximum copay of $20. In mid-2016, New York passed a broad law mandating insurance coverage without copay or any patient cost sharing for SWBUS, mammography, or MRI for the detection of breast cancer. A Connecticut bill introduced by Cappello in 2016 designed to eliminate all patient cost sharing for SWBUS failed.

The Future of Breast Density Notification

Passage of state breast density notification laws continues to gain momentum throughout the country, but patient advocates ultimately strive

Table 1
Breast density legislation

State Legislation	2009	2011	2012	2013	2014		2015	2016
Requires notification (effective date)	CT	TX	VA	CA[a]	NJ	NC	MA	OK
				AL	OR	MN	ND[a]	LA
				NY	NV	TN	MO	VT
				MD	AZ	PA	MI	SC
					HI	RI	OH	
							DE	
Suggests notification	UT, IN, ME							
Active bills	WA, IA, KY, WV, GA							
Inactive bill	CO, KS, MS, FL, NH							
Insurance coverage	CT, NY, IN, IL, NJ							
No bill introduced	ID, MT, WY, SD, NE, NM, AR, WI, IL, AK							

[a] CA and ND laws remain in effect through 1/1/19 and 7/31/17, respectively unless extended by law.

From Legislation and regulations—what is required? In: Dense breast-info an education coalition. Available at: http://densebreast-info.org/legislation.aspx. Accessed July 10, 2016.

for a consistent and strong nationwide mandate. This could be achieved by either federal legislation or federal regulation. On the legislative front, the "Breast Density and Mammography Reporting Act" has been introduced into the House of Representatives every year since 2011 by Stephen Israel (D-NY) and Rosa Delauro (D-CT). Beginning in 2014, the bill also has been introduced in the Senate by Diane Feinstein (D-CA) and Kelly Ayotte (R-NH). If federal legislation fails to gain momentum, there is also the increasingly likely possibility that the US Food and Drug Administration (FDA) may amend the patient lay letter to mandate inclusion of breast density information. This FDA panel amendment was initially approved in 2013, and a Density Reporting Amendment to the Mammography Quality Standards Act (MQSA) as a "Notice of Proposed Rulemaking" may soon be issued. Patient advocates remain cautious of any federal legislative or regulatory mandate, as the proposed language may not meet the strict criteria of providing true, clear, and strong information to women.

Issues with Breast Density Legislation

Despite the remarkable legislative success of breast density notification, barriers exist that may prevent patient–physician breast density discussion. Referring health care providers may not be knowledgeable about breast density. A study among primary care clinicians in California showed that awareness of the California breast density inform law was low, with many physicians not feeling comfortable discussing breast density-related patient questions.[18]

Patients may also not understand the breast density information written in their mammography results lay letter. Kressen, and colleagues[19] discovered a wide variation in 23 states' breast density notification content, with most having readability at high school level or above, which was higher than states' average literacy. Several studies have also demonstrated that disparities exist regarding breast density knowledge and awareness across race/ethnicity, education, and income in women living in states with breast density notification laws.[20,21] Like disparities in communicating results observed with screening mammography,[22] continued efforts are necessary to ensure adequate communication of all breast cancer screening results to all patients. Multiple educational Web sites now exist designed to provide accurate information on breast density and its clinical significance and to engage both referring Health care providers and patients.[17,23,24]

There are more than 25 million women in the United States of common screening age with dense breasts at mammography.[25] A concern of breast density reporting is the added cost of supplemental screening. If all of these patients were to undergo supplemental screening, particularly ultrasound or MRI, this could overwhelm facilities lacking equipment, infrastructure, and staff to provide high-volume supplemental screening service lines.[26] At Yale Breast Imaging, approximately 30% to 40% of women with dense breast tissue and average risk opt in for screening breast ultrasound. The lack of uniform health insurance coverage for supplemental screening may also result in disparities in health care delivery and increased anxiety for women who want to take action after being informed of their dense breast tissue, but are unable to afford additional screening.

BREAST DENSITY: CLINICAL EVIDENCE

Debate continues on the importance of dense breast tissue as an independent risk factor, which remains controversial in the literature. Many medical experts disagree on whether density alone warrants recommendation for supplemental screening.[27,28] For example, 1 study demonstrated that women with dense breast tissue are not at greater risk for dying compared with women with fatty breasts[29]; however critics of the study note that the mean length of patient follow-up was only 6.6 years, and it is known that 10 to 20 years of patient follow-up are necessary to establish accurate mortality data, because breast cancer recurrences may occur over 10 years past initial diagnosis.[30,31]

Breast Density Determination

Breast density is associated with the amount of fibroglandular tissue present on the mammogram; it is not determined by the degree of breast nodularity or firmness present on palpation and/or physical examination. No standard criteria exist for breast density determination,[32] and most commonly radiologists determine breast density by subjective visual evaluation of the amount of fibroglandular tissue relative to fat within the breast as visualized on the mammogram. Several historic subjective breast density determination methods exist, dating back to Wolfe's 1976

grading system.[33] As per the latest Breast Imaging Reporting and Data System (BI-RADS) fifth edition, breast density is defined according to 1 of 4 categories:

1. Almost entirely fatty
2. Scattered areas of fibroglandular tissue
3. Heterogeneously dense, which may obscure small masses
4. Extremely dense, which may lower the sensitivity of the mammogram[34]

Women with heterogeneous or extremely dense breast tissue are considered to have dense breast tissue, while women with fatty or scattered fibroglandular tissue are considered to have nondense breast tissue. In the previous BI-RADS version, the 4 categories of breast density were associated with quartile distribution of breast density and heterogeneous or extremely dense breast tissue considered as having at least 50% to 75% or greater than 75% fibroglandular tissue in relation to fatty tissue on the mammogram, respectively.[35] The BI-RADS fifth edition redefines breast density determination and does not rely on quartile/percentage distribution; instead, it defines breast density according to the presence of a region of confluent fibroglandular tissue that may mask and obscure an underlying cancer (**Fig. 1**).

Previous data demonstrate that breast density distribution in women living in the United States is approximately 10% fatty, 40% scattered, 40% heterogeneous, and 10% extremely dense.[34] Overall, approximately 50% of women in the United States have dense breast tissue.[34] With

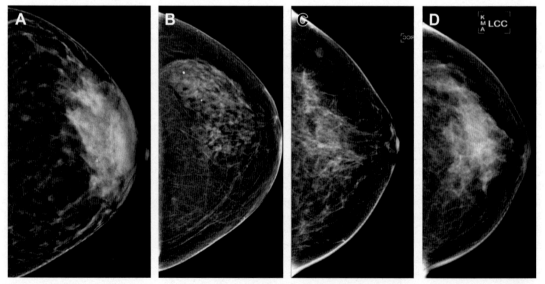

Fig. 1. (A–D) The variable appearance of heterogeneously dense breast tissue. Dense breast tissue located one area of the breast as shown in (A, B) may still mask an underlying tumor.

the new BI-RADS fifth edition breast density determination guidelines, it is possible that more women will be classified as having dense breast tissue.[32] Conversely, it is also possible that as a result of breast density notification laws, radiologists may be more likely to report breast tissue as scattered and not heterogeneously dense.[36] Dense breasts are more common in younger women, and density can decrease with age, particularly following menopause. Approximately 60% or more women under age 50 have dense breast tissue, as do 30% to 44% of women in their 60s and 25% to 36% of women in their 70s.[2,3]

Radiologists' subjective determination of breast density is imperfect and subject to inter- and intra-observer variability.[37–39] Gard and colleagues[40] demonstrated that radiologists exhibited moderate or better agreement in the their interpretation of the same examination 66% to 95% of the time, while inter-radiologist agreement was only moderate, with pairs of radiologists agreeing only 33% to 83% of the time. Using the BI-RADS fifth edition breast density rating scale, Ekpo and colleagues[41] showed substantial inter-reader agreement. Breast density determination of borderline cases can be difficult, particularly for women with mild to moderate amounts of fibroglandular tissue who can be easily assessed as either having scattered tissue or heterogeneously dense breast tissue. Training radiologists to better assess breast density using visual determination may improve overall accuracy.[42]

In response to the known variability in radiologists' subjective determination of breast density, automated computerized systems have been developed in the attempt to quantitatively measure breast density in an objective and more reproducible fashion.[32] Both visual computer-assisted semiautomated and fully automated volumetric methods exist, based on information provided by the 2-dimensional mammogram. These objective measurement tools may still be limited, because it is challenging to measure the 3-dimensional structure of the breast using 2-dimensional mammographic views, which lack depth information.[43,44] For example, breast density calculations may vary depending on breast positioning and the amount of retroglandular fat included on the mammogram, which could markedly effect breast density calculations. Other disadvantages of quantitative measurement techniques include the additional cost required to purchase these assessment programs and the possibility that existing computer algorithms may not take into account the modified breast density definitions of the BI-RADS fifth edition. Because of these limitations, automated breast density assessment tools are not universally available or widely used at this time. Although

3-dimensional data obtained from breast digital tomosynthesis, MRI, computed tomography (CT), and ultrasound may be used to determine true volumetric breast density information, these methods are also not yet used in routine clinical screening environments.[45–48]

Breast Density and Breast Cancer Risk

Mammographic density has been shown to be an independent risk factor for breast cancer, but the degree of risk is controversial due to limited research plus the historic lack of standardized breast density determination criteria. It is essential to remember that regardless of breast density and breast cancer risk, routine mammography is recommended for all women of screening age. Breast density differentiation is clinically relevant, because it is the criteria utilized by most breast density research and the basis by which patients are informed of breast density, its association with breast cancer risk, and the limitations of the mammogram.

Dense breast tissue is secondary to increased epithelial and stromal fibroglandular tissue. Most breast cancers originate from epithelial cells that line the lobules and terminal ducts within the breast, so it is logical to infer that increased epithelial cells present within dense breast tissue increase the likelihood of developing cancer.[44] Studies have shown that proliferative breast disease is a marker for increased breast cancer risk, and women with dense breast tissue have a higher likelihood of having proliferative histology seen on breast biopsy, particularly when they are associated with calcifications.[6,49]

Compared to women with predominately fatty breast tissue, women with extremely dense breasts have a 4 to 6 times increased risk for breast cancer.[6,50,51] However, only a minority of women—approximately 10%—have predominately fatty or extremely dense breast tissue. Most women in the United States have scattered fibroglandular tissue or heterogeneously dense breast tissue, each accounting for approximately 40% of the population, so relative risk among the general population may be less (Table 2). For example, comparing the majority of women with heterogeneously or extremely dense breast tissue with women with average breast density, the relative risk is only approximately 1.2 and 2.1, respectively.[57,58] Compared with other known risk factors, extremely dense breast tissue is generally considered to place a woman at intermediate risk of breast cancer (see Table 2).

Breast Density and Mammographic Sensitivity

Mammographic sensitivity is inversely proportional to breast density. Decreased mammographic

Table 2
Breast density and other risk factors for breast cancer

Author, Date	Risk Factor	Category at Risk	Comparison	Relative Risk
Boyd et al,[58] 2007	Breast density	Extremely dense	Fatty	4.6
McCormack & dos Santos Silva,[51] 2006	*Independent of age*	Extremely dense	Scattered fibroglandular	1.3–2.2
		Heterogeneously dense	Fatty	2.4–2.9
		Heterogeneously dense	Scattered fibroglandular	1.1–1.4
		Scattered fibroglandular	Fatty	2.1
Boyd et al,[4] 1995	*Dependent of age*	Extremely dense (age 40–50)	Fatty	6.1
Singletary,[52] 2003	Current age	>65 y	<65 y	5.8
Collaborative Group,[53] 2001	Family history	# Affected 1st degree relatives	No affected relatives	
		1		1.8
		2		2.9
		3		3.9
Clemmons et al,[54] 2000	Radiation exposure	Radiation for Hodgkin	No exposure	5.2
Page et al,[55] 1985	Atypical ductal hyperplasia	Prior biopsy proven ADH	No ADH	4.3
Singletary,[52] 2003	Past history breast cancer	Invasive breast cancer	No invasive breast cancer	6.8
Antoniou et al,[56] 2003	Germline mutation	BRCA 1+, ages 30–50 y	General population	33

Abbreviation: ADH, atypical ductal hyperplasia.

sensitivity occurs due to the masking effect of overlapping dense fibroglandular tissue, which is radioopaque and appears white on the mammogram, similar to most breast cancer. This is in contrast to fatty tissue, which appears as a dark gray. Complex dense tissue patterns can obscure an underlying cancer due to lack of tissue contrast, making it difficult for the radiologist to detect a suspicious abnormality.

Early studies showed that the sensitivity of film screening mammography in women with extremely dense breast tissue was 30% to 84% compared to 80% to 98% of women with fatty breast tissue.[5,59,60] Subsequent studies investigating digital mammography showed improved cancer detection in women with dense breast tissue. An early single large multicenter prospective trial demonstrated the digital mammography significantly improved diagnostic accuracy in women with dense breast tissue.[61] Likewise, data from the Breast Cancer Surveillance Consortium (BCSC) also demonstrate improved sensitivity of breast cancer of 83% in women with dense breast tissue who had digital mammography.[62]

In addition to increasing the likelihood of cancers being undetected when surrounded by dense breast tissue, the risk for interval cancer in women with dense breast tissue is markedly elevated. Interval cancers are defined as cancers that present within 12 months of a normal mammogram and tend to be larger in size, high grade, more advanced, and more likely to be associated with decrease median survival rates compared with cancers detected on screening mammography[63] (Fig. 2). Multiple studies have demonstrated an increased interval cancer risk of 6-fold and as high as even 17-fold in women with dense breast tissue compared to women with predominately fatty breast tissue,[5,58] and interval cancer rates appear similar across film-screen and digital mammography.[64]

SUPPLEMENTAL SCREENING

Increased breast cancer risk and increased interval cancers associated with increased breast density have raised the issue of providing women with dense breast tissue supplemental screening tests in addition to mammography. Supplemental screening techniques include ultrasound, tomosynthesis, MRI, and molecular breast imaging (MBI) (Table 3). Despite a supplemental cancer yield of approximately 9 cases per 1000 women screened, MBI requires an age-dependent increased radiation dose 8 to 30 times that of mammography and is not widely used in clinical practice at this time.[65,66]

Ultrasound

Screening whole breast ultrasound (SWBUS) is the most widely available supplemental screening tool in women with dense breast tissue and a negative mammogram (Fig. 3). SWBUS is practical, requires no ionizing radiation or intravenous

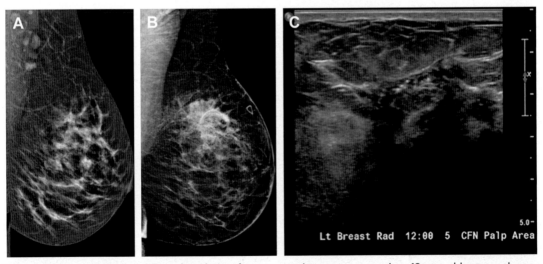

Fig. 2. (A) Left mediolateral oblique (MLO) view from a screening mammogram in a 48-year-old woman shows a complex heterogeneous dense breast tissue pattern. The mammogram was interpreted as normal, BI-RADS2. (B) Six months later, the patient returned with a palpable mass, and the left MLO revealed an irregular mass with heterogenous calcifications in the upper breast. (C) Ultrasound confirmed a corresponding irregular mass with echogenic calcifications. Ultrasound-guided CNB showed a poorly differentiated invasive carcinoma, ER/PR+, HER-, Ki-67 82%.

Table 3
Supplemental screening in dense breasts

	Incremental CDR/1000 Screens	PPV 3	Interval Cancers
Ultrasound	2–4	9%	↓50%
Magnetic resonance (+contrast)	14+	27%	↓99%
Tomosynthesis	1–2	29%	↓29%
MBI/BSG1	7–8	33%	Not determined

contrast, and is relatively inexpensive, with health care costs similar to screening mammography. Multiple single-institution and multicenter studies dating back to 1995 consistently demonstrate a cancer detection rate (CDR) of 2 to 4 cancers per 1000 women screened.[10–12,14–16,67] Most cancers detected on SWBUS are small (10 mm median size), invasive (94%), and node negative (>85%).[68]

Despite the positive outcomes and cancer sensitivity associated with SWBUS, radiology practices are variable in offering this service line to patients. Some practices routinely offer SWBUS to all of their patients with dense breast tissue, while others do not, even if their practice is located in a state with breast density legislation. Critics of SWBUS cite concerns over false-positive results, operator dependence associated with performing the

examination, and lack of randomized controlled trials proving a mortality benefit.

Specificity and positive predictive values (PPV) reported in early SWBUS studies have been low compared with mammography. In a meta-analysis across over 12 early studies, the PPV3 for biopsy was approximately 9%[68] compared with 30% to 40% PPV3 expected from mammography.[34,69] With experience, it is likely that SWBUS specificity will increase. Studies have shown that many non-simple cysts and oval circumscribed solid masses frequently encountered on SWBUS may be followed at 12 months with repeat ultrasound,[67,70,71] unlike similar masses encountered on targeted ultrasound, which are typically assessed as BI-RADS 3, probably benign requiring short-interval follow-up.[34] Recently, the ASTOUND

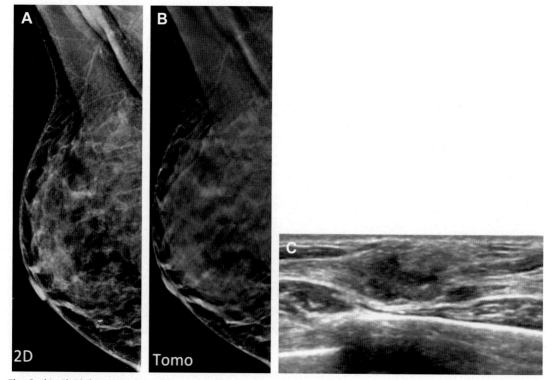

Fig. 3. (A, B) Right MLO views from a screening mammogram performed with tomosynthesis shows extremely dense breast tissue, BI-RADS 1. (C) Screening whole breast ultrasound reveals a mixed echogenic mass with indistinct margins. Ultrasound-guided core needle biopsy revealed a grade 2 infiltrating ductal cancer.

(Adjunct Screening with Tomosynthesis or Ultrasound in Women with Mammography-Negative Dense Breasts) trial, comparing adjunct screening with tomosynthesis or SWBUS, demonstrated a remarkably high SWBUS PPV3 of 48%.[72] This study included prevalent and incident SWBUS rounds, and the authors explained that the radiologists had SWBUS expertise in addition to access to comparison examinations, likely resulting in improved specificity.[72] The J-Start randomized controlled trial (RCT) showed decreased specificity among women receiving both SWBUS and mammography compared with mammography alone,[73] but it has also been shown that combined assessment of SWBUS and mammography performed on the same day can decrease mammography recall rates by 50%.[74]

Many studies reporting on SWBUS outcomes have relied on physician-performed handheld examinations. In the United States, most practices performing SWBUS rely on technologist-performed examinations, because it is not cost-effective and too time intensive for radiologists to perform the examination. Technologists performing handheld SWBUS require breast ultrasound training and experience, as well as continuous

radiologist feedback for optimal performance.[75,76] Technologist-performed examinations may have a slightly lower CDR compared with physician-performed examinations,[76] but improved SWBUS performance is associated with increased clinical experience. Equal diagnostic performance can be achieved for technologists and physicians.[77] Automated screening breast ultrasound (ABUS) is an attractive alternative to handheld SWBUS primarily because operator dependency may be reduced. A multicenter prospective trial showed that the CDR of ABUS was 2 cases per 1000 women screened, comparable to technologist-performed handheld examinations.[78] Although ABUS provides documentation of the entire breast, limitations include the need to purchase dedicated automated screening ultrasound equipment, as well as decreased sensitivity of both peripheral lesions[79] and small cancers less than 1 cm in size.[80]

Although it is highly unlikely that a long-term and broad randomized controlled SWBUS trial will ever be conducted in the United States, preliminary results of the limited RCT conducted in Japan support the clinical utility of SWBUS.[73] Furthermore, a 40% to 50% decrease in the interval cancer rate has been demonstrated among women with dense

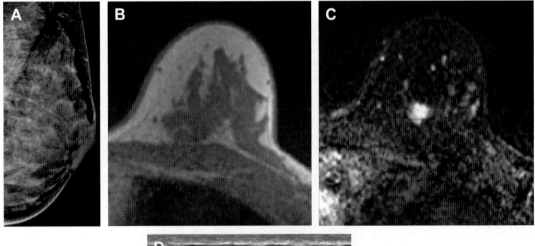

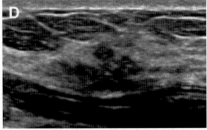

Fig. 4. (*A*) 45-year-old woman with extremely dense breast tissue on mammography, which was normal, BI-RADS2. (*B*) T1W axial MRI of the left breast also shows the fibroglandular tissue, which appears hypointense compared with the bright fat. (*C*) T1W, fat suppressed C+ axial view of the left breast reveals a suspicious enhancing mass with lobulated boarders in the left central breast. (*D*) Magnetic resonance-directed ultrasound shows a corresponding irregular hypoechoic mass. Ultrasound-guided CNB proved a moderately differentiated infiltrating ductal cancer.

breast tissue who also choose SWBUS.[68,73] Because interval cancers tend to be more aggressive late-stage tumors,[63,64] it is logical to believe that a reduction in interval cancers will improve treatment options for women and decrease breast cancer mortality.

MRI

MRI is a sensitive screening tool and is routinely offered to women with an elevated lifetime risk for breast cancer of over 20%. The high-risk screening MRI CDR yield is approximately 14 cases per 1000 women screened, regardless of breast density.[81] In the ACRIN 6666 multicenter trial that included women with dense breasts and at least 1 additional risk factor, the supplemental cancer yield of MRI was 15 cancers per 1000 women among 612 intermediate risk women who underwent in a single round of screening MRI after completing 3 annual rounds of mammography and SWBUS.[82] In a prospective observational study of 443 women at mild or moderately increased breast cancer risk and dense breast tissue, Kuhl and colleagues[83] demonstrated a cancer yield of 18.2 cases per 1000 women screened using an abbreviated MRI

acquisition. This abbreviated image acquisition protocol requires only 3 minutes scanning time, with expert reading times of less than 1 minute.[83] The sensitivity and specificity were high at 94.3% and 24.4%, while the negative predictive value (NPV) was 99.8% with no interval cancers.[83]

Screening MRI is undoubtedly a strong and sensitive screening tool (**Fig. 4**). The specificity is comparable to mammography, with screening PPV3 of approximately 27%.[81] However, current barriers including high cost, intravenous gadolinium contrast injection, and lack of widespread availability of high quality scans, prevent widespread use of screening breast MRI among the general population of women with dense breast tissue. With growing concerns regarding long-term safety issues associated with gadolinium contrast injections, early studies of noncontrast diffusion weighted imaging (DWI) as a magnetic resonance supplemental screening technique are promising, with a potential supplemental cancer yield of 8 cases per 1000 women screened.[84]

In an effort to determine the effectiveness of screening with mammography and MRI compared with mammography alone, investigators in the Netherlands are conducting an RCT in women

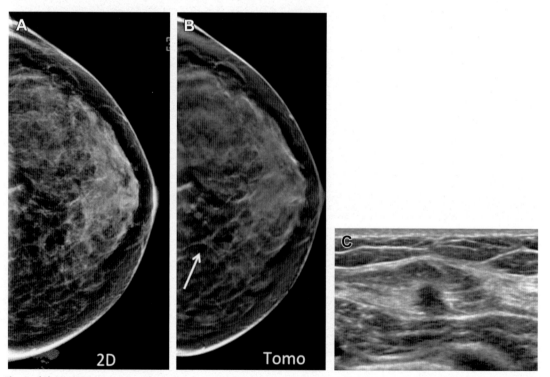

Fig. 5. (*A*) 2D FFDM CC view of a screening mammogram in a 53-year-old woman reveals heterogeneously dense breast tissue. (*B*). Tomosynthesis reveals an isodense spiculated mass (*arrow*) in the left medial breast. (*C*) Ultrasound revealed a corresponding hypoechoic mass with indistinct margins. Ultrasound-guided CNB showed a well-differentiated infiltrating ductal carcinoma. (*Courtesy of* Melissa Durand, MD, New Haven, CT.)

ages 50 to 75 years with extremely dense breast tissue, although preliminary results are not available as of this writing.[85] Early studies also indicate that increased background parenchymal enhancement present on contrast-enhanced MRI may also be predictive of breast cancer risk in addition to mammographic breast density alone, although these studies focused only high-risk women.[86,87] More studies are needed to determine the value and practicality of standard contrast-enhanced MRI, abbreviated contrast-enhanced MRI, and unenhanced rapid DWI as supplemental screening tools.

Tomosynthesis

When combined with 2-dimensional digital mammography, tomosynthesis captures images of the breast utilizing multiple thin slices. The end result is decreased summation artifacts, superior lesion detection, plus increased sensitivity and specificity across all breast densities (Fig. 5). Unlike supplemental SWBUS, tomosynthesis can decrease overall recall rates in women with dense breast tissue.[88,89] The supplemental cancer yield of tomosynthesis in addition to conventional 2-dimensional digital mammography in women with dense breast tissue is 1 to 2 cancers per 1000 women screened, lower than SWBUS and MRI.[89–92] Moreover, the benefit of tomosynthesis in women with dense breast tissue may be greatest in women with hetereogeneous compared to those with extremely dense breast tissue.[93] Tomosynthesis is well tolerated by patients, because image slices can be obtained at the same time as 2-dimensional digital using a single mammography compression. Because of its superior diagnostic performance across all breast densities, tomosynthesis will likely replace 2-dimensional screening mammography for all women. However, given that SWBUS and MRI both have a higher incremental cancer yield, these 2 modalities will likely continue to play a role in supplemental screening in addition to tomosynthesis in women with dense breast tissue, but further studies are needed.

SUMMARY

Breast density is important because of the associated increased breast cancer risk and the known limitations of mammography. Women in the United States are transitioning beyond breast cancer awareness and are now demanding more knowledge regarding the strengths and limitations of a variety of diagnostic tests available for early breast cancer detection. Patient shared decision making and patient education are essential. Breast density

inform legislation continues to gain popularity, and it is possible that a national mandate will eventually be endorsed. Radiologists and primary care physicians should be knowledgeable about the significance of breast density and the associated benefits and potential harms associated with supplemental screening. Future research will enhance knowledge regarding the clinical significance of breast density and will optimize strategies for early breast cancer detection in all women with dense breast tissue.

REFERENCES

1. Cappello NM. Decade of 'normal' mammography reports—the happygram. J Am Coll Radiol 2013; 10(12):903–8.
2. Stomper PC, D'Souza DJ, DiNitto PA, et al. Analysis of parenchymal density on mammograms in 1353 women 25-79 years old. AJR Am J Roentgenol 1996;167(5):1261–5.
3. Checka CM, Chun JE, Schnabel FR, et al. The relationship of mammographic density and age: implications for breast cancer screening. AJR Am J Roentgenol 2012;198(3):W292–5.
4. Boyd NF, Byng JW, Jong RA, et al. Quantitative classification of mammographic densities and breast cancer risk: results from the Canadian National Breast Screening Study. J Natl Cancer Inst 1995; 87(9):670–5.
5. Mandelson MT, Oestreicher N, Porter PL, et al. Breast density as a predictor of mammographic detection: comparison of interval and screen-detected cancers. J Natl Cancer Inst 2000;92:1081–7.
6. Harvey JA, Bovbjerg VE. Quantitative assessment of mammographic breast density: relationship with breast cancer risk. Radiology 2004;230(1):29–41.
7. Holland R, Hendriks JH, Mravunac M. Mammographically occult breastcancer. A pathologic and radiologic study. Cancer 1983;52:1810–9.
8. Bird RE, Wallace TW, Yankaskas BC. Analysis of cancers missed at screening mammography. Radiology 1992;184:613–7.
9. Ma LN, Fishell E, Wright B, et al. Case-control study of factors associated with failure to detect breast cancer by mammography. J Natl Cancer Inst 1992; 84:781–5.
10. Gordon PB, Goldenberg SL. Malignant breast masses detected only by ultrasound: a retrospective review. Cancer 1995;76:626–30.
11. Buchberger W, DeKoekkoek-Doll P, Springer P, et al. Incidental findings on sonography of the breast: clinical significance and diagnostic workup. AJR Am J Roentgenol 1999;173:921–7.
12. Kaplan SS. Clinical utility of bilateral whole-breast US in the evaluation of women with dense breast tissue. Radiology 2001;221:641–9.

13. Kolb TM, Lichy J, Newhouse JH. Comparison of the performance of screening mammography, physical examination and breast US and evaluation of factors that influence them: an analysis of 27,825 patient evaluations. Radiology 2002;225:165–75.

14. LeConte I, Feger C, Galant C, et al. Mammography and subsequent whole-breast sonography of non-palpable breast cancers: the importance of radiologic breast density. AJR Am J Roentgenol 2003;180:1675–9.

15. Crystal P, Strano SD, Shcharynski S, et al. Using sonography to screen women with mammographically dense breasts. AJR Am J Roentgenol 2003;181:177–82.

16. Berg WA, Blume JD, Cormack JB, et al, ACRIN 6666 Investigators. Combined screening with ultrasound and mammography vs mammography alone in women at elevated risk of breast cancer. JAMA 2008;299(18):2151–63.

17. Legislation and Regulations—what is required? In: Dense breast-info an education coalition. Available at: http://densebreast-info.org/legislation.aspx. Accessed July 10, 2016.

18. Khong KA, Hargreaves J, Aminololama-Shakeri S, et al. Impact of the California breast density law on primary care physicians. J Am Coll Radiol 2015;12(3):256–60.

19. Kressin NR, Gunn CM, Battaglia TA. Content, readability, and understandability of dense breast notifications by state. JAMA 2016;315(16):1786–8.

20. Rhodes DJ, Radecki Breitkopf C, Ziegenfuss JY, et al. Awareness of breast density and its impact on breast cancer detection and risk. J Clin Oncol 2015;33(10):1143–50.

21. Moothathu NS, Philpotts LE, Busch SH, et al. Knowledge of Density and Screening Ultrasound. Breast J 2016. [Epub ahead of print].

22. Jones BA, Reams K, Calvocoressi L, et al. Adequacy of communicating results from screening mammograms to African American and white women. Am J Public Health 2007;97(3):531–8.

23. Frequently asked questions about breast density, breast cancer risk, and the breast density notification law in California: a consensus document. In: Breast Density.Info. Available at: http://www.breastdensity.info. Accessed July 10, 2016.

24. What is dense? In: Are you dense? Available at: http://www.areyoudense.org. Accessed July 10, 2016.

25. Sprague BL, Gangnon RE, Burt V, et al. Prevalence of mammographically dense breasts in the United States. J Natl Cancer Inst 2014;106(10).

26. Bahl M, Baker JA, Bhargavan-Chatfield M, et al. Impact of breast density notification legislation on radiologists' practices of reporting breast density: a multi-state study. Radiology 2016;28:152457.

27. Lee CI, Bassett LW, Lehman CD. Breast density legislation and opportunities for patient-centered outcomes research. Radiology 2012;264(3):632–6.

28. Kerlikowske K, Zhu W, Tosteson AN, et al, Breast Cancer Surveillance Consortium. Identifying women with dense breasts at high risk for interval cancer: a cohort study. Ann Intern Med 2015;162(10):673–81.

29. Gierach GL, Ichikawa L, Kerlikowske K, et al. Relationship between mammographic density and breast cancer death in the Breast Cancer Surveillance Consortium. J Natl Cancer Inst 2012;104(16):1218–27.

30. Tabár L, Vitak B, Chen TH, et al. Swedish two-county trial: impact of mammographic screening on breast cancer mortality during 3 decades. Radiology 2011;260(3):658–63.

31. Duffy SW, Tabar L, Olsen AH. Absolute numbers of lives saved and over diagnosis in breast cancer screening, from a randomized trial and from the Breast Screening Programme in England. J Med Screen 2010;17(1):25–30.

32. Winkler NS, Raza S, Mackesy M, et al. Breast density: clinical implications and assessment methods. Radiographics 2015;35(2):316–24.

33. Wolfe J. Breast patterns as an index of risk for developing breast cancer. AJR Am J Roentgenol 1976;126:1130e7.

34. D'Orsi CJ, Sickles EA, Mendelson EB, et al. ACR BI-RADS® Atlas, Breast imaging reporting and data system. Reston (VA): American College of Radiology; 2013.

35. D'Orsi CJ, Mendelson EB, Ikeda DM, et al. Breast imaging reporting and data system: ACR BI-RADS – breast imaging atlas. Reston (VA): American College of Radiology; 2003.

36. Gur D, Klym AH, King JL, et al. Impact of the new density reporting laws: radiologist perceptions and actual behavior. Acad Radiol 2015;22(6):679–83.

37. Kerlikowske K, Grady D, Barclay J, et al. Variability and accuracy in mammographic interpretation using the American College of Radiology Breast Imaging Reporting and Data System. J Natl Cancer Inst 1998;90:1801–9.

38. Berg WA, Campassi C, Langenberg P, et al. Breast imaging reporting and data system: inter- and intra-observer variability in feature analysis and final assessment. Am J Roentgenol 2000;174:1769–77.

39. Ciatto S, Houssami N, Apruzzese A, et al. Categorizing breast mammographic density: intra- and inter-observer reproducibility of BI-RADS density categories. Breast 2005;14:269–75.

40. Gard CC, Aiello Bowles EJ, Miglioretti DL, et al. Misclassification of Breast Imaging Reporting and Data System (BI-RADS) mammographic density and implications for breast density reporting legislation. Breast J 2015;21(5):481–9.

41. Ekpo EU, Ujong UP, Mello-Thoms C, et al. Assessment of interradiologist agreement regarding

mammographic breast density classification using the fifth edition of the BI-RADS Atlas. AJR Am J Roentgenol 2016;206(5):1119–23.

42. Raza S, Mackesy MM, Winkler NS, et al. Effect of training on qualitative mammographic density assessment. J Am Coll Radiol 2016;13(3):310–5.

43. Kopans DB. Basic physics and doubts about relationship between mammographically determined tissue density and breast cancer risk. Radiology 2008;246(2):348–53.

44. Freer PE. Mammographic breast density: impact on breast cancer risk and implications for screening. Radiographics 2015;35(2):302–15.

45. Yaffe MJ. Mammographic density: measurement of mammographic density. Breast Cancer Res 2008; 10(3):209.

46. Ekpo EU, McEntee MF. Measurement of breast density with digital breast tomosynthesis—a systematic review. Br J Radiol 2014;87(1043):20140460.

47. Chen JH, Lee YW, Chan SW, et al. Breast density analysis with automated whole-breast ultrasound: comparison with 3-D magnetic resonance imaging. Ultrasound Med Biol 2016;42(5):1211–20.

48. Chen JH, Chan S, Lu NH, et al. Opportunistic breast density assessment in women receiving low-dose chest computed tomography screening. Acad Radiol 2016;23(9):1154–61.

49. Lewis MC, Irshad A, Ackerman S, et al. Assessing the relationship of mammographic breast density and proliferative breast disease. Breast J 2016; 22(5):541–6.

50. Boyd NF, Jensen HM, Cooke G, et al. Relationship between mammographic and histologic risk factors for breast cancer. J Natl Cancer Inst 1992;84: 1170–9.

51. McCormack VA, dos Santos Silva I. Breast density and parenchymal patterns as markers of breast cancer risk: a meta-analysis. Cancer Epidemiol Biomarkers Prev 2006;15(6):1159–69.

52. Singletary SE. Rating the risk factors for breast cancer. Ann Surg 2003;237(4):474–82.

53. Collaborative Group on Hormonal Factors in Breast Cancer. Familial breast cancer: collaborative reanalysis of individual data from 52 epidemiological studies including 58,209 women with breast cancer and 101,986 women without the disease. Lancet 2001;358(9291):1389–99.

54. Clemons M, Loijens L, Goss P. Breast cancer risk following irradiation for Hodgkin's disease. Cancer Treat Rev 2000;26:29.

55. Page DL, Dupont WD, Rogers LW, et al. Atypical hyperplastic lesions of the female breast: a long-term follow-up study. Cancer 1985;55(11):2698–708.

56. Antoniou A, Pharoah PD, Narod S, et al. Average risks of breast and ovarian cancer associated with BRCA1 or BRCA2 mutations detected in case Series unselected for family history: a combined analysis of 22 studies. Am J Hum Genet 2003; 72(5):1117–30 [Erratum appears in Am J Hum Genet 2003;73(3):709].

57. Sickles EA. The use of breast imaging to screen women at high risk for cancer. Radiol Clin North Am 2010;48(5):859–78.

58. Boyd NF, Guo H, Martin LJ, et al. Mammographic density and the risk and detection of breast cancer. N Engl J Med 2007;356(3):227–36.

59. Kerlikowske K, Grady D, Barclay J, et al. Effect of age, breast density, and family history on the sensitivity of first screening mammography. JAMA 1996; 276:33–8.

60. Carney PA, Miglioretti DL, Yankaskas BC, et al. Individual and combined effects of age, breast density, and hormone replacement therapy use on the accuracy of screening mammography. Ann Intern Med 2003;138(3):168–75.

61. Pisano ED, Gatsonis C, Hendrick E, et al, Digital Mammographic Imaging Screening Trial (DMIST) Investigators Group. Diagnostic performance of digital versus film mammography for breast-cancer screening. N Engl J Med 2005;353(17):1773–83.

62. Kerlikowske K, Hubbard RA, Miglioretti DL, Breast Cancer Surveillance Consortium. Comparative effectiveness of digital versus film-screen mammography in community practice in the United States: a cohort study. Ann Intern Med 2011;155(8):493–502.

63. Webb ML, Cady B, Michaelson JS, et al. A failure analysis of invasive breast cancer: most deaths from disease occur in women not regularly screened. Cancer 2014;120(18):2839–46.

64. Henderson LM, Miglioretti DL, Kerlikowske K, et al. Breast cancer characteristics associated with digital versus film-screen mammography for screen-detected and interval cancers. AJR Am J Roentgenol 2015;205(3):676–84.

65. Rhodes DJ, Hruska CB, Conners AL, et al. Journal club: molecular breast imaging at reduced radiation dose for supplemental screening in mammographically dense breasts. AJR Am J Roentgenol 2015; 204(2):241–51.

66. Hendrick RE, Tredennick T. Benefit to radiation risk of breast-specific gamma imaging compared with mammography in screening asymptomatic women with dense breasts. Radiology 2016;281(2):583–8.

67. Hooley RJ, Greenberg KL, Stackhouse RM, et al. Screening US in patients with mammographically dense breasts: initial experience with Connecticut Public Act 09-41. Radiology 2012;265(1):59–69.

68. Berg W. Screening ultrasound. In: Berg WA, Yang WT, editors. Diagnostic imaging: breast. 2nd edition. Salt Lake City (UT): Amirsys; 2014. p. 9-38–9-40.

69. Rosenberg RD, Yankaskas BC, Abraham LA, et al. Performance benchmarks for screening mammography. Radiology 2006;241(1):55–66.

70. Berg WA, Sechtin AG, Marques H, et al. Cystic breast masses and the ACRIN 6666 experience. Radiol Clin North Am 2010;48(5):931–87.

71. Barr RG, Zhang Z, Cormack JB, et al. Probably benign lesions at screening breast US in a population with elevated risk: prevalence and rate of malignancy in the ACRIN 6666 trial. Radiology 2013; 269(3):701–12.

72. Tagliafico AS, Calabrese M, Mariscotti G, et al. Adjunct screening with tomosynthesis or ultrasound in women with mammography-negative dense breasts: interim report of a prospective comparative trial. J Clin Oncol 2016;34(16):1882–8.

73. Ohuchi N, Suzuki A, Sobue T, et al. Sensitivity and specificity of mammography and adjunctive ultrasonography to screen for breast cancer in the Japan Strategic Anti-cancer Randomized Trial (J-START): a randomised controlled trial. Lancet 2016; 387(10016):341–8.

74. Tohno E, Umemoto T, Sasaki K, et al. Effect of adding screening ultrasonography to screening mammography on patient recall and cancer detection rates: a retrospective study in Japan. Eur J Radiol 2013;82(8):1227–30.

75. Berg WA, Blume JD, Cormack JB, et al. Training the ACRIN 6666 Investigators and effects of feedback on breast ultrasound interpretive performance and agreement in BI-RADS ultrasound feature analysis. AJR Am J Roentgenol 2012;199(1):224–35.

76. Berg WA, Mendelson EB. Technologist-performed handheld screening breast US imaging: how is it performed and what are the outcomes to date? Radiology 2014;272(1):12–27.

77. Tohno E, Takahashi H, Tamada T, et al. Educational program and testing using images for the standardization of breast cancer screening by ultrasonography. Breast Cancer 2012;19(2):138–46.

78. Brem RF, Tabár L, Duffy SW. Assessing improvement in detection of breast cancer with three-dimensional automated breast US in women with dense breast tissue: the SomoInsight Study. Radiology 2015; 274(3):663–73.

79. An YY, Kim SH, Kang BJ. The image quality and lesion characterization of breast using automated whole-breast ultrasound: a comparison with handheld ultrasound. Eur J Radiol 2015;84(7):1232–5.

80. Jeh SK, Kim SH, Choi JJ, et al. Comparison of automated breast ultrasonography to handheld ultrasonography in detecting and diagnosing breast lesions. Acta Radiol 2016;57(2):162–9.

81. Niell BL, Gavenonis SC, Motazedi T, et al. Auditing a breast MRI practice: performance measures for screening and diagnostic breast MRI. J Am Coll Radiol 2014;11(9):883–9.

82. Berg WA, Zhang Z, Lehrer D, et al. ACRIN 6666 investigators: detection of breast cancer with addition of annual screening ultrasound or a single screening MRI to mammography in women with elevated breast cancer risk. JAMA 2012;307(13):1394–404.

83. Kuhl CK, Schrading S, Strobel K, et al. Abbreviated breast magnetic resonance imaging (MRI): first postcontrast subtracted images and maximum-intensity projection-a novel approach to breast cancer screening with MRI. J Clin Oncol 2014;32(22):2304–10.

84. McDonald ES, Hammersley JA, Chou SH, et al. Performance of DWI as a rapid unenhanced technique for detecting mammographically occult breast cancer in elevated-risk women with dense breasts. Am J Roentgenol 2016;207(1):205–16.

85. Emaus MJ, Bakker MF, Peeters PH, et al. MR imaging as an additional screening modality for the detection of breast cancer in women aged 50-75 years with extremely dense breasts: the DENSE trial study design. Radiology 2015;277(2):527–37.

86. King V, Brooks JD, Bernstein JL, et al. Background parenchymal enhancement at breast MR imaging and breast cancer risk. Radiology 2011;260(1):50–60.

87. Dontchos BN, Rahbar H, Partridge SC, et al. Are qualitative assessments of background parenchymal enhancement, amount of fibroglandular tissue on MR images, and mammographic density associated with breast cancer risk? Radiology 2015;276(2):371–80.

88. Haas BM, Kalra V, Geisel J, et al. Comparison of tomosynthesis plus digital mammography and digital mammography alone for breast cancer screening. Radiology 2013;269(3):694–700.

89. Friedewald SM, Rafferty EA, Rose SL, et al. Breast cancer screening using tomosynthesis in combination with digital mammography. JAMA 2014;311(24):2499–507.

90. Durand MA, Haas BM, Yao X, et al. Early clinical experience with digital breast tomosynthesis for screening mammography. Radiology 2015;274(1):85–92.

91. Rose SL, Tidwell AL, Bujnoch LJ, et al. Implementation of breast tomosynthesis in a routine screening practice: an observational study. AJR Am J Roentgenol 2013;200(6):1401–8.

92. Skaane P, Bandos AI, Gullien R, et al. Comparison of digital mammography alone and digital mammography plus tomosynthesis in a population-based screening program. Radiology 2013;267(1):47–56.

93. Rafferty EA, Durand MA, Conant EF, et al. Breast cancer screening using tomosynthesis and digital mammography in dense and non dense breasts. JAMA 2016;315(16):1784–6.

Implementation of Whole-Breast Screening Ultrasonography

Melissa A. Durand, MD, MS*, Regina J. Hooley, MD

KEYWORDS

• Dense breasts • Screening breast ultrasonography • Supplementary screening

KEY POINTS

- Understanding how to implement whole-breast screening ultrasonography requires consideration of many variables.
- Education of staff, patients, and referrers is essential for smooth transitions and to ensure high-quality scanning.
- Screening ultrasonography may be hand-held or automated, and performed by physicians or technologists.
- Choosing real-time or batch reading is a balance of time and resources.
- Radiology billing codes for ultrasonography have been updated and are reviewed here.

INTRODUCTION

Conventional two-dimensional (2D) mammography in dense breasts has known limitations: early studies showed sensitivity decreasing to 30% to 48% in dense breasts compared with 80% to 98% in fatty breasts, with a more recent study showing 57.1% sensitivity in dense breasts and up to 92.7% in fatty breasts.[1–3] Dense breasts are common, with 31% to 43% of women categorized as dense at screening mammography.[4] In a study of 335 screening ultrasonography–detected cancers, 81% (272 out of 335) were not seen at mammography, even in retrospect.[5] Consequently, supplemental screening modalities such as whole-breast screening ultrasonography have been explored as complementary tools to improve performance outcomes of breast cancer screening. In addition, whole-breast ultrasonography screening is an alternative modality to MR imaging for additional screening of high-risk patients for whom MR imaging cannot be performed. Multiple studies have shown that whole-breast screening ultrasonography, as an adjunct to 2D mammography, results in detection of 3 to 4 additional cancers per 1000 women screened.[6–11]

As of this writing, 27 states have passed breast density notification laws and the public is increasingly aware of how breast density affects cancer detection and its association with increased breast cancer risk. Breast imaging centers are increasingly incorporating supplemental screening modalities, such as screening whole-breast ultrasonography (SWBUS), into their service lines. This article discusses how to implement a robust SWBUS program, from educating referrers, patients, and staff, to deciding who performs and how to perform whole-breast screening ultrasonography, and achieving efficient scheduling and billing.

Disclosure: M.A. Durand: research grant from Hologic, Inc; consultant for Hologic, Inc, and Fuji Medical. R.J. Hooley: consultant for Fuji Medical, Siemens, Hologic; royalties from Elsevier Publishing and Amirsys, Inc.
Department of Diagnostic Radiology and Biomedical Imaging, Yale University School of Medicine, 333 Cedar Street, PO Box 208042, New Haven, CT 06520-8042, USA
* Corresponding author.
E-mail address: melissa.durand@yale.edu

Radiol Clin N Am 55 (2017) 527–539
http://dx.doi.org/10.1016/j.rcl.2016.12.007
0033-8389/17/© 2016 Elsevier Inc. All rights reserved.

EDUCATION
Educating Referring Health Care Providers

More and more states are passing dense breast notification laws. Before any new law comes into effect, it is important to communicate with referring health care providers so they can be aware of upcoming changes in the law and be equipped to have informed discussions with patients. For example, outreach by breast imagers at local obstetrics-gynecology and/or internal medicine society meetings can serve as a means to review the clinical rationale behind dense breast legislation and provide an effective way to address the immediate questions and concerns from colleagues of other clinical specialties.

In addition, formal letter communication to referring providers before starting an SWBUS program may be helpful. This letter should include the breast density inform text, which is often stated in the patient's lay letter, so referring providers are aware of the level of information that will be given to their patients. It can clarify what breast density means: that density is based on the mammographic assessment, not palpation of lumpy tissue. Key benefits and risks of SWBUS, including the possibility of false-positives, can be reviewed. The importance of assessing each patient's risk status to determine the optimal supplemental screening modality for high-risk and even intermediate-risk patients can also be emphasized. Importantly, it can underscore that SWBUS is an optional supplemental screening tool, and is not intended to replace mammography.

Multiple randomized controlled trials have shown mortality reduction with mammography, and so this remains the primary screening modality for breast cancer screening.[12] Patients determined to be high risk should undergo supplemental breast MR imaging, not SWBUS.[13] Reflexive referral of all women with dense breasts for SWBUS is also discouraged. The choice to undergo SWBUS should be a shared decision involving the patient, made after open discussion of the benefits and risks of SWBUS, and is a key point to convey to referring colleagues (**Box 1**).

Educating Patients

Letter communication to all existing patients before the dense breast law enactment can also help prepare them for upcoming legislation. Once the law is in place, the patient lay letter notifies patients if they are dense and includes information on supplementary screening options. A recent study has found that some notification wordings are written at the high-school reading level and are thus too complicated for the general public to comprehend.[14] This underscores the importance of encouraging patients to have open discussions with their physicians regarding breast density.

Educating Technologists

With technologist-performed whole-breast ultrasonography, it is possible to either have a mammography technologist or an ultrasonography technologist specially trained in breast ultrasonography. Cross-training mammography technologists in breast ultrasonography can be advantageous because these technologists already possess a fundamental knowledge of breast anatomy and

---

Box 1
Key points to give referring providers when informing them of the breast notification law enactment

- Dense breast inform text (verbiage may vary depending on state).
- Screening ultrasonography is optional and usually only appropriate in patients with heterogeneously dense or extremely dense tissue.
- High-risk patients (>20%–25% lifetime breast cancer risk; BRCA1 or BRCA2 gene mutation; untested with first-degree relative with BRCA1 or BRCA2 gene mutation; radiation therapy to the chest at ages 10–30 years; Li-Fraumeni, Cowden, or Bannayan-Riley-Ruvalcaba syndrome, or first-degree relatives with one of these syndromes) should undergo annual mammography and MR imaging.[12] Women do not need both supplemental screening MR imaging and ultrasonography.
- High-risk women who cannot tolerate supplemental MR imaging screening may benefit from SWBUS.
- It is important for women to understand that dense tissue is defined by mammography, not palpation.
- Screening ultrasonography is associated with the risk of false-positive results and the possibility of requiring a biopsy of a suspicious finding that ultimately proves to be normal.
- Early detection of small, node-negative, invasive tumors may result in better treatment options and reduce the chance of developing an interval cancer, which tends to be more aggressive.

positioning and thus benefit from using mammographic information to localize findings sonographically. This approach also provides continuity of care for the patients because the same technologist can perform both examinations, and furthermore improves workflow.

There are a variety of breast sonography training and educational programs. Both the Association of Registered Diagnostic Medical Sonographers (ARDMS) and the American Registry of Radiologic Technologists (ARRT) offer clinical certification in breast sonography, although this is not specific to screening ultrasonography. The ARRT requires performance of 200 breast ultrasonography examinations within 24 months and participation in 10 ultrasonography-guided interventional procedures. Some institutions require passage of a breast ultrasonography certifying examination within 1 year of training in order for the technologist to continue to perform screening breast ultrasonography.[15] Of note, these certification programs are geared toward diagnostic sonography, not screening. Although not required, additional training specific to screening is important and varies across institutions. A breast sonographer-in-training should be proficient in targeted ultrasonography and also typically performs a minimum of 25 to 100 screening examinations with an experienced technologist before independent screening is allowed.[6,11,15–17]

If technologist-performed SWBUS is used, it may be beneficial in the early stages of implementing a program to have both the technologist and the radiologist scan each patient. With increased technologist experience, the radiologist may not need to recheck a negative examination. Periodic checks of benign findings could be made to ensure high performance, and if the technologist has a question, if there is an artifact that could mimic a cancer, or if there is a positive finding, the radiologist should recheck the study in real time.

Presently at the authors' institution, there is an in-house training program lasting 6 weeks for full-time staff and 8 weeks for part-time staff. This program includes textbook self-study covering physics, equipment operation, clinical image production/evaluation, anatomy, physiology, and pathology. A practice breast phantom is initially used to familiarize the trainee with equipment operation and scanning technique. An experienced technologist is paired with a breast sonographer-in-training for one-on-one mentorship; the sonographer-in-training progresses from observing to targeted scanning, and eventually to whole-breast screening. Although formal breast ultrasonography certification is not required for technologists to perform breast ultrasonography, a salary/financial incentive is offered for those who achieve ARRT

certification. In addition, all technologists receive constant feedback because each ultrasonography scan is reviewed together by the technologist and radiologist and any questions/concerns are addressed by rescanning the patient before the patient leaves the ultrasonography examination room. Constant feedback has been shown to increase overall diagnostic performance.[18] In this manner, benign and malignant ultrasonography findings in the breast can be consistently reviewed, reinforcing the technologists' skills (**Fig. 1**).

Educating Radiologists

As with any new modality, if radiologists are new to breast ultrasonography, a minimum of 8 hours' training is required by the Mammography Quality Standards Act (MQSA).[19] This training can be achieved through continued medical education courses or residency/fellowship training.

American College Of Radiology (ACR) requirements for diagnostic breast ultrasonography outline that non–board-certified radiologists must initially have been supervised for and/or performed and interpreted at least 300 breast ultrasonography examinations over 3 years, with at least 200 examinations in the prior 36 months to maintain skills thereafter.[20] Requirements for screening ultrasonography, although not formally defined, warrant achievement of diagnostic minimums, and ideally merit additional training and experience to ensure high performance levels.

For example, in the ACRIN (American College of Radiology Imaging Network) 6666 trial, in which screening mammography plus ultrasonography was compared with screening mammography alone in women with dense breasts, the participating radiologists were required to have interpreted 500 breast ultrasonography examinations per year within 2 years of the study, and to complete a training course on breast anatomy, physiology, the postsurgical breast, and mammographic and sonographic Breast Imaging Reporting and Data System (BI-RADS) interpretation, with before/after testing.[18] The Society of Breast Imaging has recommended that any person performing screening breast ultrasonography should meet eligibility criteria as set forth by the ACRIN 6666 trial.[21] The International Breast Ultrasound School, a physician-run, nonprofit organization incorporated in Switzerland, requires physicians to perform 500 examinations with 300 cytologic/histologic correlation cases and 50 interventional procedures.[22] For automated breast ultrasonography, both Web-based and one-on-one standardized training programs are available for radiologists to learn how to interpret images accurately.

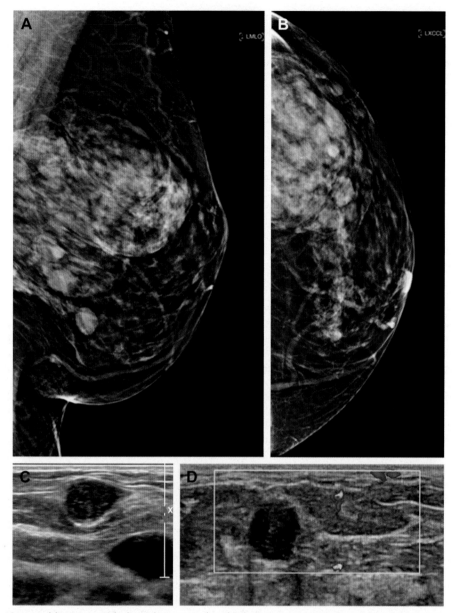

Fig. 1. A 48-year-old woman with dense breasts and multiple known cysts presented for screening mammogram and whole-breast screening ultrasonography. (*A*) Left mediolateral oblique mammogram shows multiple stable circumscribed masses and stable calcifications. (*B*) Left craniocaudal mammogram shows multiple stable circumscribed masses and stable calcifications. (*C*) Radial gray-scale ultrasonography image shows an oval solid mass anterior to a simple cyst. (*D*) Color Doppler image shows the mass contains internal vascularity. Ultrasonography-guided core needle biopsy confirmed invasive ductal carcinoma, final pathology indicating pT1cN0, stage 1A.

One of the most important learning tools is feedback: follow-up on cases recommended for biopsy and sharing of interesting cases freely and regularly can positively affect performance. Berg and colleagues[18] showed that immediate feedback on feature analysis and diagnosis improved ultrasonography interpretive skills even in experienced observers.

PERFORMANCE
Hand-Held Ultrasonography

Hand-held ultrasonography (HHUS) requires highly trained, specialized personnel and, because results are operator dependent, consistency may be variable. Physician time has also been cited as a barrier to acceptance of HHUS.

The ACRIN 6666 trial used physician-performed HHUS screening and documented an average of 19 minutes during the first year of the study.[7] Kolb and colleagues[1] previously reported an average of 4 minutes 39 seconds for physician-performed ultrasonography. In busy high-volume practices, the physician time needed to perform these examinations may not be practical or financially viable.

One solution to the demands on physician time needed for scanning is technologist-performed scanning, with real-time scanning by the interpreting radiologist as needed before final assessment. Kaplan[11] reported 10 minutes for technologist-performed examinations. Hand-held physician-performed versus ultrasonography technologist–performed versus mammography technologist–performed bilateral ultrasonography examinations has been shown to average 11.9 minutes versus 9.3 minutes versus 13.2 minutes respectively.[23]

Can technologist-performed ultrasonography SWBUS perform as well as physician-performed whole-breast US? In a meta-analysis of technologist-performed and physician-performed prevalent screening ultrasonography examinations in the United States, an average incremental cancer detection rate (ICDR) of 2.5 cancers per 1000 technologist-performed examinations was shown across 4 series (42 cancers per 16,676 examinations), which was lower than the average ICDR of 4.3 cancers per 1000 physician-performed examinations in multicenter trials (51 cancers per 11,803 examinations).[15] Although technologist-performed SWBUS does have a lower ICDR compared with physician-performed SWBUS, additional cancers are still found.

In Japan, a 2-day training program on breast sonography has been established, with tests using video and still images to evaluate trainees. In a study of this program, results of 422 physicians and 415 technologists were compared. Thirty-three out of 422 physicians were radiologists, with the rest a mix of physicians, including surgeons, gynecologists, and internists. The technologists included sonographers and radiographers. Although breast surgeons and radiologists outperformed other physicians, technologists performed significantly better compared with physicians.[24]

In another study of 412 hand-held SWBUS examinations, performed by technologists specially trained in screening ultrasonography, radiologist/technologist agreement was shown to be discordant in just 1% of cases, and only 76 required targeted evaluation by the radiologist (<20%), taking less than 5 minutes of radiologists' time.[23] This recheck time is comparable with the 3 minutes of interpretation time for automated SWBUS reported by Brem and colleagues,[25] but carries the advantage of not requiring patients with an abnormal finding to be recalled for a second examination. With appropriate training, technologist-performed screening ultrasonography, with radiologist rechecks in real time as needed, could be a reasonable balance of efficiency and accuracy.

One major benefit of real-time interpretation is that results can be given to the patient immediately without requiring additional recall. This practice decreases patient anxiety and health care costs and also removes the responsibility of the technologist to determine whether a questionable finding is real or not, which can affect documentation and image capture. Furthermore, HHUS does not require special equipment and is performed with the same ultrasonography unit used to perform targeted ultrasonography.

Automated Ultrasonography

Several automated breast ultrasonography (ABUS) systems are presently available. ABUS systems can be divided into supine-type or prone-type scanners. All supine automated systems apply gentle compression during scanning. The technologist guides the transducer to ensure good contact, but does not have to apply full scanning pressure, which may make performing ABUS easier than HHUS and cause less scanning fatigue. Although learning to perform ABUS is not as intensive as HHUS, it does take time and training to learn proper positioning and to perform examinations consistently,[26] similar to the training required to perform a high-quality mammogram.

One supine system uses a standard high-frequency ultrasonography transducer with a 5-cm footprint attached to an articulating arm. Images of the entire breast are acquired in the transverse plane and recorded as a cine video clip for the radiologist to review. This system received 510(k) US Food and Drug Administration (FDA) clearance as an adjunct to screening mammography in 2008.[27]

Another supine system uses a high-frequency, large-footprint transducer, similar in size to a mammography compression paddle. This system gained FDA approval in 2012. With this system, 3 acquisition views of each breast are obtained and the raw data are reconstructed for review on a dedicated workstation in the transverse, sagittal, and coronal planes. The coronal plane, or surgeon's view, is unique to this ABUS system and has been beneficial for detection of architectural distortion.[26]

Prone-type scanning units are still in development; although in 2014 one prone system gained 510(k) FDA clearance. In this system, the patient lies prone on the table and the breast is suspended in a warm-water bath. Data are acquired circumferentially and can be processed/reconstructed for three-dimensional rendering.[28]

Acquisition time for automated scanning can be fairly constant (~15 minutes' total examination time), which may permit more regimented scheduling.[25] In addition, because the entire breast is documented and imaged, it is feasible to perform the study after hours without a radiologist on site and studies can be read off-line.

Results of ABUS performance have been promising. In a study by Kelly and colleagues[7,29] using a standard 5.2-cm transducer on an articulating arm, an additional 3.6 cancers per 1000 women screened were found when ABUS was added to mammography, in keeping with results from the ACRIN 6666 trial using physician-performed HHUS. A study by Brem and colleagues[25] using the large 15.4-cm transducer and a dedicated ABUS unit yielded an additional 1.9 cancers per 1000 women screened. In a study of 200 cases, Giger and colleagues[30] also showed significantly improved performance and sensitivity and a nonsignificant decrease in specificity when ABUS was added to 2D mammography compared with 2D mammography alone.

However, ABUS does have some limitations. It requires investment in specialized equipment that may only be used for screening ultrasonography. The radiologist then has thousands of images to interpret: the small-footprint system creates a video clip of 2000 to 5000 images; the large-footprint system acquires up to 3000 2D images.[25,29] Interpretation initially may take up to 10 to 15 minutes to review, although with experience the time to interpret the examination may decrease to ~3 minutes per case.[26]

In addition, if a finding is made, patients may need to be recalled for targeted scanning, which may require a second patient visit and HHUS equipment. Brem and colleagues[25] showed that, of 15,318 women, 4364 women were recalled when examinations were performed with mammography and ABUS, whereas 2301 women were recalled from screening mammography alone. ABUS recall rates may decrease with increased radiologist experience, but, because mammography is already criticized for recall rates of 5% to 12%, the additional recall associated with ABUS screening is a relevant concern.[31]

Lack of contact of the transducer with the breast can produce artifacts, which can result in missed cancers. The breast periphery, especially in large breasts, can be outside the field of view of the transducer, although this area can be overlooked with HHUS as well. Color Doppler evaluation of vascularity is also not possible with ABUS. Although ultrasonography parameters may be modified in real time with HHUS to optimize imaging, the automated nature of ABUS precludes fine adjustments.[26]

Hand-Held Ultrasonography Versus Automated Breast Ultrasonography

Studies directly comparing HHUS with ABUS have been mixed. In a study of 30 BI-RADS 4 or 5 lesions, 7 malignant lesions were seen with equal confidence on HHUS and ABUS; however, 23 benign lesions were seen with greater confidence on ABUS.[32] In a study of 411 lesions, image quality of ABUS was identical or superior to HHUS in 97.1% but inferior to HHUS in 2.9%, and contact artifact was cited as a contributor to poor ABUS quality.[33] It showed that HHUS was superior for lesions located in the periphery of the breast, and for masses with irregular shapes and noncircumscribed margins. Jeh and colleagues[34] showed overall detection rates of 83.0% for ABUS and 94.2% for HHUS among 206 lesions (46 malignant, 160 benign), although detection of microcalcifications proved difficult with both ABUS and HHUS. In a study by Chang and colleagues,[35] ABUS was performed on 13 women with 14 HHUS-detected cancers. Three readers who had not performed the HHUS interpreted the ABUS examinations and only 57% to 79% of the cancers were detected with ABUS; 2 subcentimeter cancers were missed by all 3 readers.

SCHEDULING

Guidelines for frequency of screening ultrasonography examinations have not yet been established. The utility of ultrasonography is to detect small invasive cancers that may be obscured in dense breast tissue. As such, it may be reasonable to offer ultrasonography as an adjunct at the same frequency as mammography screening. At initial implementation, 45-minute dense breast ultrasonography appointments may be needed. However, with experience, appointment times can be reduced to 30 minutes.

For convenience, some patients prefer to schedule SWBUS for the same day as their mammogram. Same-day ultrasonography screening may aid in dismissing some mammographic findings as benign, thereby reducing mammographic recalls by nearly 50%.[36]

Other patients may prefer to stagger their ultrasonography screening 6 months apart from mammography screening; particularly high-risk patients who are not able to undergo MR imaging screening. Occasionally, insurance companies require documentation of mammographic breast density before approving dense breast screening ultrasonography. In these cases the ultrasonography may be performed a few weeks after the annual mammography examination. In a study of 2557 women who underwent mammography and HHUS screening, when SWBUS was performed on a different day than mammography, no significant difference was found in cancer detection, recommendations for short-interval follow-up, or biopsy based on ultrasonography findings compared with women who had SWBUS performed on the same day as mammography. However, performing both examinations on the same day can decrease mammography recalls.[36,37]

Note that SWBUS is an optional supplement to screening mammography. Patients should not feel pressured to undergo SWBUS and open discussions regarding the benefits and risks of SWBUS are key to shared decision making with the patient. Notably, if a patient undergoes high-risk supplementary screening with MR imaging, SWBUS is redundant and should not be performed.

SCANNING AND IMAGE DOCUMENTATION

Whole-breast ultrasonography performance is outlined in the ACR practice parameters: overlapping scans in 2 planes are required, with angled views behind the nipple to ensure complete coverage of the breast, using at least a 12 to 5MHz linear transducer.[20] Gain is adjusted such that subcutaneous fat is a medium gray, the field of view is set such that the pectoralis is along the far aspect of the image, and focal zone at or slightly below the area of interest. The patient is supine with the ipsilateral arm overhead and the chest supported such that the scanned area is parallel to the chest wall. The outer breast is scanned with the patient in the supine semioblique position; the remainder of the breast and retroareolar region are typically scanned with the patient in the supine position.[38]

Scanning of the axilla is considered optional. Although breast cancers may occur in accessory axillary breast tissue, which is present in 0.6% to 6% of the general population, the axilla is typically well evaluated on mammography.[39] Evaluation of the axilla may also increase scan time and result in more false-positive findings. However, including documentation the axilla can be beneficial because it reinforces the importance of scanning of the posterior breast and, with experience, the likelihood of false-positives is low.[39] In addition, the large-footprint transducer used by dedicated ABUS units is presently not designed to scan the axilla, requiring HHUS for full evaluation if the axilla was considered mandatory.

Once scanning is complete, findings should be documented, including documentation of normal tissue if no focal findings are present. As per the ACRIN 6666 trial, the recommended recorded representative images for a negative examination are defined as a minimum of 1 image of each quadrant and 1 image behind the nipple.[15] For example, negative images may be documented at the following clock positions: 12, 3, 6, and 9, as well as the retroareolar region plus/minus the axilla. A finding is documented with measurements in at least 2 dimensions (maximum diameter and orthogonal to maximum diameter), with clock position, and distance from the nipple, clearly marked. Images without calipers are also obtained. Although color Doppler images can be acquired, routine color Doppler images showing vascularity are not required.

Cysts are a common finding on SWBUS, seen in up to 47.1% of the participants of the ACRIN 6666 trial, but documentation of each cyst is not required.[40] For cases of multiple bilateral cysts, representative images may be taken of the largest cyst in each quadrant in the longest dimension without calipers.[15]

Complicated cysts in the setting of bilateral simple cysts can be categorized as benign, BI-RADS 2, and did not require short-interval follow-up in ACRIN 6666.[15] Single images of the largest complicated cysts in each quadrant, without calipers, are sufficient. A solitary complicated cyst should be recommended for short-interval follow-up, BI-RADS 3.[40] New or solitary complicated cysts, complex cystic and solid masses, and solid masses should be documented with measurements in at least 2 dimensions (maximum diameter and orthogonal to maximum diameter), clock position, and distance from the nipple clearly marked. Images without calipers are also obtained. They may include a color Doppler image, although saving routine negative color Doppler images is not required. A cine loop may be useful to provide additional detail for the radiologist's review.[15] Cysts or solid masses with suspicious findings should be categorized as BI-RADS 4, and require biopsy.

It bears repeating that, for technologist-performed HHUS, if unsure of a finding, there should be a low threshold for the radiologist to scan the area again in real time. Interpretive performance has been shown to improve with direct scanning by the radiologist; rescanning after the technologist and immediate feedback are also important factors for high performance.[18] Rechecks with the technologists also provide them with valuable educational opportunities.

RADIOLOGIST INTERPRETATION

Screening breast ultrasonography examinations may be read out in one of 2 ways. As with screening mammograms, examinations may be batch-read with patients recalled if needed for additional imaging. If automated ultrasonography is used, this reading method is most common. However, batch reading SWBUS increases patient recalls, which is one of the stated harms of breast cancer screening.

Unlike screening mammography or ABUS, HHUS patients may be aware when there is a finding, because the sonographer may pause over one region of the breast to take additional pictures. If examinations are batch-read, patients leave the department in a state of uncertainty. Alternatively, if read in real time, the radiologist may deliver a final assessment immediately. This final assessment does require an in-house radiologist and can limit mobile and after-hours screening programs. However, it carries the advantage of being able to immediately recheck patients right away without the patient being recalled, sparing them time, expense, and worry.

In addition, technologists are often faced with questions from patients whenever they document a finding. It is important for technologists to be comfortable conveying to patients that it is not their job to interpret the findings and give results. Real-time interpretation helps technologists as well because they are able to reassure patients that the radiologist will give patients their results before the patient leaves the office. Furthermore, if the mammogram is performed on the same day, real-time ultrasonography interpretation permits scanning of any questionable areas on mammography without loss of time and often can avoid a mammography recall.

REPORTING

Because SWBUS is a supplemental tool, and not a replacement for mammography, the ultrasonography should be interpreted together with the most recent screening mammogram. When screening mammography and screening ultrasonography are performed on the same patient on the same day, a single combined report, with separate paragraphs for each modality but a single combined final assessment and management plan, is recommended. BI-RADS requires breast facilities to choose whether to audit only the combined examination or the combined examination and the separate component examinations. With the latter option, the strengths and weaknesses of the 2 separate modalities may be assessed in greater detail.[41]

If SWBUS is performed on a different day than the screening mammogram, or the same interpreting physician does not read both examinations, the ultrasonography report should reference any mammographic findings.[15] Of note, final assessment of BI-RADS 0 for an otherwise normal mammogram showing only dense breast tissue in order to initiate a recall or SWBUS is inappropriate. SWBUS referral should be from the referring provider, ideally after a shared decision is reached with the patient.

BILLING

In 2015, radiology coding deleted the breast ultrasonography code 76645. In its place are 2 codes: 76641 and 76642. Procedure code 76641 represents a complete unilateral breast ultrasonography examination of all 4 quadrants and the retroareolar region. Procedure code 76642 represents a limited, unilateral focused examination. Both codes can include examination of the axilla.[42]

If both breasts are evaluated, the modifier 50 for bilateral procedure is added. With this bilateral modifier, Medicare increases reimbursement to 150% of the unilateral rate. However, Medicaid does not accept the bilateral modifier and requires separate claims for the left and right breasts.[42]

At present, the global payment for a complete examination, encompassing both the professional and technical components, can result in a gain of 21.6% compared with limited examinations. This gain is a significant change from prior nonspecific billing codes, which did not differentiate between complete and limited examinations.[42]

Private insurers have been following suit with Medicare and Medicaid practices. This change has resulted in overall higher reimbursement levels for breast ultrasonography. However, patients with private insurance may have higher copayments as a result of the new charges, or even 2 copayments if separate right/left claims for bilateral ultrasonography are made.[42]

Some states have insurance coverage laws for SWBUS; however, there is variability among them. New York and Illinois have insurance coverage laws stating that SWBUS should be performed at no charge to the insured (no copays or deductibles). In Connecticut, Indiana, and New Jersey, although insurance coverage laws are in place, patients may still be required to pay a copay or deductible.[43] Knowledge of these billing changes is important because patients may question the changes in their charges (**Table 1**).

SCREENING WHOLE-BREAST ULTRASONOGRAPHY PERFORMANCE OUTCOMES

Any institution interested in establishing a strong SWBUS program should be prepared to audit performance outcomes. SWBUS is held to the same high standards as mammography, with efforts to keep false-positive rates low and cancer detection rates high of prime importance. Knowledge of positive predictive values (PPV) for biopsies recommended (PPV2) and biopsies performed (PPV3) is essential to maintain acceptable biopsy rates and provides valuable feedback to improve interpretation.

Because SWBUS is a different modality than mammography, it does require some adjustment of audit guidelines, which is a work in progress. Presently, there is no standard for documenting a negative screening examination. In ACRIN 6666, a set of 5 images (1 image of each quadrant and retroareolar behind the nipple) was recorded for a negative examination of each breast.[15]

Audit guidelines for breast ultrasonography outlined in the 2013 edition of BI-RADS are controversial.[44] The BI-RADS guidelines state that any additional ultrasonography images obtained beyond a facility's established documentation of a negative examination count as a positive examination,[45] including additional images obtained of focal findings that are immediately determined to be benign and/or stable after thorough evaluation. Such an examination would be assessed as a BI-RADS 0, with the additional images counted as a diagnostic examination, even though the additional images confirm a negative or benign assessment. Therefore, even though the patient only had a single scan, for audit purposes the screening examination would be counted as a positive examination

and the final diagnostic assessment as negative/benign, resulting in an increased recall rate for benign findings. This auditing practice also discourages the use of orthogonal scanning. In contrast, if a technologist scans for a prolonged period of time or a repeat real-time physician-performed HHUS scan is obtained to evaluate a focal benign finding but additional images are not recorded, the examination would be assessed as negative.

Audit of ABUS is more straightforward, because any screening examination requiring the patient to return for additional hand-held evaluation would be considered a positive examination.

For both hand-held SWBUS and ABUS, a screening examination can be assessed as BI-RADS 3, not only because additional diagnostic images are taken but also because additional imaging is recommended before the next screening examination.[45] BI-RADS 4 and 5 assessments are also counted as positive examinations.

Regardless of the controversy surrounding SWBUS performance measures, radiologists must track outcomes. Monitoring PPVs for recalls and biopsies is essential. Review of biopsied lesions is an invaluable learning tool and this exercise helps to improve overall performance.

OTHER SUPPLEMENTAL SCREENING MODALITIES

SWBUS is just one of the modalities that may be considered for a supplemental screening program. Both MR imaging and digital breast tomosynthesis (DBT) are also used as adjuncts to conventional 2D screening mammography and warrant some reflection when choosing to implement SWBUS. The American Cancer Society recommends annual supplementary screening with MR imaging for women at high risk, regardless of breast density.[13] The addition of breast MR imaging screening has been shown to yield a supplemental cancer detection yield of 14.7 cancers per 1000

Table 1
Medicare payments for breast ultrasonography examinations, based on National Payment Amounts for 2016. Bilateral examinations are billed using the bilateral payment indicator (−50) and are paid at 150% of the unilateral payment

Breast Ultrasonography CPT Code	Professional Component ($)	Technical Component ($)	Global ($)
Complete unilateral (76,641)	37.24	71.61	108.85
Limited unilateral (76,642)	34.73	54.78	89.51
Complete bilateral (76,641–50)	55.86	107.42	163.28
Limited bilateral (76,642–50)	52.10	82.17	134.27

Abbreviation: CPT, Current Procedural Terminology.

women,[8] which is far higher than SWBUS yields of 3 to 4 cancers per 1000 women screened.[6–11] However, false-positives and high cost have been barriers for MR imaging acceptance. Lower-cost alternatives using an abbreviated MR imaging protocol are gaining interest and studies are underway to evaluate this possibility.[46,47]

DBT has earned acceptance because it both increases cancer detection and decreases recall rates, which is distinct from MR imaging or SWBUS.[48–50] Although incremental cancer detection is less than that of MR imaging and SWBUS, compared with 2D mammography alone, relative invasive cancer detection rates have been shown to increase by up to 41% with a simultaneous decrease in recall rates by 15%.[48–50] These dual benefits are seen in women with dense and nondense breasts and all age groups.[51–53] From a technical standpoint, DBT has been easy to incorporate because the patient is positioned the same way as for conventional 2D mammography and the images take just a few seconds obtain. The ASTOUND (Adjunct Screening With Tomosynthesis or Ultrasound in Women With Mammography-Negative Dense Breasts) trial is the first published prospective trial comparing SWBUS and DBT in women with dense breasts and negative mammograms. The ICDR for SWBUS was 7.1 per 1000, and 4.0 per 1000 for DBT, with similar false-positive rates.[54] In Rafferty and colleagues'[52] multicenter study comparing DBT plus 2D mammography with 2D mammography alone, although adding DBT benefitted both dense and nondense women, an increase in cancer detection was not significantly different for women with extremely dense breasts. This finding raises the possibility that, for women with dense breasts, supplementary screening with DBT as well as SWBUS may be reasonable.

LIMITATIONS OF SCREENING WHOLE-BREAST ULTRASONOGRAPHY IMPLEMENTATION

False-positive biopsies, as reflected by low PPVs, have been cited as a main limitation of whole-breast screening ultrasonography. The PPV of biopsies ranged from 5.2% to 6.7% for technologist-performed HHUS.[6,11,16,17] With increased experience, PPV is expected to improve.

In addition, many examinations lead to short-interval follow-up, increasing health care costs and requiring patients to return for another examination. BI-RADS 3 lesions accounted for nearly 20% of lesions (519 of 2662) after 3 rounds of screening in ACRIN 6666.[55] However, the malignancy rate of these BI-RADS 3 lesions was low at 0.8%, and only 1 had suspicious findings on short-interval follow-up. Chae and colleagues[56] similarly showed that, although BI-RADS 3 lesions were detected frequently (1783 of 12,187), just 0.7% (8 of 1164) were malignant.

Hooley and colleagues[6] detected BI-RADS 3 lesions at a rate of 20% (187 of 935 lesions), but noted that if lesions in this study, such as solitary, oval circumscribed complicated cysts, and nonsimple cysts in the setting of multiple cysts, were reclassified as benign, this would have decreased the number of BI-RADS 3 short-interval follow-up lesions by as much as 50%. In another study of 153 multiple bilateral circumscribed masses with follow-up of at least 11 months, no malignancies were found.[57] Reexamining sonographic criteria for benign and probably benign lesions may permit yearly diagnostic follow-up of BI-RADS 3 lesions detected at SWBUS. Additional studies are needed to improve performance and work-flow efficiency.

Long-term randomized clinical trials to establish a direct decrease in patient mortality are not feasible because of high financial costs and the length of time necessary to perform such trials, and have not been performed for SWBUS. However, early detection of additional small invasive cancers should improve treatment options and is expected to reduce overall morbidity and mortality. Moreover, a low interval cancer rate (<1 per 1000 per year) is a measure of screening effectiveness.

Results from the Japan Strategic Anti-cancer Randomized Trial (J-START) have recently been published.[58] Participants in this study were randomly assigned to undergo mammography and ultrasonography (36,859 patients) or mammography alone (36,139 patients) within a 2-year period. Notably, overall cancer detection was increased, with more of these cancers at lower stage when ultrasonography was added to mammography. A lower interval cancer rate (0.05% vs 0.10%) was also observed in the mammography plus ultrasonography group.

SUMMARY

Whole-breast screening ultrasonography is a beneficial supplement to screening mammography in women with dense breasts. With more breast density notification laws in effect throughout the United States, implementation of quality SWBUS programs into existing practices is more common. Varying options from hand-held or automated systems to physician-performed or technologist-performed ultrasonography exist. Sites will find each has advantages and disadvantages. The keys to the success of any program are a strong educational foundation with constructive feedback and effective communication.

REFERENCES

1. Kolb TM, Lichy J, Newhouse JH. Comparison of the performance of screening mammography, physical examination, and breast US and evaluation of factors that influence them: an analysis of 27,825 patient evaluations. Radiology 2002;225(1):165–75.

2. Mandelson MR, Oestreicher N, Porter PL, et al. Breast density as a predictor of mammographic detection: comparison of interval- and screen-detected cancers. J Natl Cancer Inst 2000;92(13):1081–7.

3. Kerlikowske K, Zhu W, Tosteson AN, et al. Identifying women with dense breasts at high risk for interval cancer: a cohort study identifying women with dense breasts at high risk for interval cancer. Ann Intern Med 2015;162(10):673–81.

4. Lee C, Bassett L, Lehman C. Breast density legislation and opportunities for patient-centered outcomes research. Radiology 2012;264(3):632–6.

5. Bae MS, Moon WK, Chang JM, et al. Breast cancer detected with screening US: reasons for nondetection at mammography. Radiology 2014;270(2):369–77.

6. Hooley RJ, Greenberg KL, Stackhouse RM, et al. Screening US in patients with mammographically dense breasts: initial experience with Connecticut Public Act 09-41. Radiology 2012;265(1):59–69.

7. Berg WA, Blume JD, Cormack JB, et al. Combined screening with ultrasound and mammography vs mammography alone in women at elevated risk of breast cancer. JAMA 2008;299(18):2151–63.

8. Berg WA, Zhang Z, Lehrer D, et al. Detection of breast cancer with addition of annual screening ultrasound or a single screening MRI to mammography in women with elevated breast cancer risk. JAMA 2012;307(13):1394–404.

9. Berg WA. Supplemental screening sonography in dense breasts. Radiol Clin North Am 2004;42(5):845–51.

10. Corsetti V, Houssami N, Ferrari A, et al. Breast screening with ultrasound in women with mammography-negative dense breasts: evidence on incremental cancer detection and false positives, and associated cost. Eur J Cancer 2008;44(4):539–44.

11. Kaplan SS. Clinical utility of bilateral whole-breast US in the evaluation of women with dense breast tissue. Radiology 2001;221(3):641–9.

12. Smith RA, Duffy SW, Gabe R, et al. The randomized trials of breast cancer screening: what have we learned? Radiol Clin North Am 2004;42:793–806.

13. Saslow D, Boetes C, Burke W, et al. American Cancer Society guidelines for breast screening with MRI as an adjunct to mammography. CA Cancer J Clin 2007;57:75–89.

14. Kressin NR, Gunn CM, Battaglia TA. Content, readability, and understandability of dense breast notifications by state. JAMA 2016;315(16):1786–8.

15. Berg WA, Mendelson EB. Technologist-performed handheld screening breast us imaging: how is it performed and what are the outcomes to date? Radiology 2014;272(1):12–27.

16. Parris T, Wakefield D, Frimmer H. Real world performance of screening breast ultrasound following enactment of Connecticut Bill 458. Breast J 2013;19(1):64–70.

17. Weigert J, Steenbergen S. The Connecticut experiment: the role of ultrasound in the screening of women with dense breasts. Breast J 2012;18(6):517–22.

18. Berg WA, Blume JD, Cormack JB, et al. Training the ACRIN 6666 investigators and effects of feedback on breast ultrasound interpretive performance and agreement in BIRADS ultrasound feature analysis. AJR Am J Roentgenol 2012;199:224–35.

19. US FDA Mammography Quality Standards Act. Available at: http://www.fda.gov/Radiation-Emitting Products/MammographyQualityStandardsActand Program/. Accessed July 22, 2016.

20. American College of Radiology Website. Breast ultrasound accreditation program requirements. Available at: http://www.acraccreditation.org/~/media/ACRAccreditation/Documents/Breast-Ultrasound/Requirements.pdf?la=en. Accessed October 18, 2016.

21. Screening breast sonography in dense breasts - SBI statements. Available at: https://www.sbi-online.org/RESOURCES/Breast_Sonography.aspx. Accessed August 23, 2016.

22. IBUS Guidelines for the ultrasonic examination of the breast. International breast ultrasound school. 2015. Available at: http://ibus.org/ibus-guidelines/. Accessed July 29, 2016.

23. Philpotts LE, Andrejeva L, Horvath L, et al. Practical aspects of technologist performed screening breast ultrasound. ARRS Annual Meeting. San Diego (CA), May 4–9, 2014.

24. Tohno E, Takahashi H, Tamada T, et al. Educational program and testing using images for the standardization of breast cancer screening by ultrasonography. Breast Cancer 2012;19(2):138–46.

25. Brem RF, Tabar L, Duffy S, et al. Assessing improvement in detection of breast cancer with three-dimensional automated breast us in women with dense breast tissue: the SomoInsight study. Radiology 2015;274(3):663–73.

26. Kaplan SS. Automated whole breast ultrasound. Radiol Clin North Am 2014;52(3):539–46.

27. Available at: https://www.accessdata.fda.gov/cdrh_docs/pdf8/K082543.pdf. Accessed August 23, 2016.

28. Available at: http://www.accessdata.fda.gov/cdrh_docs/pdf14/k142517.pdf. Accessed August 23, 2016.

29. Kelly KM, Dean J, Comulada WS, et al. Breast cancer detection using automated whole breast ultrasound and mammography in radiographically dense breasts. Eur Radiol 2010;20(3):734–42.

30. Giger ML, Inciardi MF, Edwards A, et al. Automated breast ultrasound in breast cancer screening of women with dense breasts: reader study of mammography-negative and mammography-positive cancers. AJR Am J Roentgenol 2016; 206(6):1341–50.

31. Arleo EK, Saleh M, Ionescu D, et al. Recall rate of screening ultrasound with automated breast volumetric scanning (ABVS) in women with dense breasts: a first quarter experience. Clin Imaging 2014;38(4):439–44.

32. Kuzmiak CM, Ko EY, Tuttle LA, et al. Whole breast ultrasound: comparison of the visibility of suspicious lesions with automated breast volumetric scanning versus hand-held breast ultrasound. Acad Radiol 2015;22:870–9.

33. An Y, Kim SH, Kang BJ. The image quality and lesion characterization of breast using automated whole-breast ultrasound: a comparison with handheld ultrasound. Eur J Radiol 2015;84: 1232–5.

34. Jeh SK, Kim SH, Choi JJ, et al. Comparison of automated breast ultrasonography to handheld ultrasonography in detecting and diagnosing breast lesions. Acta Radiol 2016;57(2):162–9.

35. Chang JM, Moon WK, Cho N, et al. Breast cancers initially detected by hand-held ultrasound: detection performance of radiologists using automated breast ultrasound data. Acta Radiol 2011;52(1): 8–14.

36. Tohno E, Umemoto T, Saski K, et al. Effect of adding screening ultrasonography to screening mammography on patient recall and cancer detection rates: a retrospective study in Japan. Eur J Radiol 2013; 82(8):1227–30.

37. Dave HB, Raghu M, Geisel J, et al. Should screening ultrasound be performed on the same day as mammography? ARRS Annual Meeting. San Diego (CA), 2014.

38. Hooley RJ, Scoutt LM, Philpotts LE. Breast ultrasonography: state of the art. Radiology 2013;208: 642–59.

39. Ferre R, AlSharif S, Pare M, et al. Should the axilla be included in screening US? Radiology 2015;274(2): 623–4.

40. Berg WA, Sechtin AG, Marques H, et al. Cystic breast masses and the ACRIN 6666 experience. Radiol Clin North Am 2010;48:931–87.

41. Available at: http://www.acr.org/~/media/acr/documents/pdf/qualitysafety/resources/birads/birads faqs.pdf. Accessed August 23, 2016.

42. Centers for Medicare and Medicaid services physician fee schedule search. Available at: https://www.cms.gov/apps/physician-fee-schedule/search/search-criteria.aspx. Accessed July 22, 2016.

43. Available at: http://densebreast-info.org/legislation.aspx. Accessed August 23, 2016.

44. Berg WA, Mendelson EB. How should screening breast US be audited? The patient perspective. Radiology 2014;272(2):309–15.

45. Mendelson EB, Böhm-Vélez M, Berg WA, et al. ACR BI-RADS ultrasound: Follow-up and outcome monitoring. In: ACR BI-RADS atlas, breast imaging reporting and data system. Reston (VA): American College of Radiology; 2013. p. 61.

46. Kuhl CK, Schrading S, Strobel K, et al. Abbreviated breast magnetic resonance imaging (MRI): first postcontrast subtracted images and maximum-intensity projection—a novel approach to breast cancer screening with MRI. J Clin Oncol 2014; 32(22):2304–10.

47. Available at: https://www.sbi-online.org/Portals/0/Breast%20Imaging%20Symposium%202016/Final%20Presentations/311C%20Comstock%20-%20Breast%20MRI%20New%20and%20Abbreviated%20Protocols.pdf. Accessed August 23, 2016.

48. Friedewald SM, Rafferty EA, Rose SL, et al. Breast cancer screening using tomosynthesis in combination with digital mammography. JAMA 2014; 311(24):2499–507.

49. Skaane P, Bandos AI, Gullien R, et al. Comparison of digital mammography alone and digital mammography plus tomosynthesis in a population-based screening program. Radiology 2013;267(1):47–56.

50. Ciatto S, Houssami N, Bernardi D, et al. Integration of 3D digital mammography with tomosynthesis for population breast-cancer screening (STORM): a prospective comparison study. Lancet 2013;14(7): 583–9.

51. McCarthy AM, Kontos D, Synnestvedt M, et al. Screening outcomes following implementation of digital breast tomosynthesis in a general population screening program. J Natl Cancer Inst 2014;106(11) [pii:dju316].

52. Rafferty EA, Durand MA, Conant EF, et al. Breast cancer screening using tomosynthesis and digital mammography in dense and non-dense breasts. JAMA 2016;315(16):1784–6.

53. Haas B, Kalra V, Geisel J, et al. Performance of digital breast tomosynthesis compared to conventional digital mammography for breast cancer screening. Radiology 2013;269(3):694–700.

54. Tagliafico AS, Calabrese M, Mariscotti G. Adjunct screening with tomosynthesis or ultrasound in women with mammography-negative dense breasts: interim report of a prospective comparative trial. J Clin Oncol 2016;34(16):1882–8.

55. Barr RG, Zhang Z, Cormack JB, et al. Probably benign lesions at screening breast US in a population with elevated risk: prevalence and rate of malignancy in the ACRIN 6666 trial. Radiology 2013; 269(3):701–12.

56. Chae EY, Cha JH, Shin HJ, et al. Reassessment and follow-up results of BI-RADS category 3 lesions

detected on screening breast ultrasound. AJR Am J Roentgenol 2016;206:666–72.

57. Berg WA, Zhang Z, Cormack JB, et al. Multiple bilateral circumscribed masses at screening breast US: consider annual follow-up. Radiology 2013;268(3): 673–83.

58. Ohuchi N, Suzuki A, Sobue T, et al. Sensitivity and specificity of mammography and adjunctive ultrasonography to screen for breast cancer in the Japan Strategic Anti-cancer Randomized Trial (J-START): a randomised controlled trial. Lancet 2016; 387(10016):341–8.

Breast MR Imaging in Newly Diagnosed Breast Cancer

 CrossMark

Dipti Gupta, MD[a],*, Laura Billadello, MD[b]

KEYWORDS

• MR imaging • Extent of disease • Newly diagnosed

KEY POINTS

- Several studies show the superior sensitivity of breast MR Imaging in detecting multifocal and multicentric cancer in the ipsilateral breast as well as synchronous contralateral breast cancer.
- Two prospective randomized controlled trials examined the effect of preoperative breast MR imaging on reexcision rates for patients undergoing breast conservation and did not find any benefit in the MR imaging group.
- As yet, there are no randomized studies that report clinical outcomes as a primary end point after extent of disease breast MR imaging.
- In the setting of invasive lobular carcinoma, MR imaging can better delineate extent of disease, leading to a reduction in reexcision rates in several retrospective studies.
- Other indications for extent of disease breast MR imaging include axillary metastasis with an unknown primary, assessing response to neoadjuvant chemotherapy, patients receiving partial breast irradiation, and those with subareolar and posterior tumors.

INTRODUCTION

Breast MR Imaging is the most sensitive tool for detection of breast cancer. The role of breast MR imaging in screening patients who are at an increased risk of breast cancer has been widely accepted. However, there is much debate over the utility of MR imaging in evaluation of the extent of disease in patients with newly diagnosed breast cancer. Despite this, the use of MR imaging in preoperative evaluation has steadily increased. In a retrospective study of 52,202 women, the use of preoperative MR imaging in women younger than 65 years increased annually from 2005 to 2008.[1] Similar trends are seen across hospitals, with the University of Minnesota reporting an increase in MR imaging use from 9% in 2002 to 75% in 2009[2] and Mayo clinic from 10% in 2003 to 23% in 2006.[3]

There is significant variability in the amount of MR imaging use. In a survey of the American Society of Breast Surgeons (ASBS), 41% of surgeons routinely recommended preoperative breast MR imaging with significant differences in use.[4] The surgeons in an academic practice were less likely ($P = .01$) to recommend MR imaging than those in a private practice. Wang and colleagues[5] performed a review of 56,743 women with early-stage breast cancer in the Surveillance Epidemiology End Results (SEER) database between the years 2002 and 2007 to analyze the variability of preoperative breast MR imaging

Disclosure: The authors have nothing to disclose.

[a] Department of Radiology, Feinberg School of Medicine, Northwestern University, Suite 4-2304, 250 East Superior Street, Chicago, IL 60611, USA; [b] Department of Radiology, Saint Louis University, 3635 Vista Avenue, St Louis, MO 63110, USA

* Corresponding author.

E-mail address: dgupta4@nm.org

Radiol Clin N Am 55 (2017) 541–552
http://dx.doi.org/10.1016/j.rcl.2016.12.008

use. They also found physician practice style to be a major determinant of who received preoperative breast MR imaging. This difference in the physician preference on ordering breast MR imaging examinations in the preoperative setting is likely caused by a lack of sufficient evidence-based criteria. This article discusses the current data on breast MR imaging for evaluation of extent of disease and examines its role in specific clinical scenarios.

ADDITIONAL CANCER DETECTION

Several studies show the superior sensitivity of breast MR imaging in detecting multifocal and multicentric cancer in the ipsilateral breast as well as synchronous contralateral breast cancer (Figs. 1 and 2). In a meta-analysis of 19 studies providing data for 2610 women, Houssami and colleagues[6] found that MR imaging detection of additional disease in the same breast ranged from 6% to 34%, with a median of 16%. Change in surgical management caused by MR imaging staging was collected from 13 studies and showed change to mastectomy in 8% of women and a wider excision in 11% of women. Meta-analysis of 50 studies with a total of 10,811 women by Plana and colleagues[7] yielded similar results, with additional ipsilateral breast cancer found 20% of the time and contralateral breast cancer found 5.5% of the time. Brennan and colleagues[8] also found contralateral breast cancer in 4% of patients with extent of disease MR imaging in a meta-analysis of 3253 women.

The presence of synchronous breast cancer not identified on conventional imaging has been known for some time. Histologic analysis of mastectomy specimens yields synchronous breast cancers 20% to 63% of the time.[9–12] However, it has been proved that, for early-stage breast cancer, there is no survival difference between women treated with mastectomy and those treated with breast conservation along with radiation therapy.[13,14] This finding may signify that additional mammographically occult disease is treated by radiation therapy and/or chemotherapy and may not be biologically relevant. The significance of the MR imaging–detected foci of ductal carcinoma in situ (DCIS) and small invasive cancers is thus controversial. In a retrospective review of 2021 patients who had MR imaging after newly diagnosed breast cancer, 87 multicentric cancers were detected.[15] Multicentric cancers detected only on MR imaging were invasive in 66 out of 87 patients (76%), larger than 1 cm in 18 out of 73 (25%) patients, and larger than the index cancer in 17 out of 73 (23%) patients. Invasive disease, especially when larger than 1 cm, is not likely to be adequately treated with radiation therapy and is probably clinically significant. However, the effectiveness of radiation therapy as primary treatment of breast cancer is not well studied.

SHORT-TERM OUTCOMES: SURGICAL END POINTS

An important goal of preoperative breast MR imaging is to delineate the size of the known malignancy and improve surgical reexcision rates. MR imaging is superior to physical examination and conventional imaging in assessing the size of malignant lesions in the breast.[16] However, studies have shown that MR imaging may both underestimate and overestimate tumor burden.[17,18] Some studies suggest that MR imaging more accurately correlates with tumor size with high-grade invasive and in situ disease, and underestimates tumor burden with low-grade disease.[19,20] Also, tumors larger than 2 cm are more likely to be overestimated on MR imaging.[21]

It was thought for some time that preoperative breast MR imaging would reduce the rate of positive surgical margins after a lumpectomy and thus the surgical reexcision rates. Two prospective randomized controlled trials examined the effect of preoperative breast MR imaging on reexcision rates for patients undergoing breast conservation and did not find any benefit in the MR imaging group. The COMICE (Comparative effectiveness of MR Imaging in Breast Cancer) trial was undertaken in the United Kingdom and included 1625 women who had recently been diagnosed with a primary breast malignancy. The trial found no significant difference in the reoperation rate of 19% between the group that received preoperative breast MR imaging and the group that did not.[22] The MONET (MR mammography of Nonpalpable Breast Tumors) trial randomized 418 women who had a nonpalpable suspicious mammographic or sonographic finding to receive preoperative MR imaging (207 women) versus usual care (211 women). The investigators found a paradoxic increase in the reexcision rate for positive surgical margins in the group that received preoperative MR imaging (34%) compared with the group that did not (12%).[23] Results of these studies were unexpected, but both studies had drawbacks. One of the major limitations in the COMICE trial was the lack of experience of the radiologists with interpretation of breast MR imaging. In addition, the lack of systematic use of MR imaging–guided biopsies may have decreased accurate diagnosis

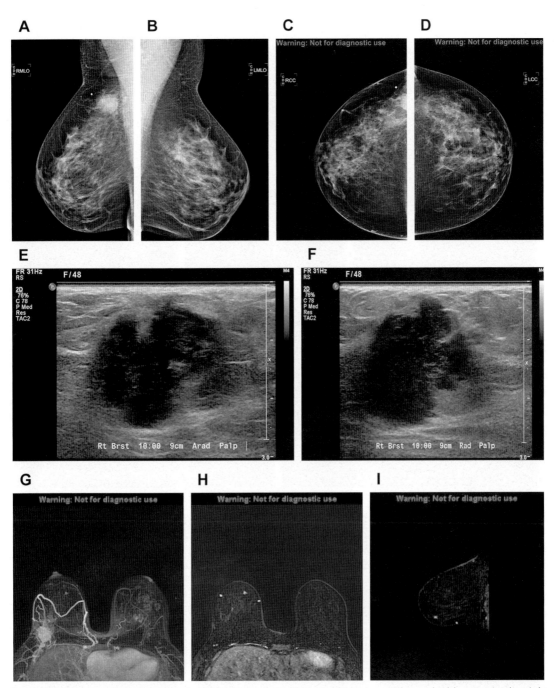

Fig. 1. Additional cancer detection: ipsilateral breast. A 48-year-old woman with a palpable mass in the right breast. Bilateral craniocaudal (CC) and mediolateral-oblique (MLO) views (*A–D*) show an irregular mass corresponding with the palpable abnormality in the right upper outer quadrant. No additional suspicious findings were identified on mammography. (*E, F*) Targeted breast ultrasonography (US) of the palpable abnormality shows an irregular, hypoechoic mass that was subsequently biopsied and yielded invasive ductal carcinoma, grade 3. Postcontrast subtraction axial maximal intensity projection (MIP) (*G*), axial (*H*), and sagittal (*I*) images show a suspicious 6-mm irregular enhancing mass in the right lower inner, anterior breast. MR imaging–guided biopsy yielded invasive ductal carcinoma (IDC), grade 2, proving multicentric disease, which led to mastectomy.

Gupta & Billadello

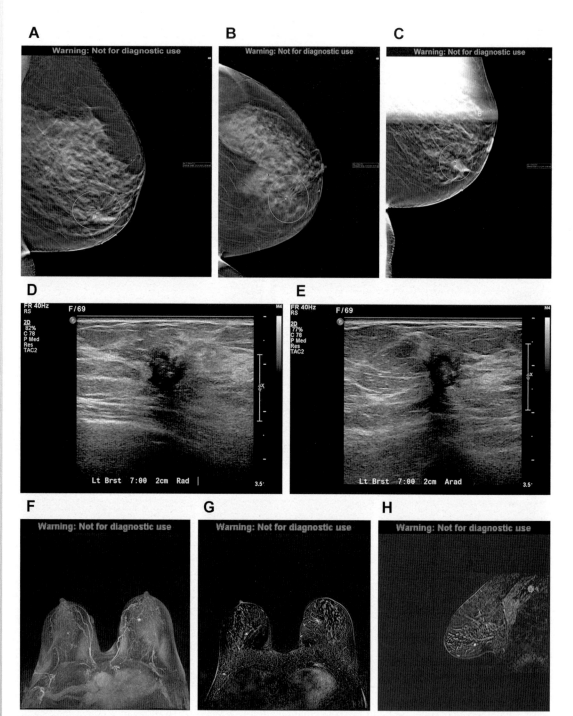

Fig. 2. Additional cancer detection: contralateral breast. Tomosynthesis CC, MLO, and spot compression (*A–C*) views of the left breast show an area of architectural distortion in the left lower inner quadrant. No other suspicious mammographic findings were identified in either breast. Radial (*D*) and antiradial (*E*) US images of the left lower inner breast show an irregular hypoechoic mass that correlates with the area of mammographic distortion. US-guided core biopsy yielded IDC, grade 1. Breast MR imaging was performed for extent of disease. On the postcontrast subtracted axial MIP image (*F*), the biopsy-proven malignancy in the left breast is seen. In addition, there is a 4-mm enhancing focus in the right central breast, which is confirmed on the axial (*G*) and sagittal (*H*) images. The focus had washout kinetics, was biopsied with MR imaging guidance, and yielded IDC, grade 1.

of additional lesions. The MONET trial had a strong selection bias in which there was a disproportionate amount of microcalcification (60% in the study group vs 25% described in the literature), likely because the lesions were nonpalpable. MR imaging is less sensitive in detecting DCIS than invasive carcinoma and therefore the effectiveness may be underestimated.

Preoperative breast MR imaging has been attributed to increased mastectomy rates, although the 2 randomized trials have shown differing results. In the COMICE trial, the avoidable mastectomy rate was 4.6 times higher in the MR imaging group. However, the MONET trial showed no difference in the rate of conversion to mastectomy after initial breast conservation surgery in the MR imaging group.

LONG-TERM OUTCOMES

Retrospective studies reporting the impact of preoperative breast MR imaging on recurrence rates after breast conservation have also shown conflicting results. Fischer and colleagues[24] reported a decrease in local recurrence 40 months after breast conservation treatment from 6.5% for patients who did not receive preoperative breast MR imaging to 1.2% for patients who underwent breast MR imaging (P<.001). However, the 2 groups in this study were poorly matched and the administration of systemic chemotherapy was not equivalent. Furthermore, the cancers in the MR imaging group were less advanced and the recurrence rate of 6.5% in the control group was higher than expected.

In contrast, in a single-center retrospective study of 756 women, Solin and colleagues[25] showed no difference in 8-year rates for local recurrence, contralateral disease, overall survival, or distant metastasis. Again, the 2 groups were poorly matched, with subjects in the group that received breast MR imaging being younger, at higher risk of recurrence (patients who had extensive disease were treated with a mastectomy and were excluded from the study), and having smaller tumors. Nearly half the women completed breast MR imaging after the initial surgical excision. Several other retrospective studies showed no decrease in ipsilateral breast tumor recurrence when preoperative breast MR imaging was performed for patients undergoing breast-conserving therapy.

Because tumor recurrence after breast conservation is linked directly to overall mortality, the impact of preoperative breast MR imaging on recurrence rates is an important end point. As yet, there are no randomized studies that report clinical outcomes as a primary end point after extent of disease breast MR imaging. Because the incidence of breast cancer recurrence is already low, it is estimated that a study investigating local recurrence as the primary end point would need to enroll between 2900 and 14,000 patients to have adequate statistical power.[26] In order to study the impact of breast MR imaging on distant recurrence or breast cancer–associated mortality, the number of patients needed in the study would be even higher.

MR IMAGING IN INVASIVE LOBULAR CARCINOMA

Invasive lobular carcinoma (ILC) represents 10% of all invasive breast cancers, and its incidence is increasing.[27] ILC cells lack cohesion and grow in a single-file pattern, infiltrating breast tissue, which makes it more difficult to detect on conventional imaging than invasive ductal carcinoma (IDC). False-negative mammograms occur at higher rates for ILC than for IDC. Even on retrospective imaging review of ILC cases, there is no suggestion of malignancy in 46% of the negative mammograms.[28] The sensitivity of mammography for the detection of ILC is only 57% to 81%[29,30] and the sensitivity of ultrasonography for the detection of ILC is only 68% to 87%.[31] By comparison, breast MR imaging is the most sensitive test for the detection of ILC, with a sensitivity of 83% to 100%, which is the same as the overall sensitivity of MR imaging for the detection of breast cancer.[29,31]

In addition to being more sensitive for the detection of ILC, breast MR imaging is better able to delineate the extent of ILC than conventional imaging. In 3 retrospective studies of patients with ILC, final surgical pathologic size and extent of disease correlate with preoperative MR imaging in 75% to 97% of patients, with ultrasonography in only 45% to 57% of cases and with mammography in only 32% to 65% of cases.[31–34] In a meta-analysis comparing preoperative MR imaging with conventional imaging, MR imaging finds additional ipsilateral malignant lesions not detected by conventional imaging in 32% of patients with ILC and contralateral malignant lesions not detected by conventional imaging in 7% of patients with ILC.[31]

Likely as a result of improved evaluation of extent of disease, preoperative MR imaging in patients with ILC is associated with a decrease in close and positive margins and, therefore, a reduced reexcision rate.[34–37] In a large retrospective study of 20,332 patients with breast cancer, including 1928 patients with ILC, preoperative MR imaging to evaluate extent of disease was associated with a 40% reduction in reexcision rate for patients with ILC.[35] Similarly, a retrospective cohort study of 267 patients with ILC undergoing breast conservation surgery showed that patients undergoing preoperative MR imaging are 3.63 times less likely to need reexcision.[37] Reduced reexcision rates were also found in a large meta-analysis of 3112 patients with breast cancer, 766 of whom had ILC. The study showed that preoperative MR imaging is associated with a reduced reexcision rate of 10.9%, compared with 18% in the control group not undergoing MR imaging, and this was statistically significant ($P = .031$).[36] However, the difference is not statistically significant after adjusting for age ($P = .09$).

Preoperative MR imaging is nearly twice as likely to change surgical management in ILC cases than in IDC. In a retrospective study of 267 patients with breast cancer who underwent preoperative MR imaging, surgical management was altered in 46% of lobular tumors compared with 24% of ductal tumors.[38] In addition, in a retrospective population-based study of 1928 patients with ILC, preoperative MR imaging did not increase the final mastectomy rate in patients with ILC.[35] There was a trend toward a lower final mastectomy rate in the MR imaging group in a retrospective study of 267 patients with ILC. In this study, patients with ILC undergoing preoperative MR imaging had a final mastectomy rate of 48% versus a final mastectomy rate of 59% in the group with conventional imaging only ($P = .098$).[37]

ROLE OF MR IMAGING IN AXILLARY METASTASIS WITH AN UNKNOWN PRIMARY

Unilateral axillary lymphadenopathy in the setting of negative diagnostic mammography is considered suspicious for ipsilateral breast cancer. If the biopsy of an axillary lymph node yields metastatic disease and conventional imaging is negative, breast MR imaging is uniformly recommended as the next step to evaluate for occult breast cancer because of the high sensitivity for invasive carcinoma (Fig. 3).[39,40]

In the past, modified radical mastectomy was the treatment of patients with axillary metastasis and negative conventional imaging. However, one-third of these patients do not have a primary breast cancer on surgical pathology of the mastectomy specimen.[41–43] Breast MR imaging, with its high sensitivity for the detection of breast cancer in both fatty and dense breasts, finds breast cancers not identified on mammography and clinical breast examination (CBE).[41]

When breast MR imaging identifies the primary breast malignancy in these patients, breast conservation becomes a treatment option. In a retrospective study of 40 women with biopsy-proven metastatic adenocarcinoma to an axillary lymph node and negative CBE and mammography, MR imaging identified the primary malignancy in 21 women, and 16 of these patients underwent breast conservation surgery.[43] Even in patients with distant metastasis, breast MR imaging can be useful to identify the occult primary breast malignancy, because it is often the safest and easiest lesion to biopsy to obtain a histologic diagnosis and molecular markers. Treatment can then be tailored, and response to treatment can be monitored. Even negative MR imaging in this setting can potentially be helpful. The high sensitivity of MR imaging for the detection of breast cancer makes it likely that a patient with negative MR imaging has either a nonbreast primary or a small tumor burden in the breast. These patients may be candidates for radiation therapy to the breast and axilla for locoregional control.[42,43]

Diagnostic evaluation with mammography or ultrasonography in patients who have suspicious axillary adenopathy should be performed before MR imaging evaluation. Ultrasonography of the axillae can exclude bilateral adenopathy, which would make a breast malignancy less likely.[39] Although primary breast cancer is the most common cause of unilateral axillary lymphadenopathy, other causes include mastitis, breast abscess, cat-scratch fever, herpes zoster, and melanoma. Clinical examination of the ipsilateral breast, axilla, arm, and hand can suggest an infectious or inflammatory cause of lymphadenopathy, if present.

Ipsilateral whole-breast ultrasonography may identify a finding suspicious for an occult primary that can be biopsied under ultrasonography guidance.[39,40] In addition, fine-needle aspiration or core biopsy of an enlarged lymph node should be performed for tissue diagnosis to confirm metastatic adenocarcinoma consistent with breast primary.

After a lymph node biopsy confirms a breast malignancy with negative mammogram and ultrasonography, MR imaging is then recommended. However, histologic proof of suspicious enhancement should be obtained before definitive surgery is performed. Options include MR imaging–guided biopsy, second-look ultrasonography with ultrasonography-guided biopsy, and MR imaging–guided wire localization for excisional biopsy.

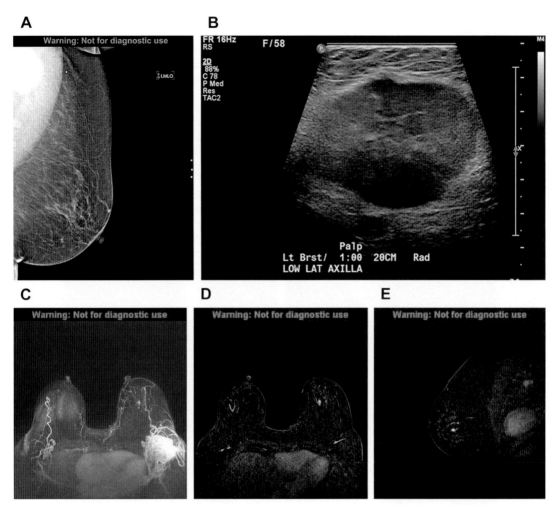

Fig. 3. Axillary metastasis with unknown primary. A 58-year-old woman presented with a palpable left axillary mass. Left MLO (*A*) and targeted US (*B*) show an enlarged lymph node with replacement of the normal fatty hilum. US-guided biopsy yielded poorly differentiated carcinoma consistent with a breast primary. Left mammography and whole-breast US did not yield any suspicious breast masses. Postcontrast subtracted axial MIP (*C*) and axial (*D*) and sagittal (*E*) images show a 1-cm enhancing mass in the left upper outer quadrant, which yielded IDC on biopsy.

MR IMAGING AND NEOADJUVANT CHEMOTHERAPY

Neoadjuvant chemotherapy (NAC) is defined as combination chemotherapy given before definitive surgical treatment, including both lumpectomy and mastectomy. It is usually given to patients with breast cancer who have large tumor masses (stage T3 or T4) or regional lymph node involvement. By shrinking the tumor to decrease tumor burden, NAC may allow some patients to undergo lumpectomy and radiation for local control, rather than mastectomy. In addition, assessment of tumor response to NAC can help guide treatment and be a prognostic indicator.

MR imaging has been shown in several studies to be superior to conventional imaging and physical examination in assessing response to NAC as well as predicting the eventual pathologic tumor size. As a part of the American College of Radiology Imaging Network (ACRIN) 6657 study in the I-SPY1 (Investigation of Serial Studies to Predict Your Therapeutic Response With Imaging and Molecular Analysis) trial, the ability of MR imaging to evaluate treatment response was examined. In 216 patients, MR imaging was superior to clinical examination in predicting both pathologic complete response and residual tumor burden, with the greatest advantage observed early in treatment.[44] In a meta-analysis of 44 studies with 2050 patients, MR imaging correctly identified residual disease after NAC with a median sensitivity of 0.92.[45] MR imaging had a higher accuracy than mammography, and was not significantly different from ultrasonography in predicting pathologic complete response. Some studies suggest that the accuracy of MR imaging in predicting response may depend on tumor phenotype, with MR imaging performing better in evaluation of triple-negative and HER2-positive breast cancers than the luminal cancers.[46,47] The use of breast MR imaging in assessing postneoadjuvant surgical treatment allows more widespread and accurate use of breast conservation (Fig. 4).

PARTIAL BREAST IRRADIATION

Whole-breast radiotherapy (WBRT) is the standard treatment after breast conservation to reduce the risk of ipsilateral breast tumor recurrence.

Whole-breast irradiation has been known to reduce the risk of recurrence by 50% to 60%. Because most recurrences occur near the tumor bed, accelerated partial breast irradiation (APBI) allows radiation of only the breast tissue at the greatest risk of recurrence. APBI shortens the conventional radiation treatment of 6 weeks to 5 days of twice-daily fractionation.[48] In addition, for certain patients with early-stage breast cancers, a single dose of radiotherapy delivered at the time of surgery, called intraoperative radiation therapy, is an option.[49]

Partial breast irradiation is optimal when treating unicentric disease. Breast MR imaging has been suggested for pretreatment evaluation of patients being considered for partial breast irradiation to

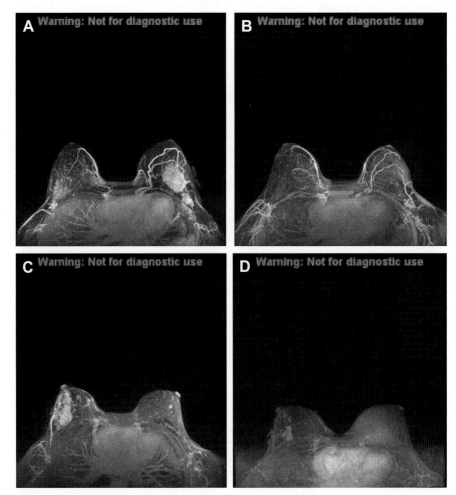

Fig. 4. Neoadjuvant chemotherapy: complete response. Postcontrast subtracted axial MIP images are shown in a 37-year-old with triple-negative breast cancer after diagnosis (A) and postneoadjuvant chemotherapy (B). There is complete response to treatment with resolution of the 6-cm irregular enhancing mass in the left upper outer breast. Neoadjuvant chemotherapy: partial response. A 28-year-old, BRCA-1–positive, patient with multicentric IDC and DCIS, grade 2, of the right breast. Postcontrast subtracted axial MIP images after chemotherapy (D) show decreased size and confluence of the biopsy-proven malignancy compared with pretreatment MR imaging (C).

evaluate for multifocal and multicentric disease. In a retrospective study of 79 patients, Godinez and colleagues[50] found mammographically occult foci of cancer in 38% of cases. In another study of 51 patients, pretreatment breast MR imaging altered patient selection for partial breast irradiation in 9.8% of candidates.[51] Until the results of ongoing randomized trials of partial breast irradiation that do not incorporate breast MR imaging into the selection criteria become available, a conservative approach to eligibility using MR imaging should be pursued.

SUBAREOLAR AND POSTERIOR TUMORS

MR imaging can be a useful tool in assessing involvement of the nipple, pectoralis muscle, and chest wall, all of which can change surgical management. Although Paget disease is uncommon,

accounting for 1% to 3% of all breast cancers, it may be undetectable on mammography in nearly half the cases.[52] MR imaging can play an important role in assessing the nipple areolar complex as well as evaluating for an underlying malignancy, especially when conventional imaging is negative (**Fig. 5**).[53]

Involvement of the chest wall can be difficult to assess on mammography or ultrasonography. The obliteration of the prepectoral fat plane by a posteriorly located tumor as well as enhancement of the pectoralis muscle suggest invasion of the pectoralis muscle.[54] Although this does not alter staging of the tumor, patients with pectoralis muscle involvement may require neoadjuvant chemotherapy or partial resection of the muscle. Invasion of the ribs, intercostal muscle, and serratus anterior muscle is consistent with chest wall involvement and affects staging. Involvement of

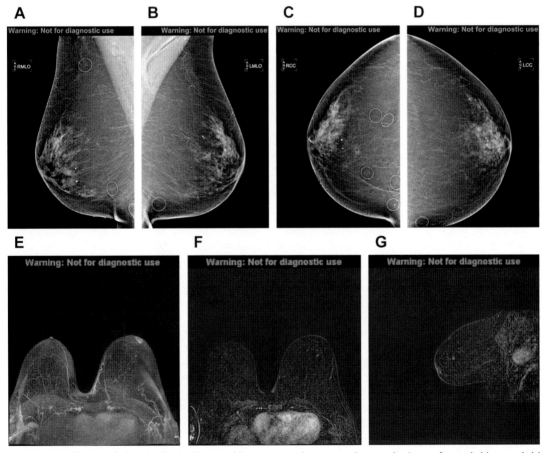

Fig. 5. Paget disease of the nipple. A 73-year-old woman underwent a dermatologist-performed skin punch biopsy of the left nipple, which yielded Paget disease. Bilateral mammography (*A–D*) and left subareolar US were negative. Postcontrast subtracted axial MIP (*E*) and axial (*F*) and sagittal (*G*) images are significant for a 5-mm mass in the left upper outer quadrant, which did not meet the threshold for kinetic analysis. Because this is the only enhancing mass in either breast in a patient with biopsy-proven Paget disease, MR imaging–guided biopsy was performed and was positive for DCIS, grade 2.

all these structures is more accurately assessed on MR imaging than either mammography or breast ultrasonography.

SUMMARY

The role of breast MR imaging in preoperative evaluation of extent of disease remains controversial. MR imaging increases detection of mammographically occult ipsilateral and contralateral disease, but the clinical impact of these incidental cancers is unknown. There are no randomized trials that study recurrence or mortality as the primary end point. Although such trials would be a huge undertaking, this missing evidence is needed before the role of extent of disease MR imaging can be outlined. There are specific clinical scenarios, such as axillary metastasis with an unknown primary malignancy and patients receiving neoadjuvant chemotherapy, in which breast MR imaging plays a clear role. However, in most cases, the decision to obtain MR imaging depends on physician practice style and patient preference.

REFERENCES

1. Breslin TM, Banerjee M, Gust C, et al. Trends in advanced imaging use for women undergoing breast cancer surgery. Cancer 2013;119(6):1251–6.
2. Miller BT, Abbott AM, Tuttle TM. The influence of preoperative MRI on breast cancer treatment. Ann Surg Oncol 2012;19(2):536–40.
3. Katipamula R, Degnim AC, Hoskin T, et al. Trends in mastectomy rates at the Mayo Clinic Rochester: effect of surgical year and preoperative magnetic resonance imaging. J Clin Oncol 2009;27(25): 4082–8.
4. Parker A, Schroen AT, Brenin DR. MRI utilization in newly diagnosed breast cancer: a survey of practicing surgeons. Ann Surg Oncol 2013;20(8): 2600–6.
5. Wang SY, Virnig BA, Tuttle TM, et al. Variability of preoperative breast MRI utilization among older women with newly diagnosed early-stage breast cancer. Breast J 2013;19(6):627–36.
6. Houssami N, Ciatto S, Macaskill P, et al. Accuracy and surgical impact of magnetic resonance imaging in breast cancer staging: systematic review and meta-analysis in detection of multifocal and multicentric cancer. J Clin Oncol 2008;26(19): 3248–58.
7. Plana MN, Carreira C, Muriel A, et al. Magnetic resonance imaging in the preoperative assessment of patients with primary breast cancer: systematic review of diagnostic accuracy and meta-analysis. Eur Radiol 2012;22(1):26–38.
8. Brennan ME, Houssami N, Lord S, et al. Magnetic resonance imaging screening of the contralateral breast in women with newly diagnosed breast cancer: systematic review and meta-analysis of incremental cancer detection and impact on surgical management. J Clin Oncol 2009;27(33): 5640–9.
9. Holland R, Veling SH, Mravunac M, et al. Histologic multifocality of Tis, T1-2 breast carcinomas. Implications for clinical trials of breast-conserving surgery. Cancer 1985;56(5):979–90.
10. Lagios MD. Multicentricity of breast carcinoma demonstrated by routine correlated serial subgross and radiographic examination. Cancer 1977;40(4): 1726–34.
11. Rosen PP, Fracchia AA, Urban JA, et al. "Residual" mammary carcinoma following simulated partial mastectomy. Cancer 1975;35(3):739–47.
12. Vaidya JS, Vyas JJ, Chinoy RF, et al. Multicentricity of breast cancer: whole-organ analysis and clinical implications. Br J Cancer 1996;74(5):820–4.
13. Fisher B, Jeong JH, Anderson S, et al. Twenty-five-year follow-up of a randomized trial comparing radical mastectomy, total mastectomy, and total mastectomy followed by irradiation. N Engl J Med 2002;347(8):567–75.
14. Fisher B, Redmond C, Fisher ER, et al. Ten-year results of a randomized clinical trial comparing radical mastectomy and total mastectomy with or without radiation. N Engl J Med 1985;312(11):674–81.
15. Iacconi C, Galman L, Zheng J, et al. Multicentric cancer detected at breast MR imaging and not at mammography: important or not? Radiology 2016; 279(2):378–84.
16. Boetes C, Mus RD, Holland R, et al. Breast tumors: comparative accuracy of MR imaging relative to mammography and US for demonstrating extent. Radiology 1995;197(3):743–7.
17. Kristoffersen Wiberg M, Aspelin P, Sylvan M, et al. Comparison of lesion size estimated by dynamic MR imaging, mammography and histopathology in breast neoplasms. Eur Radiol 2003;13(6): 1207–12.
18. Schouten van der Velden AP, Boetes C, Bult P, et al. The value of magnetic resonance imaging in diagnosis and size assessment of in situ and small invasive breast carcinoma. Am J Surg 2006;192(2): 172–8.
19. Blair S, McElroy M, Middleton MS, et al. The efficacy of breast MRI in predicting breast conservation therapy. J Surg Oncol 2006;94(3):220–5.
20. Kuhl CK, Schrading S, Bieling HB, et al. MRI for diagnosis of pure ductal carcinoma in situ: a prospective observational study. Lancet 2007; 370(9586):485–92.
21. Onesti JK, Mangus BE, Helmer SD, et al. Breast cancer tumor size: correlation between magnetic

resonance imaging and pathology measurements. Am J Surg 2008;196(6):844–8 [discussion: 849–50].

22. Turnbull L, Brown S, Harvey I, et al. Comparative effectiveness of MRI in breast cancer (COMICE) trial: a randomised controlled trial. Lancet 2010; 375(9714):563–71.

23. Peters NH, van Esser S, van den Bosch MA, et al. Preoperative MRI and surgical management in patients with nonpalpable breast cancer: the MONET - randomised controlled trial. Eur J Cancer 2011; 47(6):879–86.

24. Fischer U, Zachariae O, Baum F, et al. The influence of preoperative MRI of the breasts on recurrence rate in patients with breast cancer. Eur Radiol 2004;14(10):1725–31.

25. Solin LJ, Orel SG, Hwang WT, et al. Relationship of breast magnetic resonance imaging to outcome after breast-conservation treatment with radiation for women with early-stage invasive breast carcinoma or ductal carcinoma in situ. J Clin Oncol 2008; 26(3):386–91.

26. Houssami N, Hayes DF. Review of preoperative magnetic resonance imaging (MRI) in breast cancer: should MRI be performed on all women with newly diagnosed, early stage breast cancer? CA Cancer J Clin 2009;59(5):290–302.

27. Li CI, Anderson BO, Daling JR, et al. Trends in incidence rates of invasive lobular and ductal breast carcinoma. JAMA 2003;289(11):1421–4.

28. Krecke KN, Gisvold JJ. Invasive lobular carcinoma of the breast: mammographic findings and extent of disease at diagnosis in 184 patients. AJR Am J Roentgenol 1993;161(5):957–60.

29. Brem RF, Ioffe M, Rapelyea JA, et al. Invasive lobular carcinoma: detection with mammography, sonography, MRI, and breast-specific gamma imaging. AJR Am J Roentgenol 2009;192(2):379–83.

30. Weinstein SP, Orel SG, Heller R, et al. MR imaging of the breast in patients with invasive lobular carcinoma. AJR Am J Roentgenol 2001;176(2):399–406.

31. Mann RM, Hoogeveen YL, Blickman JG, et al. MRI compared to conventional diagnostic work-up in the detection and evaluation of invasive lobular carcinoma of the breast: a review of existing literature. Breast Cancer Res Treat 2008;107(1):1–14.

32. Rodenko GN, Harms SE, Pruneda JM, et al. MR imaging in the management before surgery of lobular carcinoma of the breast: correlation with pathology. AJR Am J Roentgenol 1996;167(6):1415–9.

33. Caramella T, Chapellier C, Ettore F, et al. Value of MRI in the surgical planning of invasive lobular breast carcinoma: a prospective and a retrospective study of 57 cases: comparison with physical examination, conventional imaging, and histology. Clin Imaging 2007;31(3):155–61.

34. McGhan LJ, Wasif N, Gray RJ, et al. Use of preoperative magnetic resonance imaging for invasive lobular cancer: good, better, but maybe not the best? Ann Surg Oncol 2010;17(Suppl 3):255–62.

35. Fortune-Greeley AK, Wheeler SB, Meyer AM, et al. Preoperative breast MRI and surgical outcomes in elderly women with invasive ductal and lobular carcinoma: a population-based study. Breast Cancer Res Treat 2014;143(1):203–12.

36. Houssami N, Turner R, Morrow M. Preoperative magnetic resonance imaging in breast cancer: meta-analysis of surgical outcomes. Ann Surg 2013;257(2):249–55.

37. Mann RM, Loo CE, Wobbes T, et al. The impact of preoperative breast MRI on the re-excision rate in invasive lobular carcinoma of the breast. Breast Cancer Res Treat 2010;119(2):415–22.

38. Bedrosian I, Mick R, Orel SG, et al. Changes in the surgical management of patients with breast carcinoma based on preoperative magnetic resonance imaging. Cancer 2003;98(3):468–73.

39. National Comprehensive Cancer Network. Occult Primary (Version 1). 2015. Available at: https://www.tri-kobe.org/nccn/guideline/occult/english/occult.pdf. Accessed August 7, 2016.

40. D'Orsi CJ, Sickles SE, Mendelson EB, et al. ACR BI-RADS® Atlas, breast imaging reporting and data system. Reston (VA): American College of Radiology; 2013.

41. Buchanan CL, Morris EA, Dorn PL, et al. Utility of breast magnetic resonance imaging in patients with occult primary breast cancer. Ann Surg Oncol 2005;12(12):1045–53.

42. Chen C, Orel SG, Harris E, et al. Outcome after treatment of patients with mammographically occult, magnetic resonance imaging-detected breast cancer presenting with axillary lymphadenopathy. Clin Breast Cancer 2004;5(1):72–7.

43. Olson JA Jr, Morris EA, Van Zee KJ, et al. Magnetic resonance imaging facilitates breast conservation for occult breast cancer. Ann Surg Oncol 2000; 7(6):411–5.

44. Hylton NM, Blume JD, Bernreuter WK, et al. Locally advanced breast cancer: MR imaging for prediction of response to neoadjuvant chemotherapy–results from ACRIN 6657/I-SPY TRIAL. Radiology 2012; 263(3):663–72.

45. Marinovich ML, Houssami N, Macaskill P, et al. Meta-analysis of magnetic resonance imaging in detecting residual breast cancer after neoadjuvant therapy. J Natl Cancer Inst 2013;105(5):321–33.

46. De Los Santos JF, Cantor A, Amos KD, et al. Magnetic resonance imaging as a predictor of pathologic response in patients treated with neoadjuvant systemic treatment for operable breast cancer. Translational Breast Cancer Research Consortium trial 017. Cancer 2013;119(10):1776–83.

47. McGuire KP, Toro-Burguete J, Dang H, et al. MRI staging after neoadjuvant chemotherapy for breast

cancer: does tumor biology affect accuracy? Ann Surg Oncol 2011;18(11):3149–54.

48. Ojeda-Fournier H, Olson LK, Rochelle M, et al. Accelerated partial breast irradiation and posttreatment imaging evaluation. Radiographics 2011; 31(6):1701–16.

49. Vaidya JS, Wenz F, Bulsara M, et al. Risk-adapted targeted intraoperative radiotherapy versus whole-breast radiotherapy for breast cancer: 5-year results for local control and overall survival from the TARGIT-A randomised trial. Lancet 2014; 383(9917):603–13.

50. Godinez J, Gombos EC, Chikarmane SA, et al. Breast MRI in the evaluation of eligibility for accelerated partial breast irradiation. AJR Am J Roentgenol 2008;191(1):272–7.

51. Horst KC, Ikeda DM, Fero KE, et al. Breast magnetic resonance imaging alters patient selection for accelerated partial breast irradiation. Am J Clin Oncol 2014;37(3):248–54.

52. Lim HS, Jeong SJ, Lee JS, et al. Paget disease of the breast: mammographic, US, and MR imaging findings with pathologic correlation. Radiographics 2011;31(7):1973–87.

53. Morrogh M, Morris EA, Liberman L, et al. MRI identifies otherwise occult disease in select patients with Paget disease of the nipple. J Am Coll Surg 2008; 206(2):316–21.

54. Morris EA, Schwartz LH, Drotman MB, et al. Evaluation of pectoralis major muscle in patients with posterior breast tumors on breast MR images: early experience. Radiology 2000;214(1):67–72.

MR Imaging
Future Imaging Techniques

Lilian C. Wang, MD

KEYWORDS

- Abbreviated breast MR imaging • Pharmacokinetic modeling • Diffusion-weighted imaging

KEY POINTS

- Abbreviated breast MR imaging protocols maintain the high diagnostic accuracy of full diagnostic protocols while minimizing the time and cost associated with traditional MR imaging examinations.
- Pharmacokinetic modeling of DCE–MR imaging data allows quantitative parameters related to vessel permeability, perfusion, and blood volume to be obtained.
- Pharmacokinetic parameters have the potential to improve diagnostic accuracy, assess response to therapy, and predict prognosis and survival in patients with breast cancer.
- Diffusion-weighted imaging is a noncontrast MR imaging technique that provides information on tissue cellularity and microstructure and has the potential to aid in the detection, diagnosis, and evaluation of treatment response for breast cancer.

Breast MR imaging, as the most sensitive imaging modality for breast cancer detection, has contributed to improved screening, diagnosis, and assessment of treatment response in patients with breast cancer.[1,2] Despite its high sensitivity, however, the specificity of MR imaging remains moderate using current clinical protocols, because malignant and benign lesions may enhance after contrast administration.[1,3] Future imaging techniques in breast MR imaging aim not only to improve accuracy for breast cancer detection but also to help predict and assess response to chemotherapy, predict survival, and better understand the biology and behavior of different molecular subtypes of breast cancer.

This article discusses evolving breast MR imaging techniques, including abbreviated breast MR imaging, pharmacokinetic modeling, and diffusion-weighted imaging (DWI). New hybrid techniques, such as PET–MR imaging, have also generated significant interest, and are discussed elsewhere in this issue.

ABBREVIATED BREAST MR IMAGING

Given its high sensitivity and ability to detect cancers occult to mammography, ultrasound, and clinical breast examination,[1–7] breast MR imaging use has increased over the past decade, particularly for high-risk screening. Limitations of this technique, however, include higher cost, longer examination time, longer interpretation time, and lower availability when compared with mammography and ultrasound.[3] With this in mind, an abbreviated breast MR imaging protocol has been introduced with the aim of decreasing these limitations, thereby increasing access to MR imaging screening.

Principles of Abbreviated MR Imaging

Although variable from institution to institution, most clinical breast MR imaging protocols are comprised of multiple precontrast and postcontrast sequences, with and without fat suppression, with emphasis on high spatial and temporal

Disclosure Statement: The author has nothing to disclose.
Department of Radiology, Prentice Women's Hospital, Northwestern University Feinberg School of Medicine, 250 East Superior Street, 4th Floor, Chicago, IL 60611, USA
E-mail address: lwang1@nm.org

Radiol Clin N Am 55 (2017) 553–577
http://dx.doi.org/10.1016/j.rcl.2016.12.009

resolution for detection and characterization of breast lesions. In general, a typical breast MR imaging examination requires up to 40 minutes for image acquisition and generates several hundred images for interpretation. In contrast, an abbreviated protocol may consist of only one precontrast and one postcontrast acquisition and their derived images (subtraction and maximum-intensity projection [MIP] images), resulting in significantly reduced imaging and reading times.[8–12] **Table 1** provides a summary of abbreviated protocols.

The rationale for using the first postcontrast sequence is the observation that cancers are best visualized during the early arterial phase after contrast injection, when contrast between the angiogenic tumor and adjacent fibroglandular tissue is greatest.[3,13] Later dynamic sequences and other pulse sequences are traditionally used for further characterization rather than detection of enhancing lesions. Some studies evaluating abbreviated MR imaging have included T2-weighted images and later postcontrast phases to evaluate their role in overall performance (**Table 2**).[9,11,12] With increased reader experience and protocols emphasizing high spatial resolution, however, the need for additional sequences for further classification may be reduced.

Current Evidence

Overall, abbreviated MR imaging has been shown to have a similar diagnostic accuracy to full diagnostic MR imaging protocols while reducing time for image acquisition and interpretation. Such data would support the use of this technique to increase access to MR imaging screening and decrease cost of existing MR imaging screening programs.

Cancer detection

In their prospective observational reader study of 443 women undergoing 606 high-risk screening MR imaging examinations, Kuhl and colleagues[8] reported a diagnostic accuracy equivalent to that of the full diagnostic protocol, with sensitivity and negative predictive value (NPV) of 100%, specificity of 94.3%, and positive predictive value (PPV) of 24.4% for their abbreviated protocol, with an incremental cancer detection rate of 18.2 per 1000. Heacock and colleagues[9] reported similar high sensitivity in their study of 107 patients with biopsy-proven unifocal breast cancer, with sensitivities ranging from 97.8% to 99.4% for the three abbreviated protocols. In a study of 100 consecutive breast MR imaging examinations in patients with biopsy-proven unicentric breast carcinoma, 96% sensitivity was reported for the first postcontrast and first postcontrast subtraction sequences, although this decreased to 93% for the subtraction MIP, which was statistically significantly inferior relative to the full diagnostic protocol.[10] In a pilot study of 48 breast MR imaging (24 normal, 12 benign, and 12 malignant), sensitivity was 86% for abbreviated protocol 1 and 89% for abbreviated protocol 2, not statistically different from performance for the full protocol.[11] Lastly, in a study of 470 patients with 185 breast lesions, Moschetta and colleagues[12] found no statistical difference in the sensitivity, specificity, diagnostic accuracy, PPV, or NPV for the abbreviated protocol compared with the standard MR imaging protocol,

Table 1
Summary of MR imaging sequences for abbreviated MR imaging protocols per study

Study/Protocol	T1 Precontrast	T1 Postcontrast First Pass	Subtraction	MIP	T1 Postcontrast Second Pass	T1 Postcontrast Third Pass	T2	STIR
Kuhl et al,[8] 2014	x	x	x	x				
Mango et al,[10] 2015	x	x	x	x				
Grimm et al,[11] 2015, AP1	x	x	(Available)				x	
Grimm et al,[11] 2015, AP2	x	x	(Available)		x		x	
Heacock et al,[9] 2016	x	x	(Available)				x	
Moschetta et al,[12] 2016	x		(Available)			x	x	x

Abbreviations: AP, abbreviated protocol; STIR, short TI inversion recovery.

Table 2
Summary table for abbreviated MR imaging studies: performance, acquisition time, and interpretation time of abbreviated and full diagnostic MR protocols

Author, Year	Study Design	Protocol/Sequences	Sensitivity, %	Specificity, %	Acquisition Time	Interpretation Time
Kuhl et al,[8] 2014	P	MIP	90.9	—	3 min	2.8 s
		AP	100	94.3	—	28 s
		Full diagnostic	100	93.9	—	—
Mango et al,[10] 2015	R	MIP	93	—	10–15 min	44 s
		First subtraction	96	—	—	—
		First postcontrast	96	—	—	—
Grimm et al,[11] 2015	R	AP1	86	52	~10 min	2.98 ± 1.86 min
		AP2	89	45	—	—
		Full diagnostic	95	52	20 min	2.95 ± 1.59 min
Heacock et al,[9] 2016	R	T1 only	97.8	—	—	14.0–25.4 s
		T1+history/priors	99.4	—	—	1–2 min
		T1+T2+history/priors	99.4	—	12 min	~15 min
		Full diagnostic	100	—	35 min	
Moschetta et al,[12] 2016	R	AP	89	91	10 min	2 min
		Full diagnostic	92	92	16 min	6 min

Abbreviations: AP, abbreviated protocol; P, prospective; R retrospective.

with sensitivity of 89%, specificity of 91%, diagnostic accuracy of 91%, PPV of 64%, and NPV of 98% for the abbreviated protocol. Examples of cancers detected using an abbreviated MR imaging protocol are shown in **Fig. 1**.

Interpretation time

Mean interpretation times for the abbreviated protocols vary from study to study (see **Table 2**). In general, the interpretation time for the abbreviated protocols is reduced compared with that for the full diagnostic protocol, mostly because of the decreased number of sequences for review. Kuhl and colleagues[8] reported an interpretation time as short as 2.8 seconds for the MIP image with an NPV of 99.8%. In the study by Mango and

colleagues,[10] mean interpretation time was 44 seconds, reduced compared with the published mean time to read a standard MR imaging of 4.7 minutes.[14] Although the reading time reported by Moschetta and colleagues[12] was longer than that reported by Kuhl and colleagues[8] and Mango and colleagues,[10] likely because of the addition of morphologic precontrast sequences, the postprocessing and reading time for the abbreviated protocol was statistically significantly shorter than that for the standard protocol.

However, in the series by Grimm and colleagues,[11] the abbreviated protocol 1 and full protocol interpretation times were similar. It was postulated that the three to four additional

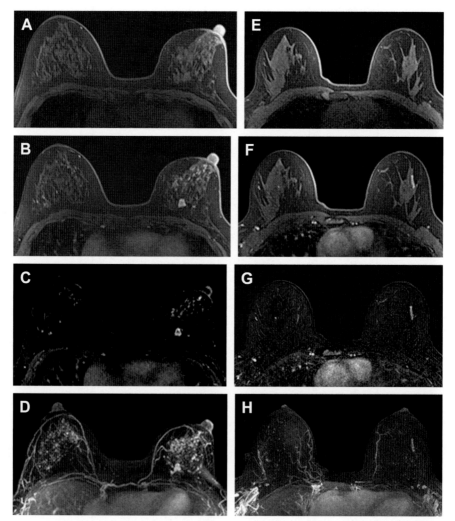

Fig. 1. Abbreviated MR imaging screening protocol showing precontrast (*A, E*), first postcontrast (*B, F*), first postcontrast subtraction (*C, G*), and MIP (*D, H*) images for two different patients undergoing high-risk screening MR imaging. Images for patient 1 (*A–D*) demonstrate an irregular rim-enhancing mass at 9:00 in the left breast representing grade 3 invasive ductal carcinoma and ductal carcinoma in situ (DCIS). Images for patient 2 (*E–H*) demonstrate a linear area of nonmass enhancement at 2:00 in the left breast with pathology of grade 2 DCIS.

sequences in the full protocol (non-fat-saturated T1 and two to three dynamic postcontrast sequences) may not be routinely used for clinical decision making, or that readers may have spent more time reviewing the available sequences in the abbreviated protocol to be confident in their interpretations.

Of note, one study reported shorter interpretation times for masses compared with nonmass enhancement and decreased interpretation time with increased initial enhancement ratio (mean percentage increase in signal between the precontrast and first postcontrast series).[9] They also observed that initial enhancement ratio correlated significantly with increasing tumor grade and with invasive rather than in situ disease. Although the study size was small, the data suggest that the abbreviated protocol may preferentially detect higher grade cancers.

The decrease in interpretation time enables the possibility of batch MR imaging screening akin to mammographic screening. In the study by Kuhl and colleagues,[8] 61% of examinations were negative on MIP and could have been completed with a reading time less than 3 seconds. In the remaining 31% of cases where significant enhancement was seen on the MIP, the abbreviated protocol was used to establish a diagnosis within a reading time of less than 30 seconds. The authors stated that this compares favorably with times published for batch reading of screening mammograms, which range between 60 and 120 seconds.[15,16]

The time investment for abbreviated MR imaging also compares favorably with screening breast ultrasound. In the American College of Radiology Imaging Network breast ultrasound screening trial (ACRIN 6666), the average ultrasound examination time was reported to be 19 minutes; yet, the addition of a single screening MR imaging study doubled the cancer yield in the same group of women, with similar supplemental cancer yield as that reported in Kuhl's abbreviated MR imaging study.[6,8,17]

Considerations

Eliminating additional sequences in the full diagnostic protocol may limit interpretation and affect potential recall rates in screening breast MR imaging. As with screening mammography, indeterminate findings at screening MR imaging would be recalled for additional diagnostic evaluation for further characterization. For example, with additional sequences in the diagnostic setting, the presence of T2 hyperintensity could be used to help assess a finding as benign, whereas the presence of T1 non-fat-saturated images may be helpful in the evaluation of fat necrosis or intramammary lymph nodes.[3,13,18,19]

In their study, Kuhl and colleagues[8] found that more than one-third of probably benign findings on the abbreviated protocol images could be downgraded to benign after interpreting the full diagnostic protocol, obviating short-term follow-up. Three of the studies of abbreviated MR imaging included T2-weighted sequences within their abbreviated MR imaging protocols.[9,11,12] Although T2-weighted sequences did not improve reader cancer detection in the Heacock series,[9] two of three readers reported significantly increased confidence in lesion evaluation with its inclusion.

The benefit of kinetic information, derived from multiple postcontrast series, is lacking in most abbreviated protocols and may necessitate recall for diagnostic MR imaging evaluation. Grimm and colleagues[11] found that the addition of the second postcontrast series for lesion kinetic analysis did not affect reader sensitivity or specificity. This may be supported by previous work indicating that fewer postcontrast sequences may not significantly impact diagnostic accuracy.[20] In addition, rather than using the first postcontrast sequence, Moschetta and colleagues[12] used the third postcontrast sequence without impacting diagnostic accuracy.

Another consideration in the adoption of abbreviated MR imaging is that published studies use expert readers; therefore, preliminary results may not be transferrable to community practice. However, if abbreviated MR imaging is adopted into clinical screening programs, reader expertise would increase over time, just as with mammography screening programs. Minimum standards for reader qualification could be introduced to ensure that the benefits of abbreviated MR imaging are realized while minimizing false positives caused by reader inexperience.

Lastly, the logistics of implementing an abbreviated MR imaging screening program are yet to be established. Although use of the full diagnostic protocol may reduce the number of BI-RADS 3 assessments at screening, it is unclear if this justifies the extra costs associated with the acquisition and interpretation of the full diagnostic protocol, or whether positive findings on abbreviated MR imaging could be managed clinically in the same way as those seen on the full diagnostic protocol. In addition, with new concerns regarding gadolinium deposition within the brain, patients may be reluctant to undergo additional diagnostic MR imaging evaluation for findings detected on abbreviated MR imaging. The cost of the abbreviated MR imaging also needs to be addressed, and should be competitively priced with other supplemental screening modalities. Prospective clinical trials are needed to validate abbreviated MR imaging as a viable alternative to the standard MR imaging examination.

Summary of Abbreviated MR Imaging

Abbreviated breast MR imaging protocols maintain the high diagnostic accuracy of full diagnostic protocols while minimizing the time and cost associated with traditional MR imaging examinations. Although larger prospective studies are needed to confirm benefit, the data show great promise in using this technique to make MR imaging screening available to a larger population of women.

PHARMACOKINETIC MODELING

Dynamic contrast-enhanced (DCE) MR imaging detects the uptake and washout of gadolinium over time. Gadolinium-based contrast agents (GBCA) shorten the T1 relaxation time, increasing signal intensity on fast T1-weighted images as measured in a voxel or region of interest (ROI), followed by a return to the native relaxation time as the gadolinium returns to the vascular space. Through appropriate imaging acquisition and pharmacokinetic modeling of DCE–MR imaging data, quantitative parameters related to vessel permeability, perfusion, and blood volume are obtained. Use of such quantitative information may have the potential to improve breast cancer detection and provide predictive, prognostic, and pharmacodynamic biomarkers of treatment response.

Principles of Pharmacokinetic Modeling

Pharmacokinetic modelling offers a quantitative approach to analyzing the distribution of GBCA in relation to the vascularity of breast lesions. After injection of GBCA, the contrast agent flows passively from the blood plasma through capillary walls into the extracellular extravascular space.[21] This distribution of contrast forms the basis for pharmacokinetic modelling of the passage of gadolinium. By combining and analyzing data from multiple images, and by assuming particular mathematical relationships between images through various models, measurements of intrinsic tissue properties are performed.

There are several models that describe the exchange of contrast agent between different body compartments. The simplest and most commonly used model is the two-compartment Tofts model, where the two compartments are blood plasma

and extracellular extravascular space, and where the tissue extravascular space is assumed to be well-mixed and homogeneous.[22] From this model, the concentration of contrast agent in the tissue $C_t(T)$ is given by:

$$C_t(T) = K^{trans} \int_0^T C_p(t) \exp\left(-(K^{trans}/v_e)(T-t)\right) dt$$
$$+ v_p c_p(T)$$

where C_t and C_p denote the concentration of GBCA in the tissue space and blood plasma, respectively; K^{trans} is the GBCA transfer rate constant; v_e is the extravascular, extracellular volume fraction; and v_p is the plasma volume fraction.[21]

To generate a map of K^{trans}, v_e, or v_p, estimates of C_t and C_p (or vascular input function [VIF]) as a function of time are needed. Because C_t and C_p are not measured directly, a conversion from the measured signal intensity to the concentration time courses must be performed.[23] To make this transformation, a precontrast T1 map and T1-weighted images during and after the injection of GBCA are required. The precontrast T1 map is used to calibrate the postcontrast T1-weighted images to estimate a T1 time course for each voxel. The T1 time course is then converted to a concentration of GBCA time course. The GBCA concentration curves for tissue and blood, measured indirectly from the MR imaging data, are then fitted to the previously mentioned equation to estimate pharmacokinetic parameters, listed in **Table 3**.

As outlined by the Radiological Society of North America Quantitative Imaging Biomarkers Alliance (QIBA), analysis of DCE–MR imaging data is carried out in the following steps[24]:

1. Generate a native tissue T1 map using the variable flip angle data
2. When required, apply time-series motion correction to the dynamic data
3. Convert DCE–MR imaging signal intensity data, SI(t) to gadolinium concentration
4. Calculate a VIF
5. Identify the region or regions of interest in the dynamic data
6. Calculate the DCE–MR imaging biomarker parameters, K^{trans} and $IAUGC_{BN}$

Because K^{trans} mainly reflects blood vessel perfusion and permeability, it is expected that malignant lesions will have larger K^{trans} values than benign lesions because of angiogenesis. Per consensus of the QIBA DCE–MR imaging committee, K^{trans} and $IAUGC_{BN}$ are the quantitative end points to be used in the application of DCE–MR

Table 3
Pharmacokinetic parameters

K^{trans}	Forward volume transfer constant (rate constant between blood plasma and extravascular extracellular space), expressed as min^{-1}
v_e	Extravascular extracellular space volume per unit volume of tissue
k_{ep}	Reverse volume transfer constant (rate constant between extravascular extracellular space and blood plasma) = K^{trans}/v_e, expressed as min^{-1}
$IAUGC_{BN}$	Blood normalized initial area under the gadolinium concentration curve = area under the concentration curve from the baseline timepoint (timepoint immediately preceding the change in gadolinium concentration intensity) up to 90 s post bolus arrival within the tumor divided by the area under the vascular input function curve, up to 90 s post the baseline timepoint within the vessel

imaging in the development of antiangiogenic and antivascular therapies. For some anticancer agents, such as vascular endothelial growth factor receptor–targeted agents, evidence of substantially reduced K^{trans} and $IAUGC_{BN}$ is necessary, but not sufficient, for a significant reduction in tumor size.[24]

Technical Considerations

Native tissue T1 mapping
A map of precontrast T1 values for the imaged slab is needed to help convert changes in signal intensity to gadolinium concentration. The slice locations, orientation, and resolution of the precontrast T1 images should be identical to those in the dynamic series to allow for coregistration for subsequent calculations. If there is concern for inaccuracies in T1 mapping and/or coregistration of initial T1 values to the dynamic data, a conversion look-up table could be used, which does not require the T1 mapping data. Fat content can alter apparent baseline and postcontrast T1 values and the use of fat saturation should be consistent throughout the examination.[24]

Spatial versus temporal resolution
Optimizing DCE acquisition involves finding an optimal balance between spatial and temporal resolution. The modeling described previously requires that the GBCA time course be sampled sufficiently fast to measure the input parameters. If the temporal resolution is not high enough, there can be significant bias in the resulting pharmacokinetic parameters. Because of the high spatial resolution required for clinical MR imaging interpretation, pharmacokinetic parameters are not routinely measured, because sequence acquisitions are not obtained at the high temporal resolution needed for pharmacokinetic modeling (QIBA recommends a temporal resolution of <10 seconds).[24] Advanced acquisition techniques that allow faster measurement, such as parallel imaging, undersampling, or view sharing, have been developed to help optimize the balance between temporal and spatial resolution.[23]

Contrast agent concentration
Pharmacokinetic analysis requires knowledge of the GBCA concentration in the tissue of interest and the VIF, which are estimated from the signal intensity time course after GBCA injection. Accurate GBCA concentration estimates require higher flip angles than are typically used in diagnostic MR imaging protocols. The Radiological Society of North America QIBA DCE–MR imaging Technical Committee recommends flip angles of 25° to 35° to minimize saturation effects, although this could lead to decreased signal-to-noise ratio (SNR) when compared with clinical imaging protocols.[24]

Vascular input function
The bias associated with pharmacokinetic estimates relies heavily on the choice of the VIF. Measurement of individual VIF is technically challenging because of need for high temporal sampling and can be difficult because of bolus dispersion, partial volume effects, inflow effects, and nonlinearity between signal and concentration.[23,24] One alternative is to use population-based, averaged VIF for specific injection parameters. Another method is to use so-called reference region models, where concentration-time-course in a reference region, such as muscle, is measured.[25] By assigning literature values of hemodynamic parameters in this reference region, it is possible to derive the respective parameters of the tissue of interest.[23–25]

Other Considerations

There are several other factors to consider when implementing pharmacokinetic modeling. This includes repeatability/reproducibility of measurements, such that changes in values are attributable to treatment changes rather than variations in measurement. The method of data summary, such as report of the average of a parameter (ie, K^{trans}) from a ROI drawn around the tumor, may not be optimal because information on tumor heterogeneity and spatial location is lost. Furthermore, direct comparison between quantitative parameters and lesion size, as per Response Evaluation Criteria in Solid Tumors (RECIST) criteria, may be difficult, because accurate measurement of the longest lesion diameter would require acquisition favoring a high spatial rather than temporal resolution.

Current Evidence

Breast cancer detection and characterization
Studies have shown that pharmacokinetic modeling can improve accuracy of breast cancer detection with DCE–MR imaging (Table 4).[26–31] Furman-Haran and coworkers[26] reported a progressive increase in microvascular perfusion parameters from benign fibrocystic changes to ductal carcinoma in situ (DCIS) and invasive ductal carcinoma. K^{trans} was the best predictor for distinguishing benign and fibrocystic changes from invasive ductal carcinoma, yielding 93% sensitivity and 96% specificity. Gibbs and colleagues[27] reported a diagnostic accuracy of 0.92 by combining postcontrast images with the dynamic data in a

Table 4
Summary of studies using MR imaging pharmacokinetic parameters for lesion classification

Author	N	MR Imaging Parameter	AUC (95% CI)
Gibbs et al,[27] 2004	43 women (32 malignant, 17 benign)	Max enhancement index	0.62 + 0.09 (0.45–0.79)
		Amplitude	0.74 + 0.07 (0.59–0.88)
		Exchange rate	0.74 + 0.08 (0.59–0.90)
		Washout	0.56 + 0.09 (0.39–0.73)
		Distribution volume	0.57 + 0.09 (0.40–0.75)
		MR_{diag} and ER_1[a] (all)	0.87 + 0.05 (0.77–0.97)
		MR_{diag} and ER_1 (9-pixel)	0.87 + 0.05 (0.78–0.97)
		MR_{diag} and exchange rate	0.92 + 0.03 (0.86–0.99)
Schabel et al,[28] 2010	93 lesions (60 benign, 5 atypical, 28 malignant)	K^{trans}/k_{ep}	0.92
		k_{ep}	0.89
		K^{trans}	0.88
		v_e	0.81
		v_p	0.79
Huang et al,[29] 2011	92 lesions (20 malignant, 72 benign)	K^{trans}	0.987 (0.971–1.000)[b]
		v_e	0.648 (0.509–0.787)[b]
		k_{ep}	0.958 (0.914–1.000)[b]
El Khouli et al,[30] 2011	101 lesions (68 malignant, 33 benign)	K^{trans}	0.76
		v_e	0.58
		k_{ep}	0.92
Veltman et al,[31] 2008	102 lesions (68 malignant, 34 benign)	K^{trans} (reader 1)	0.82 (0.735–0.905)[c]
		K^{trans} (reader 2)	0.82 (0.739–0.909)[c]
		v_e (reader 1)	0.78 (0.682–0.873)[c]
		v_e (reader 2)	0.77 (0.670–0.866)[c]
		k_{ep} (reader 1)	0.72 (0.609–0.828)[c]
		k_{ep} (reader 2)	0.74 (0.629–0.841)[c]
Furman-Haran et al,[26] 2005	89 lesions (44 benign, 45 malignant)	K^{trans}	Not reported
		k_{ep}	Not reported
		v_e	Not reported

Abbreviations: AUC, area under the receiver operating characteristic curve; CI, confidence interval.
[a] ER_1 = relative enhancement at 1 min.
[b] Shutter-speed approach.
[c] Values for the fast dynamic analysis.

logistic regression analysis, compared with 69% for interpretation of high-resolution postcontrast images alone. The best individual parameter calculated from the dynamic images was the exchange rate constant, which revealed a diagnostic accuracy of 0.74 ± 0.08. In their series, Schabel and colleagues[28] found that lesion classification based on K^{trans} and K_{ep} gave the greatest accuracy, with an area under the receiver operating characteristic (AUC) curve of 0.915, sensitivity of 91%, and specificity of 85%, compared with 88% and 68%, respectively, in a study of clinical breast MR imaging in a similar patient population. Similarly, Huang and colleagues[29] demonstrated that the use of shutter-speed DCE–MR imaging improved diagnostic accuracy; K^{trans} using the shutter-speed approach had significantly higher diagnostic specificity than standard approach K^{trans} (88.6% vs 77.8%) at 100% sensitivity. **Fig. 2** illustrates examples of DCE–MR imaging

anatomic images with corresponding reformatted maps of K^{trans} and k_{ep} for six patients with varying pathology.[28]

El Khouli and colleagues[30] evaluated the incremental value of pharmacokinetic analysis of DCE–MR imaging compared with conventional breast MR imaging (morphology plus kinetic curve type) in characterizing lesions as malignant or benign at 3-T. They found a significant association between K^{trans} and k_{ep} and the diagnosis of benign versus malignant pathology, with malignant lesions exhibiting higher K^{trans} and k_{ep} values compared with benign lesions. The use of pharmacokinetic modeling or kinetic curve assessment in conjunction with high-resolution breast MR imaging offered similar improvement in diagnostic performance. Inclusion of pharmacokinetic parameters showed modest improvement in performance, with AUC of 0.88 to 0.89 compared with 0.85 for lesion margin and enhancement pattern alone.[30]

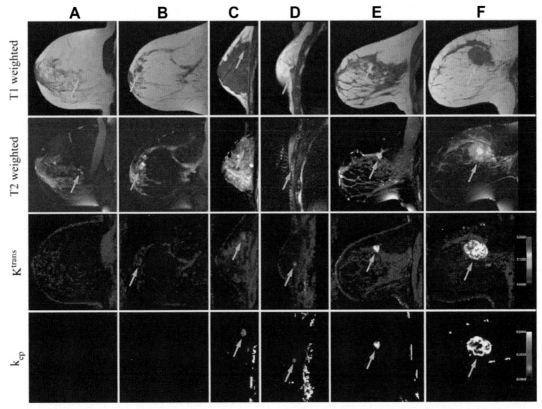

Fig. 2. T1 and fat-saturated T2-weighted images are shown for six study patients (A–F), along with the corresponding sagittal reformatted maps of K^{trans} (in 1/min) and k_{ep} (in 1/min). T1-weighted images are plotted in the first row, fat-saturated T2-weighted images in the second row, K^{trans} in the third row, and k_{ep} in the fourth row. The approximate location of the biopsied lesion is indicated by arrow in each panel. Patient A was diagnosed with mammary fibrosis, patients B and C with benign fibroadenoma, patient D with ductal carcinoma in situ, and patients E and F with invasive ductal carcinoma. (*From* Schabel MC, Morrell GR, Oh KY, et al. Pharmacokinetic mapping for lesion classification in dynamic breast MRI. J Magn Reson Imaging 2010;31:1374; with permission.)

Lastly, Veltman and colleagues[31] found that pharmacokinetic parameters derived from fast dynamic scanning (high temporal resolution of 4.1 seconds) were a valuable additional tool for differentiation between benign and malignant lesions. The pharmacokinetic parameters were significantly higher for the malignant group compared with benign lesions. Although the diagnostic performance for the fast dynamic analysis was not significantly different from the slow dynamic analysis (high spatial resolution images recorded at a temporal resolution of 86 seconds), the combination of the slow and fast dynamic analyses resulted in a significant improvement of diagnostic performance with an AUC of 0.93 and 0.90 for the two readers. K^{trans} was found to be the best individual parameter with a diagnostic accuracy of 0.82.

Response to therapy

In addition to improving breast cancer detection, pharmacokinetic modeling is used to assess response to therapy through quantitative end points, such as K^{trans} and $IAUGC_{BN}$, which may serve as pharmacodynamic biomarkers of treatment response.[24] Antiangiogenesis agents act through altering the vasculature and reducing tumor blood flow/permeability. As such, DCE–MR imaging represents an MR imaging–based method to assess the tumor microvascular environment by tracking the kinetics of contrast agent through the lesion of interest. Unlike conventional end points for treatment response, such as tumor dimension (RECIST criteria), pharmacokinetic modeling has the potential to allow for earlier and more specific indications of response to treatment, even before changes in morphology and size are evident.

Several studies have reported that pharmacokinetic parameters can predict response to treatment.[32–44] In the series by Pickles and colleagues,[32] a highly significant reduction in K_{trans} and k_{ep} ($P<.001$) was noted for responders between the pretreatment and early treatment time points, whereas v_e significantly increased during the same time period for nonresponders ($P<.001$). Hayes and colleagues[33] reported a reduction in K^{trans} after one cycle of treatment more frequently in eventual responders than nonresponders, and Wasser and coworkers[34] reported a reduction in k_{ep} after the first cycle of therapy in patients showing posttreatment tumor regression after the third cycle. Another study of 25 women undergoing neoadjuvant chemotherapy reported that K^{trans} and size were equally sensitive in identifying patients who would gain no clinical or pathologic benefit after two cycles of treatment.[35] Similarly, Li and colleagues[36] reported that pharmacokinetic parameters had the potential to be prognostic biomarkers for disease-free and overall survival. In their study, higher posttreatment K^{trans} and larger posttreatment $IAUCG_{60}$ were significant predictors of worse disease-free survival and worse overall survival, with K^{trans} an independent indicator of overall survival. **Figs. 3** and **4** provide examples of transfer constant changes in responders versus nonresponders.[32]

In a study of 28 patients with breast cancer who received six cycles of neoadjuvant 5-fluorouracil, epirubicin, and cyclophosphamide chemotherapy, DCE–MR imaging was performed before and after two cycles of treatment to assess whether DCE–MR imaging after two cycles could predict final clinical and pathologic response. A change in K^{trans} was found to be the best predictor of pathologic nonresponse (receiver operating characteristic curve, 0.93; sensitivity, 94%; specificity, 82%), correctly identifying 94% of nonresponders and 73% of responders. The authors concluded that changes in DCE–MR imaging after two cycles of anthracycline-based neoadjuvant chemotherapy can predict final clinical and pathologic response.[37]

Another study examined whether DCE–MR imaging pharmacokinetic parameters obtained before and during chemotherapy could predict pathologic complete response (pCR) in 84 patients with locally advanced breast cancer, and the impact of breast cancer subtypes on diagnostic accuracy. The authors found that DCE–MR imaging derived pharmacokinetic parameters can predict response status to neoadjuvant chemotherapy. With respect to cancer subtypes, K^{trans} was found to better predict pCR for triple-negative breast cancers, but no pharmacokinetic parameter could predict response for the ER+/HER2-group. Improved response prediction with quantitative DCE–MR imaging for the triple-negative subtype could be related to the high vascularization of this subgroup. The authors concluded that stratification of patients into breast cancer subtypes is important to better tailor imaging evaluation of response to therapy, with patients with triple-negative cancers more likely to benefit from DCE–MR imaging evaluation compared with those in the ER+/HER2-group.[38] **Fig. 5** illustrates changes in size and K^{trans} for an ER+/HER2 nonresponder and a triple-negative responder.[38]

Despite these promising results, additional studies evaluating the use of pharmacokinetic parameters as early response predictors have had mixed results.[35,45–48] Yu and colleagues[45] found

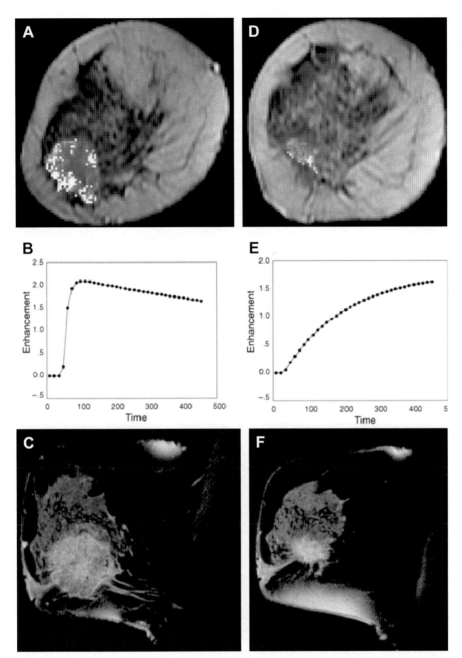

Fig. 3. Responder K^{trans} parametric maps (*A, D*) fitted enhancement curves (*B, E*) and high resolution 3D T1 SPGR (*C, F*) images for a responding patient at time point A [TPA] (*A, B, C*) and time point B [TPB] (*D, E, F*). Notice the reduced number of high value (*white*) pixels at the early time point K^{trans} parameter map as opposed to the baseline study. Baseline enhancement curve is of a malignant phenotype whereas early enhancement curve has a very gradual uptake usually associated with a less aggressive phenotype. (*From* Pickles MD, Lowry M, Manton DJ, et al. Role of DCE MRI in monitoring early response of locally advanced breast cancer to neoadjuvant chemotherapy. Breast Cancer Res Treat 2005;91:5; with permission.)

that early tumor size change after one cycle of neoadjuvant chemotherapy was a better response predictor than K^{trans} or k_{ep}, with AUCs differentiating between responders and nonresponders of 0.88, 0.63, and 0.77, respectively. No statistically significant difference was seen in changes in K^{trans} between responders and nonresponders.[45] Manton and colleagues[46] reported that none of the early changes in pharmacokinetic parameters (K^{trans}, v_e, and k_{ep}) after two treatment cycles

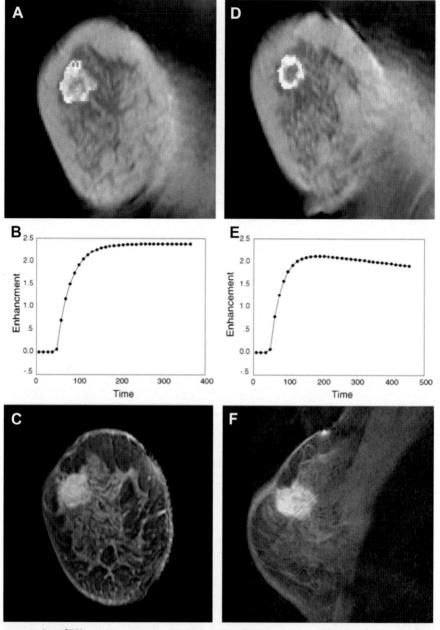

Fig. 4. Non-responder K^{trans} parametric maps (*A, D*) fitted enhancement curves (*B, E*) and high resolution 3D T1 SPGR (*C, F*) images for a non-responding patient at TPA (*A, B, C*) and TPB (*D, E, F*). Notice the increased number of high value (*white*) pixels at the TPB K^{trans} parameter map as opposed to the TPA study. Additionally the enhancement curve at the early time point is of a more malignant phenotype with a higher wash-out rate than the baseline study. (*From* Pickles MD, Lowry M, Manton DJ, et al. Role of DCE MRI in monitoring early response of locally advanced breast cancer to neoadjuvant chemotherapy. Breast Cancer Res Treat 2005;91:6; with permission.)

correlated with final tumor volume response after six cycles of therapy. Similarly, Padhani and colleagues[35] reported that none of the early changes in median values of K^{trans}, v_e, or k_{ep} after one cycle of treatment predicted tumor response, although changes in K^{trans} after two cycles of treatment were equally accurate for predicting absence of pathologic response as the change in tumor size. Table 5 provides a summary of studies examining pharmacokinetic parameters for evaluation of treatment response to neoadjuvant chemotherapy.[32–48]

Non responder   **Responder**

Pretreatment (EX1)   During treatment (EX2)   Pretreatment (EX1)   During treatment (EX2)

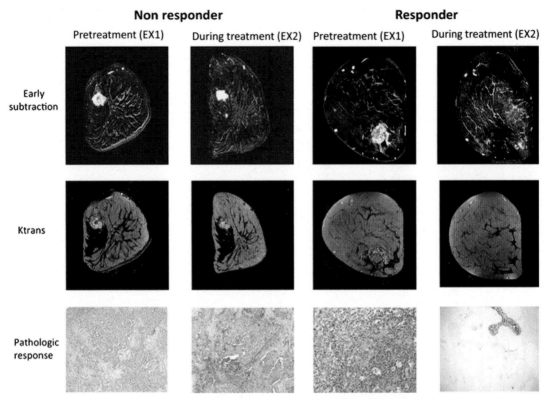

Early subtraction

Ktrans

Pathologic response

Fig. 5. The images show changes in size and transfer constant K^{trans} for ER+/HER2− in a 52-year-old nonresponder and a triple-negative 43-year-old responder, both with infiltrating ductal carcinoma. The first row shows coronal T1-weighted postcontrast anatomic early subtraction images. The second row shows the corresponding transfer constant color maps. The third row shows photomicrographs (hematoxylin-eosin, original magnification × 400). The columns show pretreatment and during treatment images for the nonresponder (*columns 1* and *2*) and responder (*column 3* and *4*). (*From* Drisis S, Metens T, Ignatiadis M, et al. Quantitative DCE-MRI for prediction of pathological complete response following neoadjuvant treatment for locally advanced breast cancer: the impact of breast cancer subtypes on the diagnostic accuracy. Eur Radiol 2016;26:1482; with permission.)

Limitations

Currently, pharmacokinetic modeling is not performed in routine clinical practice for several reasons. First, the high temporal resolution required for pharmacokinetic modeling has historically resulted in compromised spatial resolution. In addition, inadequate temporal sampling can lead to errors in VIF, which in turn affect K^{trans} and v_p. Other potential limitations include variability in technique caused by differences in manufacturers, MR pulse sequences, field strength, contrast agent relaxivity and binding, choice of tracer-kinetic model, method used to estimate GBCA concentration from signal intensities, and measurement of VIF. Such variability makes comparison of results from clinical studies difficult. Standardization of imaging protocols and data analysis is needed to help establish DCE parameters as pharmacokinetic biomarkers. With this in

mind, the RNSA QIBA DCE–MR Imaging Technical Committee has defined basic standards for DCE–MR imaging measurements and quality control to enable consistent and reliable measurement of pharmacodynamic parameters across clinical sites.

Summary of Pharmacokinetic Modeling

Pharmacokinetic modelling of DCE–MR imaging data allows quantitative parameters related to vessel permeability, perfusion, and blood volume to be obtained. Appropriate choice of pulse sequence, acquisition parameters, temporal sampling requirements, and knowledge of technical pitfalls is needed to allow for accurate calculation of parameters derived from accepted pharmacokinetic models. Pharmacokinetic parameters have the potential to improve diagnostic accuracy, assess response to therapy, and predict

Table 5
Summary of studies evaluating MR imaging pharmacokinetic parameters to assess response to neoadjuvant chemotherapy

Author, Year	Study Design	N	Breast Cancer Types	Chemotherapy Regimen	Time of Early Response Assessment	MR Imaging Parameter	AUC
Hayes et al,[33] 2002	R	15	NR	Mitoxantrone and methotrexate or epirubicin, cisplatin, and 5-FU, or cyclophosphamide and doxorubicin	1 cycle	K^{trans} v_e Max GBCA concentration	NR NR NR
Wasser et al,[34] 2003	R	21	IDC, ILC, mixed	Epirubicin and paclitaxel	4 cycles	k_{ep} Amplitude	NR NR
Pickles et al,[32] 2005	R	68	IDC, ILC, NOS, tubular	Epirubicin, cyclophosphamide, 5-FU	Median 54 d (36–153 d)	Tumor volume K^{trans} (ROI hot spot) k_{ep} (ROI hot spot) v_e (ROI hot spot)	0.649 0.631 0.604 0.673
Padhani et al,[35] 2006	P	25	IDC, ILC, NOS, mixed, other	Mitoxantrone and methotrexate or epirubicin, cisplatin, and 5-FU, or cyclophosphamide and doxorubicin	1 cycle 2 cycles	Tumor size K^{trans} Tumor size K^{trans}	0.90[a] 0.76[b] 0.93[a] 0.94[b]
Manton et al,[46] 2006	P	46	IDC, ILC, NOS	Epirubicin, cyclophosphamide, and 5-FU	2 cycles	K^{trans} K_{ep} v_e Tumor volume Water T2	NR NR NR 0.80 0.79
Yu et al,[45] 2007	R	29	NR	2–4 cycles of doxorubicin, cyclophomasphamide followed by paclitaxel, carboplatin with trastuzumab for HER2+ patients	1 cycle	Tumor size K^{trans} k_{ep}	0.88 0.63 0.77

Study		N	Histology	Treatment	Timing	Parameter	Value
Ah-See et al,[37] 2008	P	28	IDC, ILC, breast cancer NOS	6 cycles of 5-FU, epirubicin, cyclophosphamide	2 cycles (6 wk)	Tumor size	0.68
						Median K^{trans}	0.93
						k_{ep}	NR
						v_e	NR
						GBCA concentration	NR
						rBV	NR
						rBF	NR
						Mean transit time	NR
Baek et al,[47] 2009	P	35	IDC, ILC	2 cycles doxorubicin, cyclophosphamide then 2 cycles of doxorubicin, cyclophosphamide or paclitaxel, carboplatin Trastuzumab for HER2+	1–2 cycles (2–4 wk), 3–4 cycles (6–8 wk)	Tumor size	0.66, 0.90
						K^{trans}	0.65, 0.79
						k_{ep}	0.66, 0.79
Yu et al,[43] 2010	P	33	IDC, DCIS	Perarubicin, cytoxan, taxinol or perarubicin, cytoxan, 5-FU	2 cycles (6 wk)	Tumor volume	NR
						K^{trans}	NR
						v_e	NR
						Peak enhancement ratio	NR
Li et al,[44] 2010	P	31	NR	5-FU, epirubicin, cyclophosphamide or docetaxel	2 cycles (6 wk)	Tumor size	0.86
						K^{trans}	0.84
						k_{ep}	0.90
						v_e	0.59
						$R2^a$	0.62
						$IAUGC_{60}$	0.83
Li et al,[36] 2011	P	62	IDC, ILC, other or NOS	5-FU, epirubicin, cyclophosphamide or adriamycin, cyclophosphamide; 30 patients received docetaxel	2 cycles	K^{trans}	NR
						k_{ep}	NR
						$IAUGC_{60}$	NR
Cho et al,[48] 2014	P	48	IDC	Docetaxel, doxorubicin or doxorubicin, cyclophosphamide followed by docetaxel	2 wk after cycle 1	Tumor size	NR
						Tumor volume	NR
						Parametric resp. maps	0.77
						K^{trans}	NR
						k_{ep}	NR
						v_e	NR

(continued on next page)

Table 5
(continued)

Author, Year	Study Design	N	Breast Cancer Types	Chemotherapy Regimen	Time of Early Response Assessment	MR Imaging Parameter	AUC
Li et al,[39] 2015	P	42	Invasive >1 cm in size	Doxorubicin, cyclophosphamide, taxol or cisplatin, taxol or taxotere, carboplatin Trastuzumab for HER2+	1 cycle	Longest dimension	0.57
						ADC	0.82
						K^{trans}	0.68
						k_{ep}	0.76
						v_e	0.54
						v_p	0.61
						K_{ep}/ADC	0.88
Drisis et al,[38] 2016	R	84	IDC, ILC, mixed	5-FU, epirubicin, cyclophosphamide or docetaxel, cyclophosphamide or combination of anthracyclines and taxanes Trastuzumab for HER2+	2–3 cycles	K_{trans}	0.79
						v_e	0.74
						D_{max} (max diameter)	0.80
Tudorica et al,[40] 2016	P	28	IDC, ILC	4 cycles of doxorubicin, cyclophosphamide, followed by 4 cycles of taxane or 6 cycles of combination of all three Trastuzumab for HER2+	1 cycle	K^{trans}	0.967
						k_{ep}	0.957
						v_e	0.880

Abbreviations: ADC, apparent diffusion coefficient; 5-FU, fluorouracil; IDC, invasive ductal carcinoma; ILC, invasive lobular carcinoma; NOS, not otherwise specified; NR, not reported; P, prospective; R, retrospective; rBF, relative blood flow; rBV, relative blood volume.

[a] For size change analysis, an increase, no change, or decrease in size of less than 15% was used.

[b] For K^{trans} range change analysis, an increase, no change, or decrease of less than 11% was used.

prognosis and survival. Implementation of pharmacokinetic modeling techniques into clinical practice requires high spatiotemporal resolution breast MR imaging sequences. Standardization of both imaging protocols and data analysis is needed to establish DCE parameters as pharmacokinetic biomarkers and to allow for comparison of data across clinical sites.

DIFFUSION-WEIGHTED IMAGING

DWI is a noncontrast MR imaging technique that provides qualitative and quantitative evaluation of breast lesions. With a short scan time, DWI may be performed as an adjunct to DCE–MR imaging to improve diagnostic accuracy or as an alternative to gadolinium-enhanced MR evaluation in patients at risk for nephrogenic systemic sclerosis. Studies have shown that apparent diffusion coefficient (ADC) values derived from DWI can assist in differentiating benign and malignant lesions and in identifying early response in tumors undergoing neoadjuvant chemotherapy. There is also promise in using DWI as a noncontrast adjunct screening modality in women with dense breast parenchyma.

Principles of Diffusion-Weighted Imaging

DWI provides information regarding cell density and tissue microstructure by measuring the random motion of free water protons (Brownian motion).[49,50] In vivo, the diffusion of water molecules is inversely proportional to tissue cellularity and cell membrane integrity. Cancers, because of high cell density and intact cell membranes, tend to restrict the diffusion of water. Conversely, in tissues with low cellularity or compromised cell membranes, water diffusion is less restricted because water molecules may freely diffuse into the extracellular space and across cell membranes.

The faster the water molecules diffuse, the greater the attenuation and the weaker the corresponding signal intensity. Thus signal intensity is typically higher in a region with restricted diffusion, such as tumor. However, visual assessment of signal intensity on DWI is complicated by the fact that signal intensity is dependent on diffusion and T2 relaxation time, that is, the T2 shine-through effect. For example, a cyst may be misinterpreted as having restricted diffusion, although DCE–MR imaging images would confirm a benign, nonenhancing cyst. The quantitative ADC map overcomes the effect of T2 shine-through. Breast malignancies generally exhibit restricted diffusion on DWI, with ADC values being significantly lower in malignant lesions versus normal breast tissue and benign lesions.[49–52]

DWI enables qualitative and quantitative evaluation of breast lesions. Qualitatively, areas of restricted diffusion appear as high signal intensity on DWI images and low signal intensity on the ADC map.[49–52] Quantitative ADC analysis is performed by drawing an ROI on the ADC map and calculating the mean value for all pixels within the ROI. Appropriate placement of the ROI may be facilitated by use of DCE–MR imaging (**Fig. 6**). For accurate diagnosis, DWI interpretation must be performed in context with additional information provided in the DCE–MR imaging examination.

Technical Considerations

To obtain good-quality DWI images and accurate ADC measures, good shimming and suppression of fat signal are essential. The optimal technique for fat suppression may vary between scanners. Protocols must also be optimized for adequate SNR by balancing spatial resolution and appropriate diffusion sensitizations (or b values). In addition, the choice of b value directly affects the quantitative analysis of the ADC. At lower b values, T2-weighted signal is emphasized, whereas at higher b values the contribution from the diffusion coefficient alone is emphasized. Therefore, high b values (>500 s/mm^2) are recommended for breast DWI, although the optimal maximum b value has not yet been established. Although higher b values may be preferred for lesion conspicuity and detection, their use may reduce sensitivity for small lesions because of lower SNR.[53]

Current Evidence

Current research evaluating the use of DWI in breast imaging is promising. Areas in which DWI may add value to current breast MR imaging techniques include increasing diagnostic accuracy of DCE–MR imaging by aiding in the differentiation of benign and malignant breast lesions, identifying early treatment effects in tumors treated with neoadjuvant chemotherapy, and as a noncontrast alternative to breast MR imaging screening.

Differentiation of benign and malignant lesions

Several studies have reported differences in ADC values for benign and malignant lesions.[49,51–57] In general, the ADC of malignant lesions is lower than that of benign lesions, reflecting restricted water diffusion and increased cellularity. A meta-analysis of 12 studies evaluating DWI on 1.5-T scanners reported that ADC evaluation is useful in differentiating benign and malignant breast tumors, with an overall sensitivity of 89% and specificity of 77%.[54] Because ADC values are

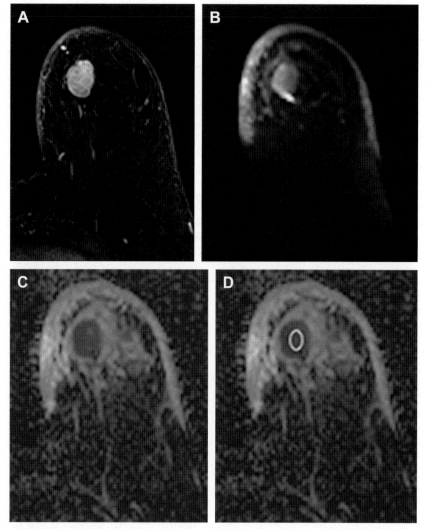

Fig. 6. DWI interpretation strategy. A 50-year-old woman with biopsy-proven left breast malignancy. (*A*) Postcontrast subtraction image demonstrates a 2.7-cm mass at 6:00 in the left breast consistent with biopsy-proven grade 3 invasive ductal carcinoma and DCIS. Corresponding (*B*) DWI at b value of 600 s/mm² and (*C*) ADC map qualitatively show an area of restricted diffusion, seen as high signal intensity on DWI and low signal intensity on ADC. (*D*) Quantitative analysis is performed by drawing an ROI in the area of interest on the ADC map.

dependent on the b factor, and given heterogeneity of studies and breast tumors, a specific ADC threshold value to differentiate benign and malignant lesions has not been established. Examples of false positives on DWI include intraductal papillomas, atypical ductal hyperplasia, intramammary lymph nodes, bleeding, and infection; false negatives include mucinous carcinomas (Fig. 7).[53–57]

The addition of DWI to DCE–MR imaging can improve diagnostic accuracy.[57–60] In a study of 83 suspicious MR imaging–detected breast lesions, the addition of ADC criteria to DCE–MR imaging resulted in increased PPV of 47%

compared with 37% for DCE–MR imaging alone.[57] Dijkstra and colleagues[58] reported that quantitative DWI implemented after DCE–MR imaging significantly improved specificity for BI-RADS 3 and 4 breast lesions, with a combined sensitivity of 99.1%, specificity of 34.8%, and NPV of 92.9%. Similarly, El Khouli and colleagues[59] showed that ADC contributed significantly to improve discrimination of benign and malignant lesions in a multivariate model incorporating DCE–MR imaging morphologic and kinetic factors, reducing the false-positive rate from 36% to 24%. Yabuuchi and colleagues[60] reported improved sensitivity of 92% and specificity of

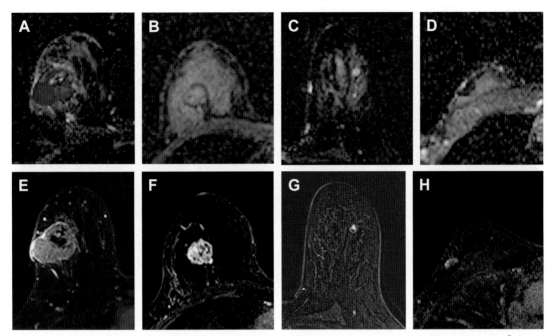

Fig. 7. Comparison of ADC values of benign and malignant lesions, obtained using a b value of 800 s/mm², for (A) invasive ductal carcinoma (0.86 × 10⁻³ mm²/s), (B) mucinous carcinoma (2.24 × 10⁻³ mm²/s), (C) papilloma (2.04 × 10⁻³ mm²/s), and (D) fibroadenoma (1.69 × 10⁻³ mm²/s). Corresponding postcontrast axial subtracted images for each lesion are seen in *row 2* (*E–H*, respectively).

86% when combining DWI and DCE–MR imaging. The authors also found that malignant masses had lower ADC values than malignant nonmass lesions and that optimal diagnostic performance was achieved by using separate criteria for mass and nonmass lesions.

Tumor detection

In addition to improving diagnostic accuracy of MR imaging, DWI has potential as an alternate tool for noncontrast breast screening. Because malignant tumors are more cellular than normal tissue, they often appear hyperintense to surrounding tissues on DWI (Fig. 8). In a study of 118 mammographically and clinically occult breast lesions, Partridge and colleagues[61] found that 89% of malignancies were hyperintense on DWI, with lower ADC values for malignant compared with benign lesions. In their study of 70 women with breast malignancies, Kuroki-Suzuki and co-workers[62] reported similar sensitivity of DWI and short TI inversion recovery criteria compared with DCE–MR imaging for detecting cancers. Baltzer and colleagues[63] also reported comparable sensitivity and specificity between DCE–MR imaging and unenhanced sequences (T2-weighted images and DWI) for breast cancer detection. In their reader study, McDonald and coworkers[64] reported that DWI can identify mammographically

occult cancers in elevated-risk women with dense breasts, with a sensitivity of 45%, specificity of 91%, PPV of 62%, and NPV of 83%. Similarly, in the reader study by Yabuuchi and colleagues,[65] DWI was more accurate than mammography, with an AUC for mean receiver operating characteristic curve of 0.73 compared with 0.64 for mammography. Such data show potential for using DWI as an adjunct to mammography without the costs and toxicity associated with DCE–MR imaging.

However, DWI cannot detect all lesions identified by DCE–MR imaging (Fig. 9). In a blinded reader study of 42 lesions, 42% of malignant breast lesions identified on DCE–MR imaging were not visible on DWI.[65] Tozaki and Fukuma[66] also reported that 32% of nonmass DCIS could not be detected on DWI. Further study is needed to determine whether sensitivity can be improved with higher field strengths to increase SNR or spatial resolution.

Tumor characterization

Current literature suggests that DWI may also be helpful for characterizing malignancies. Several studies have reported correlations between ADC values and tumor grade and hormone receptor status. It has been reported that high-grade invasive cancers have lower ADC values compared

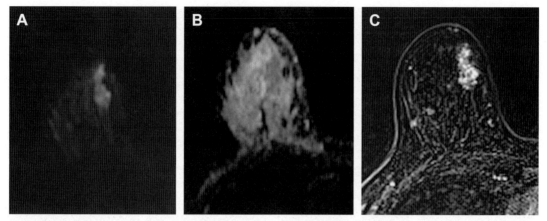

Fig. 8. Tumor detection with DWI. A 49-year-old woman with grade 2 DCIS in the upper central right breast. (*A*) DWI shows an area of restricted diffusion (high signal intensity compared with noncancerous tissue) with corresponding low signal intensity on (*B*) ADC map, with ADC value of 1.3×10^{-3} mm^2/s. (*C*) Corresponding postcontrast subtracted image demonstrating segmental nonmass enhancement.

with intermediate- or low-grade cancers and DCIS.[67,68] In their study of 192 cancers, Martincich and colleagues[69] found a correlation between ADC and receptor status, with ADC significantly higher in ER-negative versus ER-positive tumors and HER2-enriched tumors demonstrating the highest median ADC value. Jeh and colleagues[70] also reported a significant correlation between ADC values and ER expression and HER2 expression, whereas Choi and colleagues[71] reported that low ADC values were correlated with positive expression of ER, PR, and increased Ki-67 index. Higher ADC values have been reported in triple-negative tumors compared with other subtypes,[72]

likely related to intratumoral necrosis and decreased cellularity.

In addition to characterizing invasive carcinomas, DWI may have a role in distinguishing low- and high-grade DCIS, which could have significant impact in customizing treatment of patients with newly diagnosed DCIS. Studies have reported higher ADC values for DCIS compared with invasive carcinoma.[56,73,74] Furthermore, Iima and colleagues[73] reported a negative correlation between ADC values and DCIS grade. In their series of 74 pure DCIS lesions, Rahbar and colleagues[74] found that low-grade DCIS had higher visibility and contrast-ratio values compared with

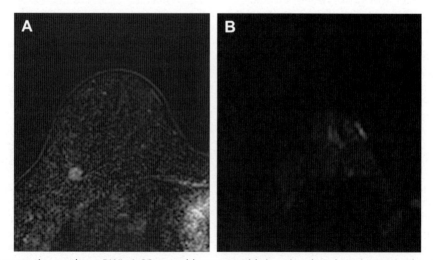

Fig. 9. False-negative result on DWI. A 26-year-old woman with invasive ductal carcinoma in the upper outer right breast. (*A*) Axial postcontrast subtraction image demonstrates an irregular enhancing mass in the upper outer breast without evidence of restricted diffusion on corresponding DWI (*B*).

high-grade DCIS, although there were no differences in ADC values.

Response to therapy

The potential of DWI for predicting treatment response to neoadjuvant therapy is an active area of investigation. In contrast to traditional DCE–MR imaging features and assessment of tumor size, DWI may allow earlier and more accurate evaluation of treatment response by reflecting changes in tumor cellularity and membrane integrity leading to increased water diffusion and ADC values. Several studies have reported that increases in ADC occur earlier than changes in lesion size with treatment.[75–77] In addition, ADC values (baseline and change) were shown to be predictive of clinical response.[76,78,79] In their study of 31 patients undergoing neoadjuvant chemotherapy, Fangberget and colleagues[80] reported that mid-treatment ADC was predictive of pCR (**Fig. 10**). Lastly, Woodhams and colleagues[81] investigated the utility of DWI to detect residual disease before surgery. They found DWI to be 97% sensitive and 89% specific in detecting residual disease in 69 patients post neoadjuvant chemotherapy, compared with 93% sensitivity and 56% specificity for DCE–MR imaging.

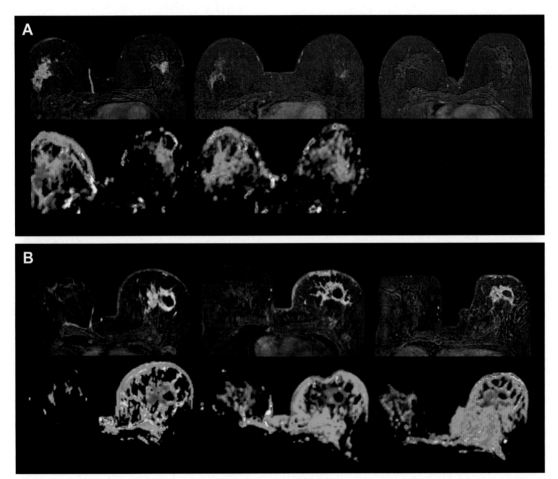

Fig. 10. Axial greyscale subtraction MR images and color-coded ADC maps from a patient obtaining pCR (*A*) and a patient not responding to neoadjuvant chemotherapy (*B*) before treatment (*left column*), after four cycles of neoadjuvant therapy (*middle column*), and before surgery (*right column*). Both patients had locally advanced invasive ductal carcinoma grade 3. The responding patient showed a 55% reduction in longest tumor diameter at MR imaging after four cycles of neoadjuvant chemotherapy. In the nonresponding patient tumor diameter increased by 5%. Tumor ADC increased by 155% between Tp0 (0.80×10^{-3} mm^2/s) and Tp1 (2.01×10^{-3} mm^2/s) in the responding patient, but remained unchanged in the nonresponder (1.21×10^{-3} mm^2/s and 1.35×10^{-3} mm^2/s at Tp0 and Tp1, respectively). (*From* Fangberget A, Nilsen LB, Hole KH, et al. Neoadjuvant chemotherapy in breast cancer-response evaluation and prediction of response to treatment using dynamic contrast-enhanced and diffusion-weighted MR imaging. Eur Radiol 2011;21(6):1193; with permission.)

Although such data show promise in using DWI to evaluate for treatment response, ADC was not shown to be predictive of clinical response in other studies.[46,81,82] These differences may be attributable to differences in ADC measurement, study populations, lesion pathology, and patient selection. Larger studies are needed to validate the use of ADC as a predictive biomarker.

Limitations

There are several limitations to the implementation of DWI in routine clinical practice. Because there is no consensus for an accepted range of b values for DWI, generalizable recommendations for ADC threshold values cannot be made, with cutoff values between malignant and benign lesions ranging from 1.1 to 1.6×10^{-3} mm^2/s.[54] In addition, ADC values are highly dependent on imaging acquisition and analysis methods used, with wide variation reported in the literature. Underlying pathophysiologic features of the lesions can also affect ADC values. Technical considerations, including artifacts caused by susceptibility, chemical shift, or distortion, can impair lesion visibility on DWI and ADC measurement. The low spatial resolution of DWI may also impair detection of small cancers and characterization of lesion morphology, although this may be improved with higher SNR seen with higher magnetic field strength. Further studies are warranted to identify standards for acquisition, display, and integration of DWI to allow for improved diagnostic accuracy.

Summary of Diffusion-Weighted Imaging

DWI is a noncontrast MR imaging technique that provides information on tissue cellularity and microstructure and has the potential to aid in the detection, diagnosis, and evaluation of treatment response for breast cancer. Malignant lesions show restricted diffusion, with high signal intensity on DWI and low ADC values. False positives on DWI include intraductal papillomas, atypical ductal hyperplasia, intramammary lymph nodes, bleeding, and infection; false negatives include mucinous carcinoma. The choice of b values affects lesion signal intensity at DWI and the quantitative analysis of ADC values. DWI may provide an alternate tool for noncontrast breast cancer screening. DWI may offer earlier and more precise information for predicting treatment response to neoadjuvant chemotherapy and assessing residual disease.

SUMMARY

Advancements in breast MR imaging techniques, such as abbreviated MR imaging, pharmacokinetic modeling, and DWI, provide valuable new capabilities for breast MR imaging. Although further study is needed to facilitate their implementation in routine clinical practice, current data suggest that these developments have the ability to improve detection, diagnostic accuracy, and treatment monitoring for breast cancer.

REFERENCES

1. DeMartini W, Lehman C. A review of current evidence-based clinical applications for breast magnetic resonance imaging. Top Magn Reson Imaging 2008;19:143–50.
2. Lehman CD. Clinical indications: what is the evidence? Eur J Radiol 2012;81(S1):S82–4.
3. Kuhl C. The current status of breast MR imaging. Part I. Choice of technique, image interpretation, diagnostic accuracy, and transfer to clinical practice. Radiology 2007;244:356–78.
4. Sardanelli F, Podo F, Santoro F, et al. Multicenter surveillance of women at high genetic breast cancer risk using mammography, ultrasonography, and contrast-enhanced magnetic resonance imaging (the High Breast Cancer Risk Italian 1 study): Final results. Invest Radiol 2011;46:94–105.
5. Kuhl CK, Schrading S, Leutner CC, et al. Mammography, breast ultrasound, and magnetic resonance imaging for surveillance of women at high familial risk for breast cancer. J Clin Oncol 2005;23:8469–76.
6. Berg WA, Zhang Z, Lehrer D, et al. Detection of breast cancer with addition of annual screening ultrasound or a single screening MRI to mammography in women with elevated breast cancer risk. JAMA 2012;307:1394–404.
7. Lehman CD, Isaacs C, Schnall MD. Cancer yield of mammography, MR, and US in high-risk women: prospective multi-institution breast cancer screen study. Radiology 2007;244(2):381–8.
8. Kuhl C, Schrading S, Strobel K, et al. Abbreviated breast magnetic resonance imaging (MRI): first postcontrast subtracted images and maximum-intensity projection - a novel approach to breast cancer screening with MRI. J Clin Oncol 2014;32:2304–10.
9. Heacock L, Melsaether AN, Heller SL, et al. Evaluation of a known breast cancer using an abbreviated breast MRI protocol: correlation of imaging characteristics and pathology with lesion detection and conspicuity. Eur J Radiol 2016;85(4):815–23.
10. Mango VL, Morris EA, Dershaw DD, et al. Abbreviated protocol for breast MRI: are multiple sequences needed for cancer detection? Eur J Radiol 2015;84:65–70.
11. Grimm LJ, Soo MS, Yoon S, et al. Abbreviated screening protocol for breast MRI: a feasibility study. Acad Radiol 2015;22(9):1157–62.

12. Moschetta M, Telegrafo M, Rella L, et al. Abbreviated combined MR protocol: a new faster strategy for characterizing breast lesions. Clin Breast Cancer 2016;16(3):207–11.

13. Mann RM, Kuhl C, Kinkel K, et al. Breast MRI: guidelines from the European Society of breast imaging. Eur Radiol 2008;18:1307–18.

14. Lehman CD, Blume JD, DeMartini WB, et al. Accuracy and interpretation time of computer-aided detection among novice and experienced breast MRI readers. AJR Am J Roentgenol 2013;200:W683–9.

15. Garg AS, Rapelyea JA, Rechtman LR, et al. Full-field digital mammographic interpretation with prior analog versus prior digitized analog mammography: time for interpretation. Am J Roentgenol 2011;196:1436–8.

16. Tchou PM, Haygood TM, Atkinson EN, et al. Interpretation time of computer-aided detection at screening mammography. Radiology 2010;257:40–6.

17. Berg WA, Blume JD, Cormack JB, et al. Combined screening with ultrasound and mammography vs mammography alone in women at elevated risk of breast cancer. JAMA 2008;299:2151–63.

18. Kuhl C, Klaschik S, Mielcarek P, et al. Do T2-weighted pulse sequences help with the differential diagnosis of enhancing lesions in dynamic breast MRI? J Magn Reson Imaging 1999;9:187–96.

19. Arponen O, Masarwah A, Sutela A, et al. Incidentally detected enhancing lesions found in breast MRI: analysis of apparent diffusion coefficient and T2 signal intensity significantly improves specificity. Eur Radiol 2016;26(12):4361–70.

20. Partridge SC, Stone KM, Strigel RM, et al. Breast DCE-MRI: influence of postcontrast timing on automated lesion kinetics assessments and discrimination of benign and malignant lesions. Acad Radiol 2014;21:1195–203.

21. Tofts PS, Brix G, Buckley DL, et al. Estimating kinetic parameters from dynamic contrast enhanced T(1)-weighted MRI of a diffusable tracer: standardized quantities and symbols. J Magn Reson Imaging 1999;10:223–32.

22. Tofts PS, Kermode AG. Measurement of the blood-brain barrier permeability and leakage space using dynamic MR imaging. 1. Fundamental concepts. Magn Reson Med 1991;17:357–67.

23. Yankeelov TE, Arlinhaus LA, Li X, et al. The role of magnetic resonance imaging biomarkers in clinical trials of treatment response in cancer. Semin Oncol 2011;38(1):16–25.

24. DCE-MRI Technical Committee. DCE-MRI Quantification Profile, Quantitative Imaging Biomarkers Alliance. Version 1.0. Publicly Reviewed Version. QIBA; 2012. Available at: RSNA.org/QIBA.

25. Yankeelov TE, Luci JJ, Lepage M, et al. Quantitative pharmacokinetic analysis of DCE-MRI data without an arterial input function: a reference region model. Magn Reson Imaging 2005;23(4):519–29.

26. Furman-Haran E, Schechtman E, Kelcz F, et al. Magnetic resonance imaging reveals functional diversity of the vasculature in benign and malignant breast lesions. Cancer 2005;104(4):708–18.

27. Gibbs P, Liney GP, Lowry M, et al. Differentiation of benign and malignant sub-1 cm breast lesions using dynamic contrast enhanced MRI. Breast 2004;13:115–21.

28. Schabel MC, Morrell GR, Oh KY, et al. Pharmacokinetic mapping for lesion classification in dynamic breast MRI. J Magn Reson Imaging 2010;31:1371–8.

29. Huang W, Tudorica LA, Li X, et al. Discrimination of benign and malignant breast lesions by using shutter-speed dynamic contrast-enhanced MR imaging. Radiology 2011;261(2):394–403.

30. El Khouli RH, Macura KJ, Kamel IR, et al. 3-T dynamic contrast-enhanced MRI of the breast: pharmacokinetic parameters versus conventional kinetic curve analysis. AJR Am J Roentgenol 2011;197:1498–505.

31. Veltman J, Stoutjesdijk M, Mann R, et al. Contrast-enhanced magnetic resonance imaging of the breast: the value of pharmacokinetic parameters derived from fast dynamic imaging during initial enhancement in classifying lesions. Eur Radiol 2008;18:1123–33.

32. Pickles MD, Lowry M, Manton DJ, et al. Role of DCE MRI in monitoring early response of locally advanced breast cancer to neoadjuvant chemotherapy. Breast Cancer Res Treat 2005;91:1–10.

33. Hayes C, Padhani AR, Leach MO. Assessing changes in tumour vascular function using dynamic contrast-enhanced magnetic resonance imaging. NMR Biomed 2002;15:154–63.

34. Wasser K, Klein SK, Fink C, et al. Evaluation of neoadjuvant chemotherapeutic response of breast cancer using dynamic MRI with high temporal resolution. Eur Radiol 2003;13:80–7.

35. Padhani AR, Hayes C, Assersohn L, et al. Prediction of clinicopathologic response of breast cancer to primary chemotherapy at contrast-enhanced MR imaging: initial clinical results. Radiology 2006;239:361–74.

36. Li SP, Makris A, Beresford MJ. Use of dynamic contrast-enhanced MR imaging to predict survival in patients with primary breast cancer undergoing neoadjuvant chemotherapy. Radiology 2011;260(1):68–78.

37. Ah-See M, Makris A, Taylor NJ, et al. Early changes in functional dynamic magnetic resonance imaging predict for pathologic response to neoadjuvant chemotherapy in primary breast cancer. Clin Cancer Res 2008;14:6580–9.

38. Drisis S, Metens T, Ignatiadis M, et al. Quantitative DCE-MRI for prediction of pathological complete response following neoadjuvant treatment for locally

advanced breast cancer: the impact of breast cancer subtypes on the diagnostic accuracy. Eur Radiol 2016;26:1474–84.

39. Li X, Abramson RG, Arlinghaus LR, et al. Multiparametric magnetic resonance imaging for predicting pathological response after the first cycle of neoadjuvant chemotherapy in breast cancer. Invest Radiol 2015;50(4):195–204.

40. Tudorica A, Oh KY, Chui SY, et al. Early prediction and evaluation of breast cancer response to neoadjuvant chemotherapy using quantitative DCE-MRI. Transl Oncol 2016;9(1):8–17.

41. Prevos R, Smidt ML, Tjan-Heijnen VCG, et al. Pretreatment differences and early response monitoring of neoadjuvant chemotherapy in breast cancer patients using magnetic resonance imaging: a systematic review. Eur Radiol 2012;22:2607–16.

42. Marinovich ML, Sardinelli F, Ciatto S, et al. Early prediction of pathologic response to neoadjuvant therapy in breast cancer: systematic review of the accuracy of MRI. Breast 2012;21(5):669–77.

43. Yu Y, Jiang Q, Miao Y, et al. Quantitative analysis of clinical dynamic contrast-enhanced MR imaging for evaluating treatment response in human breast cancer. Radiology 2010;257(1):47–55.

44. Li SP, Taylor NJ, Makris A, et al. Primary human breast adenocarcinoma: imaging and histologic correlates of intrinsic susceptibility-weighted MR imaging before and during chemotherapy. Radiology 2010;257(3):643–52.

45. Yu HJ, Chen J, Mehta RS, et al. MRI measurements of tumour size and pharmacokinetic parameters as early predictors of response in breast cancer patients undergoing neoadjuvant anthracycline chemotherapy. J Magn Reson Imaging 2007;26:615–23.

46. Manton DJ, Chaturvedi A, Hubbard A, et al. Neoadjuvant chemotherapy in breast cancer: early response prediction with quantitative MR imaging and spectroscopy. Br J Cancer 2006;94:427–35.

47. Baek HM, Chen JH, Nie K, et al. Predicting pathologic response to neoadjuvant chemotherapy in breast cancer using MR imaging and quantitative 1H MR spectroscopy. Radiology 2009;251(3):653–62.

48. Cho N, Im SA, Park IA, et al. Breast cancer: early prediction of response to neoadjuvant chemotherapy using parametric response maps for MR imaging. Radiology 2014;272(2):385–96.

49. Partridge SC. Future applications and innovations of clinical breast magnetic resonance imaging. Top Magn Reson Imaging 2008;19:171–6.

50. Koh DM, Collins DJ. Diffusion-weighted MRI in the body: applications and challenges in oncology. AJR Am J Roentgenol 2007;188(6):1622–35.

51. Guo Y, Cai YQ, Cai ZL, et al. Differentiation of clinically benign and malignant breast lesions using diffusion-weighted imaging. J Magn Reson Imaging 2002;16:172–8.

52. Woodhams R, Matsunaga K, Iwabuchi K, et al. Diffusion-weighted imaging of malignant breast tumors: the usefulness of apparent diffusion coefficient (ADC) value and ADC map for the detection of malignant breast tumors and evaluation of cancer extension. J Comput Assist Tomogr 2005;29:644–9.

53. Brandao AC, Lehman CD, Partridge SC. Breast magnetic resonance imaging: diffusion-weighted imaging. Magn Reson Imaging Clin N Am 2013;21: 321–36.

54. Tsushima Y, Takahashi-Taketomi A, Endo K. Magnetic resonance (MR) differential diagnosis of breast tumors using apparent diffusion coefficient (ADC) on 1.5-T. J Magn Reson Imaging 2009;30(2):249–55.

55. Parsian S, Rahbar H, Allison KH, et al. Nonmalignant breast lesions: ADCs of benign and high-risk subtypes assessed as false-positive at dynamic enhanced MR imaging. Radiology 2012;265(3): 696–706.

56. Woodhams R, Matsunaga K, Kan S, et al. ADC mapping of benign and malignant breast tumors. Magn Reson Med Sci 2005;4:35–42.

57. Partridge SC, DeMartini WB, Kurland BF, et al. Quantitative diffusion-weighted imaging as an adjunct to conventional breast MRI for improved positive predictive value. AJR Am J Roentgenol 2009;193(6):1716–22.

58. Dijkstra H, Dorrius MD, Wielema M, et al. Quantitative DWI implemented after DCE-MRI yields increased specificity for BI-RADS 3 and 4 breast lesions. J Magn Reson Imaging 2016;44(6):1642–9.

59. El Khouli RH, Jacobs MA, Mezban SD, et al. Diffusion-weighted imaging improves the diagnostic accuracy of conventional 3.0-T breast MR imaging. Radiology 2010;256:64–73.

60. Yabuuchi H, Matsuo Y, Kamitani T, et al. Non-mass-like enhancement on contrast-enhanced breast MR imaging: lesion characterization using combination of dynamic contrast-enhanced and diffusion-weighted MR images. Eur J Radiol 2010;75(1): e126–32.

61. Partridge SC, Demartini WB, Kurland BF, et al. Differential diagnosis of mammographically and clinically occult breast lesions on diffusion-weighted MRI. J Magn Reson Imaging 2010;31:562–70.

62. Kuroki-Suzuki S, Kuroki Y, Nasu K, et al. Detecting breast cancer with non-contrast MR imaging: combining diffusion-weighted and STIR imaging. Magn Reson Med Sci 2007;6(1):21–7.

63. Baltzer PA, Benndorf M, Dietzel M, et al. Sensitivity and specificity of unenhanced MR mammography (DWI combined with T2-weighted TSE imaging, ueMRM) for the differentiation of mass lesions. Eur Radiol 2010;20(5):1101–10.

64. McDonald ES, Hammersley JA, Chou SHS, et al. Performance of DWI as a rapid unenhanced

technique for detecting mammographically occult breast cancer in elevated-risk women with dense breasts. AJR Am J Roentgenol 2016;207:205–16.

65. Yabuuchi H, Matsuo Y, Sunami S, et al. Detection of non-palpable breast cancer in asymptomatic women by using unenhanced diffusion-weighted and T2-weighted MR imaging: comparison with mammography and dynamic contrast-enhanced MR imaging. Eur Radiol 2011;21(1):11–7.

66. Tozaki M, Fukuma E. 1H MR spectroscopy and diffusion-weighted imaging of the breast: are they useful tools for characterizing breast lesions before biopsy? AJR Am J Roentgenol 2009;193:840–9.

67. Razek AA, Gaballa G, Denewer A, et al. Invasive ductal carcinoma: correlation of apparent diffusion coefficient value with pathological prognostic factors. NMR Biomed 2010;23:619–23.

68. Costantini M, Belli P, Rinaldi P, et al. Diffusion weighted imaging in breast cancer: relationship between apparent diffusion coefficient and tumour aggressiveness. Clin Radiol 2010;65:1005–12.

69. Martincich L, Aglietta M, Regge D, et al. Correlations between diffusion-weighted imaging and breast cancer biomarkers. Eur Radiol 2012;22(7):1519–28.

70. Jeh SK, Kim SH, Kim HS, et al. Correlation of the apparent diffusion coefficient value and dynamic magnetic resonance imaging findings with prognostic factors in invasive ductal carcinoma. J Magn Reson Imaging 2011;33:102–9.

71. Choi SY, Chang YW, Park HJ, et al. Correlation of the apparent diffusion coefficiency values on diffusion-weighted imaging with prognostic factors for breast cancer. Br J Radiol 2012;85(1016):e474–9.

72. Youk JH, Son EJ, Chung J, et al. Triple-negative invasive breast cancer on dynamic contrast-enhanced and diffusion-weighted MR imaging: comparison with other breast cancer subtypes. Eur Radiol 2012;22(8):1724–34.

73. Iima M, Le Bihan D, Okumura S, et al. Apparent diffusion coefficient as an MR imaging biomarker of low-risk ductal carcinoma in situ: a pilot study. Radiology 2011;260(2):364–72.

74. Rahbar H, Partridge SC, Eby PR, et al. Characterization of ductal carcinoma in situ on diffusion weighted breast MRI. Eur Radiol 2011;21:2011–9.

75. Pickles MD, Gibbs P, Lowry M, et al. Diffusion changes precede size reduction in neoadjuvant treatment of breast cancer. Magn Reson Imaging 2006;24:843–7.

76. Sharma U, Danishad KK, Seenu V, et al. Longitudinal study of the assessment by MRI and diffusion-weighted imaging of tumor response in patients with locally advanced breast cancer undergoing neoadjuvant chemotherapy. NMR Biomed 2009;22:104–13.

77. Theilmann RJ, Borders R, Trouard TP, et al. Changes in water mobility measured by diffusion MRI predict response of metastatic breast cancer to chemotherapy. Neoplasia 2004;6:831–7.

78. Iacconi C, Giannelli M, Marini C, et al. The role of mean diffusivity (MD) as a predictive index of the response to chemotherapy in locally advanced breast cancer: a preliminary study. Eur Radiol 2010;20:303–8.

79. Park SH, Moon WK, Cho N, et al. Diffusion-weighted MR imaging: pretreatment prediction of response to neoadjuvant chemotherapy in patients with breast cancer. Radiology 2010;257:56–63.

80. Fangberget A, Nilsen LB, Hole KH, et al. Neoadjuvant chemotherapy in breast cancer-response evaluation and prediction of response to treatment using dynamic contrast-enhanced and diffusion-weighted MR imaging. Eur Radiol 2011;21(6):1188–99.

81. Woodhams R, Kakita S, Hata H, et al. Identification of residual breast carcinoma following neoadjuvant chemotherapy: diffusion-weighted imaging – comparison with contrast-enhanced MR imaging and pathologic findings. Radiology 2010;254:357–66.

82. Nilsen L, Fangberget A, Geier O, et al. Diffusion weighted magnetic resonance imaging for pretreatment prediction and monitoring of treatment response of patients with locally advanced breast cancer undergoing neoadjuvant chemotherapy. Acta Oncol 2010;49(3):354–60.

Breast PET/MR Imaging

Amy Melsaether, MD[a],*, Linda Moy, MD[b]

KEYWORDS

- PET/MR imaging • Breast MR imaging • Breast PET • Breast PET/MR imaging • Multiparametric
- Breast cancer • Whole-body PET/MR imaging

KEY POINTS

- PET/MR imaging is a flexible hybrid technology that can be customized with any PET tracer or MR imaging sequence. For localized breast PET/MR imaging examinations, 18F-FDG-PET and DCE-MR imaging data sets are typically acquired, often also with DWI.
- For whole-body PET/MR imaging examinations in the setting of breast cancer, 18F-FDG-PET data are acquired with contrast-enhanced MR imaging, DWI, and additional T2-weighted sequences.
- In breast PET/MR imaging examinations, PET and MR imaging provide complimentary information that can yield increased sensitivity for satellite lesions and axillary lymph node metastases over either examination alone.
- In breast PET/MR imaging examinations, multiple PET- and MR imaging–derived parameters are being investigated for their abilities to predict and assess response to treatments.
- In whole-body imaging, PET/MR imaging is more sensitive than PET/CT for lesion detection, especially for lesions in the bone, liver, and breast, and requires approximately half of the radiation required for PET/CT.

INTRODUCTION

New hybrid imaging technology brings together the molecular sensitivity of PET, the high-contrast anatomic imaging of MR imaging, and depending on the pulse sequences used, the functional imaging capabilities of MR imaging, in a single PET/MR exam. PET and MR imaging each already play central roles in breast cancer imaging, MR imaging predominantly as a focused examination, screening for and evaluating the extent of disease pretherapy and posttherapy,[1] and PET predominantly as a whole-body examination, assessing for distant metastases during initial staging and later surveillance.[2,3] However, PET, specifically positron emission mammography, is also used in focused breast examinations[4] and whole-body MR imaging has also been used in imaging metastatic spread.[5,6] PET and MR images of the breast have been fused[7–10] to investigate potential benefits of combining these modalities. Now, PET/MR imaging hybrid scanners, depending on the model, simultaneously or sequentially acquire and coregister PET and MR imaging data. These simultaneous scans are being put to use in patients with breast cancer not only for disease detection, but also elucidating imaging biomarkers, which may eventually guide treatments and predict prognoses. This article provides an overview of breast and whole-body examination feasibility and techniques, summarizes PET and MR imaging of the breast for lesion detection, outlines current investigations into multiparametric PET/MR imaging of the breast, looks at PET/MR imaging in the setting of neoadjuvant chemotherapy (NAC), and reviews the pros and cons of PET/MR whole-body imaging in the setting of metastatic or suspected metastatic breast cancer.

No disclosures, either author.
a Department of Radiology, New York University School of Medicine, 160 East 34th Street, 3rd Floor, New York, NY 10016, USA; b Department of Radiology, Center for Advanced Imaging Innovation and Research (CAI(2)R), New York University School of Medicine, 160 East 34th Street, 3rd Floor, New York, NY 10016, USA
* Corresponding author.
E-mail addresses: amy.melsaether@nyumc.org; amymgiroux@gmail.com

Radiol Clin N Am 55 (2017) 579–589
http://dx.doi.org/10.1016/j.rcl.2016.12.011

PET/MR IMAGING FEASIBILITY AND PROTOCOLS
Technical Feasibility

Accurate quantitation of radiotracer activity via standardized uptake values (SUVs) in PET imaging is highly important, especially for comparing between examinations, and requires reliable attenuation correction. Computed tomography (CT) attenuation correction is based on tissue density information (Hounsfield units) provided by CT.[11] MR imaging, however, does not rely on tissue density in generating signal and therefore PET/MR imaging required a new method for attenuation correction, one that addressed the patient's attenuation map and attenuation maps for MR imaging hardware, such as coils. Techniques for MR imaging–based attenuation correction include the Dixon sequence–derived segmentation method, which assigns attenuation coefficients after tissue identification using standard reference values,[12,13] and an atlas-based method, which corrects images using a template data set.[13] The segmentation method is currently in use by commercial scanners.

For breast examinations, generating attenuation correction maps for breast coils was an early issue. Fortunately, feasibility studies integrating 4- and now 16-channel breast coils into a simultaneous PET/MR imaging system (Biograph mMR, Siemens Healthcare, Erlangen, Germany) have shown technical success with accurate SUV quantification and high MR image quality.[14,15] Successful prone hybrid breast imaging has also been demonstrated with sequential PET/MR imaging (Philips Ingenuity, Philips Healthcare, Cleveland, OH).[16]

SUV values derived from PET/MR imaging via MR imaging–based attenuation correction and from PET/CT via CT-based attenuation correction have shown strong correlations in breast cancer metastases[17,18] and mostly moderate correlations in normal tissues,[17–22] validating the use of PET/MR imaging–derived SUV values in breast cancer imaging. The stronger correlations in metastases may relate, at least in part, to lesser washout in metastases compared with normal tissues because PET/MR imaging was performed after PET/CT in these studies. Finally, although correlations between PET/MR imaging and PET/CT-derived SUV values are high in breast cancer metastases, SUV values should not be compared between longitudinal PET/CT and PET/MR imaging examinations in the same patient because they are similar but not identical examinations.

Tracers

In breast cancer imaging, fluorine-18 fluorodeoxyglucose (^{18}F-FDG), which images cellular glucose uptake,[23] is the tracer most commonly used for localized and whole-body examinations. Typically, breast cancer cells are more metabolically active and demonstrate higher glucose uptake than their background organs, thus allowing for lesion detection.

[18]F sodium fluoride (Na-F), a bone-specific radiotracer, has also been administered in patients with breast cancer[24,25] to look for bony metastatic disease. In a recent study by Piccardo and colleagues,[24] ^{18}F-NaF PET/CT demonstrated higher sensitivity (100%) for osseous lesions than ^{18}F-FDG PET/CT (72%). However, none of the ^{18}F-FDG PET/CT-negative patients went on to have disease progression during the follow-up period. Moreover, ^{18}F-FDG SUV mean and whole-body bone metabolic burden were independently and significantly associated with overall survival, whereas none of the ^{18}F-NaF PET/CT parameters were associated with overall survival. This study suggests ^{18}F-FDG has a closer relationship with biologically active breast cancer than does ^{18}F-NaF, likely because ^{18}F-FDG uptake into skeletal metastases is thought to be predominantly within breast cancer tumor cells, whereas ^{18}F-NaF uptake reflects osseous blood flow and bone remodeling[26] and may provide positive results in the setting of osseous remodeling following chemotherapy.

Breast cancer can be homogenous or change gene expression patterns over time. This could be because of a variety of reasons including a response to therapy, or have metastases with biologies that differ from the index lesion. Therefore, several additional tracers in development are particularly exciting for their potential to noninvasively assess therapeutic targets, such as hormone receptors[27,28] and human epidermal growth factor receptor 2 (HER2).[29–31] This in turn helps improve individualized treatments. Additional tracers that may become useful in breast cancer imaging target gastrin-releasing peptide receptors, cellular proliferation, membrane lipid synthesis, and amino acid transport and are well reviewed by Tabouret-Viaud and coworkers.[32]

Suggested Protocols

Following a pre-examination fast of at least 4 hours, an ^{18}F-FDG injection of approximately 555 MBq is performed followed by a rest for 45 minutes in a darkened, quiet room before beginning imaging. For localized breast PET/MR imaging, the patient is then placed in prone position in a dedicated breast coil. PET acquisition can either begin after the 45-minute resting period or, if dynamic PET data are desired, the injection can occur on the scanner and imaging can begin at the time of injection. For simultaneous PET/MR imaging, PET data acquisition can be performed throughout the entire examination and therefore is not the rate-limiting factor. MR imaging sequences run during PET/MR imaging vary according to desired information. Typically, routine dynamic contrast-enhanced (DCE) MR imaging sequences including a T2-weighted fat-suppressed, T1-weighted non-fat-suppressed, a precontrast fat-suppressed T1-weighted radial three-dimensional (3D) gradient echo sequence, and up to four postcontrast fat-saturated T1-weighted radial 3D gradient echo sequences are run. Diffusion-weighted imaging (DWI) sequences and modified postcontrast sequences can also be run and processed to assess additional parameters, such as diffusion and perfusion, and are described later. Three-dimensional proton MR spectroscopic imaging (3D 1H-MRSI) has also been performed in the setting of breast PET/MR imaging.[33]

For whole-body breast MR imaging in the setting of breast cancer, fasting time, injection dose, and resting time is similar to a focused breast examination. The examination is performed in supine position with dedicated PET/MR imaging head and flexible body matrix coils and most often consists of six to seven stations from thighs to vertex, depending on the height of the patient. PET data are acquired for at least 2 minutes per station (or for the duration of the station) when the examination is begun around 45 minutes postinjection and as such, the MR imaging sequences are usually the rate-limiting factor for whole-body

examinations. If PET/MR imaging is performed after PET/CT or after a local breast PET/MR imaging (without an additional FDG injection), PET data can be acquired for longer time periods, up to about 7 minutes per station, to mitigate signal loss caused by tracer clearance. The MR imaging sequences run at each station can vary. The authors find it useful to image from the thighs to the vertex to allow for MR imaging contrast injection during the liver station, which allows for noncontrast T1-weighted images of the bony pelvis and contrast-enhanced T1-weighted liver and brain images. More detailed potential whole-body PET/MR imaging structures are presented in **Table 1**.

MR IMAGING AND PET IN LOCALIZED BREAST EXAMINATIONS

As our most sensitive examination,[34,35] breast MR imaging is commonly used to screen women at high risk, to assess disease extent, to evaluate response to chemotherapy, to assess for occult breast cancers in the setting of axillary metastases, and to problem solve difficult cases.[1] Like all breast imaging modalities, MR imaging yields false-positive results, which require expensive, invasive, and ultimately unnecessary biopsies. On its own, PET/CT is not adequately sensitive for breast cancers, in one study detecting only 30 of 44 invasive cancers 2 cm or less.[36] This low sensitivity is in keeping with the low spatial resolution of PET/CT, which varies according to device, but is approximately 5 to 6 mm full width at half maximum.[32]

Table 1
Suggested MR imaging sequences by station for whole-body PET/MR imaging in the setting of breast cancer

Station	T1-Weighted Sequences	T2-Weighted Sequences
All	Coronal 3D gradient echo for creation of DIXON-based μ-map	Coronal high-speed turbo spin echo T2
Bone/pelvis	Radial 3D gradient echo, noncontrast preferred, or T1 DIXON (fat-containing lesions)	Axial high-speed turbo spin echo, or Axial 3 b-value DWI
Liver/abdomen	Radial 3D fat-suppressed gradient echo with or without contrast	Axial high-speed turbo spin echo, axial 3 B-value DWI, possible axial fat-saturated T2 (fat-containing lesions)
Lung/thorax	Radial 3D fat-suppressed gradient echo with or without contrast	
Brain/head	Postcontrast magnetization prepared rapid gradient echo Precontrast 3D gradient echo useful for hemorrhage	T2 postcontrast FLAIR (leptomeningeal disease)

Comparison and Fusion

When comparing [18]FDG-PET/CT with breast MR imaging for the identification of breast cancers, MR imaging demonstrates increased sensitivity,[7,37,38] especially in subcentimeter lesions,[10,39,40] nonmass lesions,[10] and lobular cancers.[37] Moreover, DCE-MR imaging has been shown to be more sensitive alone than when combined with PET.[7,10,41]

However, Pinker and coworkers[33] further explored PET and MR imaging fusion, using simultaneously acquired PET and multiparametric MR imaging including DCE, DWI, and 3D 1H-MRSI data in 53 malignant and 23 benign breast lesions categorized as BI-RADS 0, 4, or 5 on initial mammographic or sonographic imaging. In contrast to studies using only DCE-MR imaging and PET data, the authors found that all four PET and MR imaging parameters together provided the highest area under the curve (AUC) of 0.935 (0.835–1), and that this AUC was significantly higher than AUCs for DCE–MR imaging or PET alone and for DCE–MR imaging combined with DWI, 3D 1H-MRSI, or PET. The authors' criteria for a positive examination were clear: with three parameters, two or more positive sequences; with four parameters, three or more positive sequences; or, in the case of two positive parameters, a positive DCE-MR imaging sequence. Had this categorization been applied to the tumors in the previously described series, unnecessary biopsies would have been reduced by 50% as compared with DCE–MR imaging alone (three of six biopsies) and by up to 38% as compared with DCE–MR imaging and one additional parameter (3 of 8–10 biopsies).

PET and MR Imaging in Local Staging

When performing examinations for extent of disease, detecting multifocality and nodal disease becomes important. MR imaging has been shown to be more sensitive but less specific than PET/CT[37,38,42] or PET alone for multifocality,[43] whereas PET/CT has generally been shown to have a higher sensitivity for axillary nodal metastases.[38,42,43] PET and MR imaging have demonstrated similar performance for the detection of internal mammary adenopathy.[44] MR imaging and PET/MR imaging have been shown to be more likely than PET/CT to determine the correct maximum diameter of the tumor (T stage), which may be useful in surgical and oncologic planning.[38] Hybrid PET/MR imaging may be of particular use in this extent-of-disease setting, where the increased sensitivity of MR imaging for multifocal disease and the increased sensitivity of PET for axillary nodal disease could come together in a single examination.

Correlating PET and MR Imaging Parameters and Prognostic Factors

PET/dynamic contrast enhancement

A couple of groups have explored relationships between metabolism and perfusion, looking at SUVmax, metabolic tumor volume, total lesion glycolysis, and a PET-derived heterogeneity factor and K trans, a volume transfer coefficient reflecting vascular permeability, Kep, a flux rate constant, and Ve, an extracellular volume ratio reflecting vascular permeability; and the relationships between these parameters and prognostic factors (**Fig. 1**).

Kim and colleagues[45] found an inverse correlation between SUVmax and Ve, where increased glucose metabolism was seen in higher cellularity tumors. On further review of that same group of patients, An and colleagues[46] found that the inverse correlation between SUVmax and Ve held in nontriple negative breast cancers (TNBC), as did a positive correlation between SUVmax and Kep, whereas in TNBC, no correlations between perfusion and metabolic parameters were seen, possibly because of the smaller sample size (n = 17). This group also looked at recurrence-free survival and found that patients with more heterogeneous FDG uptake had worse recurrence-free survival than patients with less heterogeneous tumors.[45] In a smaller study, Margolis and colleagues[47] found that metabolic tumor volume inversely correlated with Kep and K trans and that metastatic burden correlated positively with K trans and SUVmax and negatively with Kep.

PET/diffusion-weighted imaging

The relationships between SUV uptake, apparent diffusion coefficient (ADC) values, and histologic and prognostic factors have been investigated by several groups, with mixed results. Some studies have shown an inverse correlation between SUV and ADC in cancers,[40,48] whereas others have not.[49–51] SUVmax has been shown to positively correlate with many prognostic factors including tumor size,[48–51] nuclear/histologic grade,[48–51] higher Ki67,[40,48,52] TNM staging,[48] TNBC tumor type,[40,51] lymph node positivity,[48,49,51] ER-,[48,49,51] PR-,[48,51] and HER2+ status.[48,49] ADC shows fewer relationships, but has been correlated with PR+,[50] ER+,[51] and HER2- cancers,[50,51] and with tumor size, Ki67 expression, histologic subtype, the presence of axillary metastases, and TNM staging.[48] Karan and colleagues,[49] however, saw no correlations between ADC median and many of these metrics. Low ADC and high SUVmax have been associated with vascular invasion.[40,49] SUVmax correlated

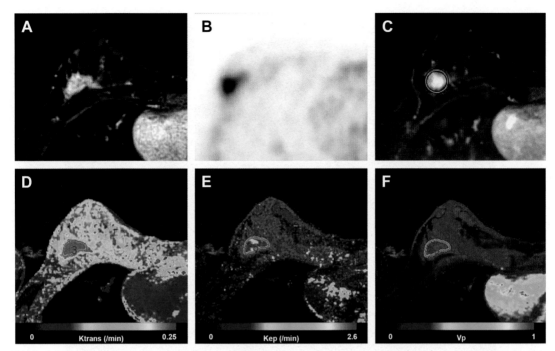

Fig. 1. A 39-year-old woman with ER, PR, and HER2 positive right breast invasive ductal carcinoma. ER, estrogen receptor; PR, progesterone receptor. (A) Axial postcontrast MR imaging shows a 2.5-cm enhancing mass consistent with the known carcinoma. (B) PET axial images demonstrate a corresponding FDG-avid mass. (C) PET/MR imaging fused images. (D–F) Ktrans, kep, and Vp color maps superimposed on axial postcontrast images. Color bar ranges are represented as follows: Ktrans, −0.09 to 0.25 min-1; kep, 0.06 to 2.61 min-1; and Vp, 0% to 1.24%. These values are consistent with a malignant lesion.

inversely with progression-free survival and overall survival.[50] The stronger and more numerous correlations between SUVmax and prognostic factors and survival suggest PET may be of particular interest in predicting clinical outcomes.

PET and MR Imaging and Neoadjuvant Chemotherapy

During therapy

PET/CT and MR imaging have also been investigated in the setting of NAC. Of particular focus has been whether PET or MR imaging during NAC is more useful in predicting pathologic complete response (pCR) and outcome. Now, however, how PET and MR imaging metrics can be used together is of increasing interest (Fig. 2).

Most studies comparing PET and MR imaging aimed at predicting pCR (performed during NAC) show changes in PET and MR metrics, but slightly improved performance with SUVmax in predicting response. Pahk and colleagues[52] looked at patients specifically with luminal B-type breast cancer and found PET imaging outperformed MR imaging because a change in SUV of 69% provided a sensitivity of 86% and a specificity of 100% whereas an MR imaging–based change in

size of 38% provided sensitivity of 64% and specificity of 71%. Similarly, Tateishi and colleagues[53] found that PET (% of original SUVmax) and MR imaging metrics (% of original Kep and % of original area under the time intensity curve at 90 seconds) predicted response to therapy, but that change in SUVmax was the most accurate. Combining modalities and clinical factors, Pengel and colleagues[54] found that age, breast cancer subtype, % change in SUVmax, and % change in largest tumor diameter on MR imaging predicted near pCR. This group then combined metrics and found that changes in SUVmax and tumor diameter together with breast cancer subtype yielded the highest AUC. Looking at outcomes, Lim and colleagues[55] found that lesser declines in SUV (41% threshold), MR slope (−6% threshold), lesser increases in ADC (11% threshold), and ER negativity were associated with poorer disease-free survival. Patients meeting thresholds for lesser declines in SUV and MR slope had a much higher recurrence rate (78%) than those that did not (13%).

In less conventional imaging, Jacobs and colleagues[56] compared sodium (^{23}Na) MR imaging with PET/CT and DCE–MR imaging and found that tissue sodium concentrations increased in all

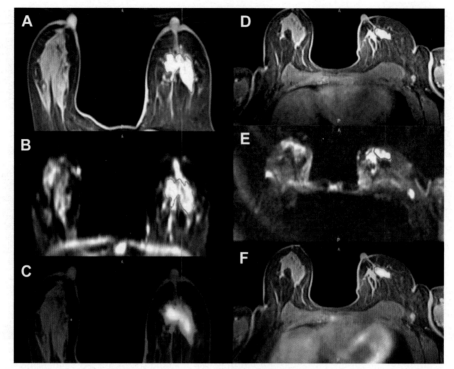

Fig. 2. Preneoadjuvant and postneoadjuvant chemotherapy on PET/MR imaging. A 53-year-old woman with a 3.5-cm invasive ductal carcinoma. (*A*) Axial postcontrast MR imaging shows a 3.8-cm enhancing mass consistent with the known carcinoma. (*B*) Diffusion image (B value 800) demonstrates a hyperintense mass. (*C*) PET/MR imaging fused images. Posttreatment images demonstrate the cancer has decreased in size. (*D*) Axial postcontrast MR imaging shows a 1.6-cm enhancing mass consistent with the known carcinoma. (*E*) Diffusion image (B value 800) demonstrates a hyperintense mass. (*F*) PET/MR imaging fused images.

partial responders and decreased in the single nonresponder, thereby providing better differentiation between partial and nonresponders than MR imaging tumor volumes or SUV max, which decreased similarly in partial responders and nonresponders. Cho and colleagues[57] compared 1H-MRSI with PET and found mean % reductions for total choline, SUV max, SUV peak, and total lesion glycolysis were greater in the pCR group than in non-pCR group, but no cutoff values were identified. Here, AUC was similar between reduction in MR imaging and PET-related variables.

After therapy
When assessing residual disease after NAC and before surgery, PET and MR imaging metrics seem to be complimentary, with PET generally providing greater sensitivity and MR imaging generally providing greater specificity. In a 2016 meta-analysis performed by Liu and colleagues,[58] data from 382 patients in six studies demonstrated sensitivity and specificity of 65% and 88% and 86% and 72% for MR imaging and PET, respectively, for pCR. Park and colleagues,[59] whose patient population was included in the analysis, also

found that DWI had 100% sensitivity for pCR when a 55% increase in ADC was used at a cutoff. In an effort toward multiparametric analysis, An and colleagues[60] looked at DCE–MR imaging, DWI–MR imaging, and PET/CT and found increased specificity and negative predictive value when either DCE–MR imaging or DWI was combined with PET as compared with PET alone. More information is needed in terms of how the two modalities are optimally combined to understand and to assess response to NAC.

In that direction, Partridge and colleagues[61] looked at dynamic PET measures including 18F FDG transport rate (K1) and metabolism flux constant (ki) and DCE–MR imaging measures including peak enhancement (PE), signal enhancement ratio (SER), and tumor volume. They found that changes in glucose delivery were correlated with changes in vascularity (SER) and that ki correlated with SER, PE, and tumor volume. Decreases in K1, ki, PE, and SER were greater for patients with pCR as compared with those with residual disease. In the future, studies like this may help clinicians better understand therapeutic processes, such as drug delivery and uptake, and it is hoped propel clinicians toward the goal of increasingly personalized medicine.

WHOLE-BODY PET/MR IMAGING

PET/MR imaging is particularly interesting as a possible improvement over PET/CT oncologic whole-body imaging because MR imaging provides improved lesion detection in the brain, breast, liver, kidneys, and bones as compared with CT. CT detects more pulmonary lesions, especially less than 1 cm,[62,63] although the clinical importance of pulmonary lesions missed on PET/MR imaging is still unclear.[63]

In whole-body imaging for breast cancer, PET/MR imaging has been shown to provide improved sensitivity over PET/CT[6,64,65] or PET alone,[43] particularly for breast cancers,[64] liver metastases,[64] and bone metastases[6,64,65] (Figs. 3 and 4). PET/MR imaging has also been shown to detect brain metastases.[64] Despite outperforming PET/CT, whole-body PET/MR imaging still lags behind prone positioned dedicated breast PET/MR imaging for breast cancer detection, in one

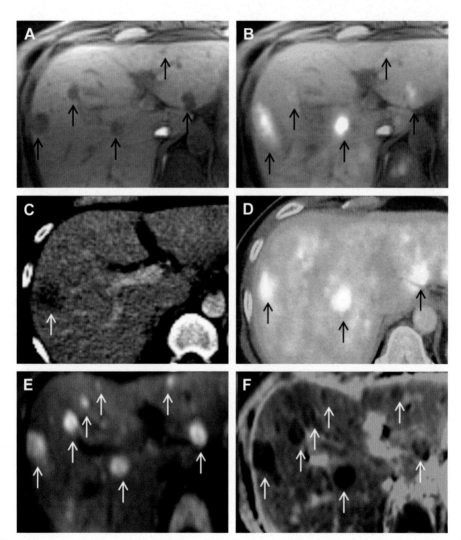

Fig. 3. Liver metastases seen best on PET/MR imaging: 56-year-old patient with a history of right breast invasive ductal cancer and known liver metastases. (*A*) Contrast-enhanced T1-weighted image demonstrates multiple metastases (*arrows*) with increased FDG uptake also readily visible on the (*B*) fused T1-weighted and PET image (*arrows*). (*C*) Contrast-enhanced CT image only clearly shows a single metastasis (*arrow*). (*D*) Although the fused PET/CT image shows additional hypermetabolic lesions (*arrows*), high background hepatic FDG uptake makes detection more difficult than on PET/MR imaging (*B*). (*E, F*) Corresponding DWI image and ADC map from the PET/MR image demonstrate even more metastases (*arrows*) with restricted diffusion (high signal on DWI and low signal on the corresponding ADC map) than seen on the (*A*) T1-weighted or (*B*) T1/PET images.

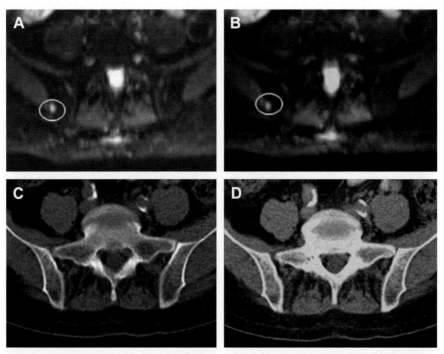

Fig. 4. A single osseous metastasis, the only evidence of metastatic disease, seen only on PET/MR imaging. A 75-year-old woman with a history of left invasive ductal cancer, status postmastectomy, imaged for surveillance. (*A*) Diffusion-weighted imaging shows this metastasis as a focus of restricted diffusion in the right ilium (*circle*), which demonstrates mild FDG uptake on the (*B*) fused T1-weighted/PET image (*circle*). (*C*) CT and (*D*) fused PET/CT images show no evidence of disease at the same location.

study seeing only 40% (4 of 10) of subcentimeter breast cancers seen on the dedicated breast examination.[40]

When separated out by sequence, DCE-MR imaging has been shown to be most useful for breast and brain lesions, DWI has been shown to be most useful for liver and bone metastases, and PET has been shown to be most useful for lymph node metastases.[64] These variable strengths highlight the advantage of multimodality imaging. In particular, combining PET and DWI may be important because PET has been shown to greatly improve the specificity of DWI in whole-body imaging.[66] In addition, omitting the whole-body CT from the PET examination can decrease the radiation dose by half.[64] These data suggest a wider role for PET/MR imaging in breast cancer staging and surveillance, particularly in young patients and in patients undergoing serial examinations.

SUMMARY

In focused breast and whole-body settings, PET/MR imaging can bring metabolic, anatomic, spectroscopic, and diffusion- and perfusion-based data together in a single examination that is directed at detecting and/or further understanding breast cancer. In local staging, PET and MR imaging seem to be complimentary with MR imaging providing greater accuracy for satellite lesions and PET providing greater sensitivity for axillary nodes. In imaging metastatic disease, PET and MR imaging are again complimentary, with MR imaging providing high sensitivity and PET tempering the relatively low specificity of DWI. Looking ahead, the multiparametric imaging possible with PET/MR imaging may provide new biomarkers, which it is hoped will help to personalize treatments and to provide more prognostic information. Additionally, as MR imaging techniques and radiotracers continue to be developed, the possibilities will continue to expand, granting a very bright future.

REFERENCES

1. Lehman CD, Mahoney M, Newell M, et al, for the American College of Radiology. ACR Practice Parameter for the performance of contrast-enhanced magnetic resonance imaging (MRI) of the breast. Reston (VA): American College of Radiology; 2014.
2. Kamel EM, Wyss MT, Fehr MK, et al. [18F]-Fluorodeoxyglucose positron emission tomography in

patients with suspected recurrence of breast cancer. J Cancer Res Clin Oncol 2003;129:147–53.

3. Moon DH, Maddahi J, Silverman DH, et al. Accuracy of whole-body fluorine-18-FDG PET for the detection of recurrent or metastatic breast carcinoma. J Nucl Med 1998;39:431–5.

4. Berg WA. Nuclear breast imaging: clinical results and future directions. J Nucl Med 2016;57(Suppl 1):46S–52S.

5. Dietzel M, Zoubi R, Burmeister HP, et al. Combined staging at one stop using MR mammography: evaluation of an extended protocol to screen for distant metastasis in primary breast cancer. Initial results and diagnostic accuracy in a prospective study. Rofo 2012;184:618–23.

6. Sawicki LM, Grueneisen J, Schaarschmidt BM, et al. Evaluation of ^{18}F-FDG PET/MRI, ^{18}F-FDG PET/CT, MRI, and CT in whole-body staging of recurrent breast cancer. Eur J Radiol 2016;85:459–65.

7. Moy L, Noz ME, Maguire GQ Jr, et al. Role of fusion of prone FDG-PET and magnetic resonance imaging of the breasts in the evaluation of breast cancer. Breast J 2010;16:369–76.

8. Dmitriev ID, Loo CE, Vogel WV, et al. Fully automated deformable registration of breast DCE-MRI and PET/CT. Phys Med Biol 2013;58:1221–33.

9. Atuegwu NC, Li X, Arlinghaus LR, et al. Longitudinal, intermodality registration of quantitative breast PET and MRI data acquired before and during neoadjuvant chemotherapy: preliminary results. Med Phys 2014;41:052302.

10. Bitencourt AG, Lima EN, Chojniak R, et al. Can 18F-FDG PET improve the evaluation of suspicious breast lesions on MRI? Eur J Radiol 2014;83:1381–6.

11. Visvikis D, Costa DC, Croasdale I, et al. CT-based attenuation correction in the calculation of semi-quantitative indices of [18F]FDG uptake in PET. Eur J Nucl Med Mol Imaging 2003;30:344–53.

12. Zaidi H, Montandon ML, Slosman DO. Magnetic resonance imaging-guided attenuation and scatter corrections in three-dimensional brain positron emission tomography. Med Phys 2003;30:937–48.

13. Hofmann M, Bezrukov I, Mantlik F, et al. MRI-based attenuation correction for whole-body PET/MRI: quantitative evaluation of segmentation- and atlas-based methods. J Nucl Med 2011;52:1392–9.

14. Aklan B, Paulus DH, Wenkel E, et al. Toward simultaneous PET/MR breast imaging: systematic evaluation and integration of a radiofrequency breast coil. Med Phys 2013;40:024301.

15. Dregely I, Lanz T, Metz S, et al. A 16-channel MR coil for simultaneous PET/MR imaging in breast cancer. Eur Radiol 2015;25:1154–61.

16. Ratib O, Schwaiget M, Beter T, editors. Atlas of PET/MR imaging in oncology. Heidelberg (Germany): Springer; 2013.

17. Pace L, Nicolai E, Luongo, et al. Comparison of whole-body PET/CT and PET/MRI in breast cancer patients: lesion detection and quantitation of 18F-deoxyglucose uptake in lesions and in normal organ tissues. Eur J Radiol 2014;83:289–96.

18. Pujara AC, Raad RA, Ponzo F, et al. Standardized uptake values from PET/MRI in metastatic breast cancer: an organ-based comparison with PET/CT. Breast J 2016;22:264–73.

19. Al-Nabhani KZ, Syed R, Michopoulou S, et al. Qualitative and quantitative comparison of PET/CT and PET/MR imaging in clinical practice. J Nucl Med 2014;55:88–94.

20. Drzezga A, Souvatzoglou M, Eiber M, et al. First clinical experience with integrated whole-body PET/MR: comparison to PET/CT in patients with oncologic diagnoses. J Nucl Med 2012;53:845–55.

21. Heusch P, Nensa F, Schaarschmidt B, et al. Diagnostic accuracy of whole-body PET/MRI and whole-body PET/CT for TNM staging in oncology. Eur J Nucl Med Mol Imaging 2015;42:42–8.

22. Huellner MW, Appenzeller P, Kuhn FP, et al. Whole-body nonenhanced PET/MR versus PET/CT in the staging and restaging of cancers: preliminary observations. Radiology 2014;273:859–69.

23. Lim HS, Yoon W, Chung TW, et al. FDG PET/CT for the detection and evaluation of breast diseases: usefulness and limitations. Radiographics 2007; 27(Suppl 1):S197–213.

24. Piccardo A, Puntoni M, Morbelli S, et al. 18F-FDG PET/CT is a prognostic biomarker in patients affected by bone metastases from breast cancer in comparison with 18F-NaF PET/CT. Nuklearmedizin 2015;54:163–72.

25. Jambor I, Kuisma A, Ramadan S, et al. Prospective evaluation of planar bone scintigraphy, SPECT, SPECT/CT, 18F-NaF PET/CT and whole body 1.5T MRI, including DWI, for the detection of bone metastases in high risk breast and prostate cancer patients: SKELETA clinical trial. Acta Oncol 2016; 55:59–67.

26. Czernin J, Satyamurthy N, Schiepers C. Molecular mechanisms of bone 18F-NaF deposition. J Nucl Med 2010;51:1826–9.

27. Katzenellenbogen JA. Designing steroid receptor-based radiotracers to image breast and prostate tumors. J Nucl Med 1995;36:8S–13S.

28. Gemignani ML, Patil S, Seshan VE, et al. Feasibility and predictability of perioperative PET and estrogen receptor ligand in patients with invasive breast cancer. J Nucl Med 2013;54:1697–702.

29. Dijkers EC, Oude Munnink TH, Kosterink JG, et al. Biodistribution of 89Zr-trastuzumab and PET imaging of HER2-positive lesions in patients with metastatic breast cancer. Clin Pharmacol Ther 2010;87:586–92.

30. Gaykema SB, Schröder CP, Vitfell-Rasmussen J, et al. 89Zr-trastuzumab and 89Zr-bevacizumab

PET to evaluate the effect of the HSP90 inhibitor NVP-AUY922 in metastatic breast cancer patients. Clin Cancer Res 2014;20:3945–54.

31. Gaykema SB, de Jong JR, Perik PJ, et al. (111)Intrastuzumab scintigraphy in HER2-positive metastatic breast cancer patients remains feasible during trastuzumab treatment. Mol Imaging 2014;13.

32. Tabouret-Viaud C, Botsikas D, Delattre BM, et al. PET/MR in breast cancer. Semin Nucl Med 2015; 45:304–21.

33. Pinker K, Bogner W, Baltzer P, et al. Improved differentiation of benign and malignant breast tumors with multiparametric 18fluorodeoxyglucose positron emission tomography magnetic resonance imaging: a feasibility study. Clin Cancer Res 2014; 20:3540–9.

34. Kuhl C, Weigel S, Schrading S, et al. Prospective multicenter cohort study to refine management recommendations for women at elevated familial risk of breast cancer: the EVA trial. J Clin Oncol 2010;28:1450–7.

35. Berg WA, Zhang Z, Lehrer D, et al, ACRIN 6666 Investigators. Detection of breast cancer with addition of annual screening ultrasound or a single screening MRI to mammography in women with elevated breast cancer risk. JAMA 2012;307:1394–404.

36. Avril N, Rosé CA, Schelling M, et al. Breast imaging with positron emission tomography and fluorine-18 fluorodeoxyglucose: use and limitations. J Clin Oncol 2000;18:3495–502.

37. Jung NY, Kim SH, Kim SH, et al. Effectiveness of breast MRI and (18)F-FDG PET/CT for the preoperative staging of invasive lobular carcinoma versus ductal carcinoma. J Breast Cancer 2015;18:63–72.

38. Grueneisen J, Nagarajah J, Buchbender C, et al. Positron emission tomography/magnetic resonance imaging for local tumor staging in patients with primary breast cancer: a comparison with positron emission tomography/computed tomography and magnetic resonance imaging. Invest Radiol 2015; 50:505–13.

39. Magometschnigg HF, Baltzer PA, Fueger B, et al. Diagnostic accuracy of (18)F-FDG PET/CT compared with that of contrast-enhanced MRI of the breast at 3 T. Eur J Nucl Med Mol Imaging 2015;42:1656–65.

40. Kong EJ, Chun KA, Bom HS, et al. Initial experience of integrated PET/MR mammography in patients with invasive ductal carcinoma. Hell J Nucl Med 2014;17:171–6.

41. Heusner TA, Hahn S, Jonkmanns C, et al. Diagnostic accuracy of fused positron emission tomography/magnetic resonance mammography: initial results. Br J Radiol 2011;84:126–35.

42. Ergul N, Kadioglu H, Yildiz S, et al. Assessment of multifocality and axillary nodal involvement in early-stage breast cancer patients using 18F-FDG

PET/CT compared to contrast-enhanced and diffusion-weighted magnetic resonance imaging and sentinel node biopsy. Acta Radiol 2015;56: 917–23.

43. Taneja S, Jena A, Goel R, et al. Simultaneous wholebody 18F-FDG PET-MRI in primary staging of breast cancer: a pilot study. Eur J Radiol 2014;83:2231–9.

44. Jochelson MS, Lebron L, Jacobs SS, et al. Detection of internal mammary adenopathy in patients with breast cancer by PET/CT and MRI. AJR Am J Roentgenol 2015;205:899–904.

45. Kim TH, Yoon JK, Kang DK, et al. Correlation between F-18 fluorodeoxyglucose positron emission tomography metabolic parameters and dynamic contrast-enhanced MRI-derived perfusion data in patients with invasive ductal breast carcinoma. Ann Surg Oncol 2015;22:3866–72.

46. An YS, Kang DK, Jung YS, et al. Tumor metabolism and perfusion ratio assessed by 18F-FDG PET/CT and DCE-MRI in breast cancer patients: correlation with tumor subtype and histologic prognostic factors. Eur J Radiol 2015;84:1365–70.

47. Margolis NE, Moy L, Sigmund EE, et al. Assessment of aggressiveness of breast cancer using simultaneous 18F-FDG-PET and DCE-MRI: preliminary observation. Clin Nucl Med 2016;41:e355–61.

48. Kitajima K, Yamano T, Fukushima K, et al. Correlation of the SUVmax of FDG-PET and ADC values of diffusion-weighted MR imaging with pathologic prognostic factors in breast carcinoma. Eur J Radiol 2016;85:943–9.

49. Karan B, Pourbagher A, Torun N. Diffusion-weighted imaging and (18) F-fluorodeoxyglucose positron emission tomography/computed tomography in breast cancer: correlation of the apparent diffusion coefficient and maximum standardized uptake values with prognostic factors. J Magn Reson Imaging 2016;43:1434–44.

50. Baba S, Isoda T, Maruoka Y, et al. Diagnostic and prognostic value of pretreatment SUV in 18F-FDG/PET in breast cancer: comparison with apparent diffusion coefficient from diffusion-weighted MR imaging. J Nucl Med 2014;55:736–42.

51. Choi BB, Kim SH, Kang BJ, et al. Diffusion-weighted imaging and FDG PET/CT: predicting the prognoses with apparent diffusion coefficient values and maximum standardized uptake values in patients with invasive ductal carcinoma. World J Surg Oncol 2012;10:126.

52. Pahk K, Kim S, Choe JG. Early prediction of pathological complete response in luminal B type neoadjuvant chemotherapy-treated breast cancer patients: comparison between interim 18F-FDG PET/CT and MRI. Nucl Med Commun 2015;36: 887–91.

53. Tateishi U, Miyake M, Nagaoka T, et al. Neoadjuvant chemotherapy in breast cancer: prediction of

pathologic response with PET/CT and dynamic contrast-enhanced MR imaging–prospective assessment. Radiology 2012;263:53–63.

54. Pengel KE, Koolen BB, Loo CE, et al. Combined use of ^{18}F-FDG PET/CT and MRI for response monitoring of breast cancer during neoadjuvant chemotherapy. Eur J Nucl Med Mol Imaging 2014;41:1515–24.

55. Lim I, Noh WC, Park J, et al. The combination of FDG PET and dynamic contrast-enhanced MRI improves the prediction of disease-free survival in patients with advanced breast cancer after the first cycle of neoadjuvant chemotherapy. Eur J Nucl Med Mol Imaging 2014;41:1852–60.

56. Jacobs MA, Ouwerkerk R, Wolff AC, et al. Monitoring of neoadjuvant chemotherapy using multiparametric, [23]Na sodium MR, and multimodality (PET/CT/MRI) imaging in locally advanced breast cancer. Breast Cancer Res Treat 2011;128:119–26.

57. Cho N, Im SA, Kang KW, et al. Early prediction of response to neoadjuvant chemotherapy in breast cancer patients: comparison of single-voxel (1) H-magnetic resonance spectroscopy and (18)F-fluorodeoxyglucose positron emission tomography. Eur Radiol 2016;26:2279–90.

58. Liu Q, Wang C, Li P, et al. The role of (18)F-FDG PET/CT and MRI in assessing pathological complete response to neoadjuvant chemotherapy in patients with breast cancer: a systematic review and meta-analysis. Biomed Res Int 2016;2016:3746232.

59. Park SH, Moon WK, Cho N, et al. Comparison of diffusion-weighted MR imaging and FDG PET/CT to predict pathological complete response to neoadjuvant chemotherapy in patients with breast cancer. Eur Radiol 2012;22:18–25.

60. An YY, Kim SH, Kang BJ, et al. Treatment response evaluation of breast cancer after neoadjuvant chemotherapy and usefulness of the imaging parameters of MRI and PET/CT. J Korean Med Sci 2015;30:808–15.

61. Partridge SC, Vanantwerp RK, Doot RK, et al. Association between serial dynamic contrast-enhanced MRI and dynamic 18F-FDG PET measures in patients undergoing neoadjuvant chemotherapy for locally advanced breast cancer. J Magn Reson Imaging 2010;32:1124–62.

62. Rauscher I, Eiber M, Fürst S, et al. PET/MR imaging in the detection and characterization of pulmonary lesions: technical and diagnostic evaluation in comparison to PET/CT. J Nucl Med 2014;55:724–9.

63. Raad RA, Friedman KP, Heacock L, et al. Outcome of small lung nodules missed on hybrid PET/MRI in patients with primary malignancy. J Magn Reson Imaging 2016;43:504–11.

64. Melsaether AN, Raad RA, Pujara AC, et al. Comparison of whole-body (18)F FDG PET/MR imaging and whole-body (18)F FDG PET/CT in terms of lesion detection and radiation dose in patients with breast cancer. Radiology 2016;281(1):193–202.

65. Catalano OA, Nicolai E, Rosen BR, et al. Comparison of CE-FDG-PET/CT with CE-FDG-PET/MR in the evaluation of osseous metastases in breast cancer patients. Br J Cancer 2015;112:1452–60.

66. Heusner TA, Kuemmel S, Koeninger A, et al. Diagnostic value of diffusion-weighted magnetic resonance imaging (DWI) compared to FDG PET/CT for whole-body breast cancer staging. Eur J Nucl Med Mol Imaging 2010;37:1077–86.

Update on Preoperative Breast Localization

Mary K. Hayes, MD

KEYWORDS

- Malignant neoplasm • Breast • Wire localization (WL, WNL)
- Radioactive seed localization I125 (RSL) • SCOUT RADAR • MAGSEED • Wire-free localization
- Targeted axillary dissection (TAD) • Radiofrequency identification (RFID)

KEY POINTS

- Preoperative same-day wire localization (WL) using mammography, ultrasound, MR imaging, and computed tomographic (CT) guidance aids surgical excision of nonpalpable breast lesions.
- Non–wire localization devices (I125 RSL, SCOUT RADAR, MAGSEED, and RFID) may provide an alternative means to mark and aids surgical excision of nonpalpable breast lesions and axillary lymph nodes up to 5 to 30 days preoperatively under mammography, ultrasound, and CT guidance.
- Non–wire deployment systems via MR guidance are not yet available; non–wire nonradioactive devices are MR conditional.
- Non–wire devices have potential for longer-term preoperative localization in patients who undergo neoadjuvant breast cancer treatment.

▶ Video content accompanies this article at http://www.radiologic.theclinics.com.

Breast-conserving surgery is a safe and effective method to treat early breast cancer (Video 1).[1-7] A successful breast-conserving treatment program requires multidisciplinary communication and planning between the surgeon, radiologist, and other specialists. The goal is to safely remove the target tissue with adequate surgical margins (SM), avoid unnecessary resection of healthy breast tissue, and provide a good cosmetic outcome without compromising survival. This article reviews image-guided tools for preoperative breast/axillary node localization, and the radiologist's role in the multidisciplinary breast care team.

CURRENT PROCEDURES

Conservative breast surgical treatment programs rely on image guidance devices and skills of the radiologist and surgeon. **Table 1** summarizes various localization methods reviewed by Corsi and colleagues.[8] They reported that because no single localization tool or technique proved better for achieving adequate SM, when advantages and disadvantages of each were taken into account, each multidisciplinary surgical team should adopt the most effective localization and margin assessment technique based on the skills and technologies available. Since then, additional non–wire preoperative localization devices were US Food and Drug Administration (FDA) cleared. These non–wire devices have noninferior breast cancer surgical outcomes compared with wires.[9-13] In the United States, preoperative wire needle localization (WL) and non–wire localization are accepted standard methods to guide intraoperative surgical excision of nonpalpable breast lesions.

Disclosure Statement: The author's hospital received research support from Hologic, Inc (IRB MH#2012.048 and MH#2014.036). The author's employer receives research support from Cianna Medical (IRB MH#2016.078). The author has served on a scientific advisory panel for Hologic and Cianna Medical.
Women's Imaging, Radiology Associates of Hollywood, Sheridan-Envision, Department of Radiology, Memorial Healthcare System, 3rd Floor, 3501 Johnson Street, Hollywood, FL 33021, USA
E-mail address: mhayes@mhs.net

Table 1
Summary of various localization methods

Localization Technique	Clear Margin Rate	Disadvantages
WL	71%–87%	Wire dislodgment, vasovagal episodes, pneumothorax
Carbon marking	81%	Foreign-body reactions that may mimic malignancy
Radio-guided occult lesion localization	75%–94%	Expense, need for nuclear medicine laboratory, intraoperative tools for surgeons, intraductal injection of 99 Technetium disperses radiotracer
Clip marker localization	90%–92%	Clip migration and need for surgeon training
Hematoma ultrasound guided localization (HUG)	89%–97%	Need for surgeon training, DCIS rarely seen unless visible by clip marker or hematoma
Clip marker localization	90%–92%	Clip migration and need for surgeon training
HUG	89%–97%	Need for surgeon training, DCIS rarely seen unless visible by clip marker or hematoma
Cavity shave	91%–94%	Longer operative times; margin assessment tools needed
RSL	Noninferior to WL	Stringent nuclear regulatory rules on access, monitoring, storage, transportation, and disposal of I125 seeds

Concurrent developments in 2014 to 2016 in techniques with breast radiology non–wire localization tools for nonpalpable breast and axillary lymph nodes, as well as the updated definitions of adequate breast surgery margins from the American Society of Breast Surgeons, each offer improved ways to optimize re-excision rates, mastectomy rates, and cosmetic outcomes for patients with breast cancer.[12–15] The 10 tools reported by the American Society of Breast Surgeons multidisciplinary consensus panel to minimize adverse surgical outcomes of increased mastectomy rates and poor cosmetic outcomes are listed in **Box 1**.

Preoperative Image-Guided Localization Procedure

Regardless of the imaging guidance method or specific needle wire/non–wire device used, all localization procedures share specific preprocedure and postprocedure steps.

Preprocedure review
Preprocedure review of the imaging and pathology reports and any clip placed during the diagnostic biopsy should be completed. Placement of a biopsy tissue marker clip (CLIP) is routine for image-guided breast biopsies and is mandated when a lesion is mammographically occult, when a lesion is difficult to visualize on post–biopsy imaging, and when it is necessary to confirm that the proper lesion has been sampled. Clip placement is useful when neoadjuvant chemotherapy

is contemplated and to correlate findings with other imaging modalities.[16,17]

The reviewer should assess the original extent of disease compared with the visible residual disease and the accuracy of biopsy clip placement at the target lesion. The preoperative localization target may be residual breast disease, biopsy clip, or post–biopsy hematoma. The radiologist should determine the best image-guidance method, the localization device, and coordinate any additional relevant schedules such as the operating room (OR) start time and lymphoscintigraphy injection.

Postprocedure, preoperative communication
Postprocedure, preoperative communication between the radiologist and the surgeon optimizes care. Common communication involves annotation of the images. A supplementary telephone call may be needed based on the surgeon's preference and patient details that may influence their approach. When feasible, marking the skin directly over the nonpalpable breast lesion and noting the skin-to-lesion depth with the patient in the supine operative position, can aid the surgeon.

Postprocedure, intraoperative communication
Postprocedure, intraoperative communication of the specimen radiograph findings should be expedited. Noncompression, 2-view specimen radiograph confirms the removal of the target lesion and can provide some information regarding the surgical excision and margins.[16] Tumor

Box 1
Ten tools to minimize adverse surgical outcomes of increased mastectomy rates and poor cosmetic outcomes

1. Preoperative diagnostic imaging should include full-field digital mammography and supplementary imaging to include ultrasound as needed.

2. Minimally invasive breast biopsy for breast cancer diagnosis.

3. Multidisciplinary discussions to include radiology, pathology, surgery, and radiation and medical oncology.

4. Localization of nonpalpable breast lesions via RSL, intraoperative ultrasound, or wire localization to direct lesion excision.

5. Oncoplastic techniques can reduce the need for reoperation in anatomically suitable patients.

6. Specimen orientation of 3 or more margins.

7. Specimen radiograph with surgeon intraoperative review.

8. Consider cavity shave margins in patients with T2 or greater tumor size or T1 with extensive intraductal carcinoma.

9. Intraoperative pathology assessment of lumpectomy margins may help decrease re-excisions when feasible.

10. Compliance with the SSO-ASTRO margin guideline to not routinely reoperate for close margins with *"No Tumor on Ink"* in patients with invasive cancer.

Postprocedure assessment of radiology-pathology concordance and communication
Postprocedure assessment of radiology-pathology concordance and communication is the final step of preoperative localization. The radiologist performs the radiology-pathology concordance assessment, issues a final radiology report with follow-up recommendations, and confirms receipt of the final report. The treating breast surgeon issues all final results and recommendations directly to the patient in order to provide a single clear uniform postoperative treatment plan.

Localization Devices: Wire Needle Localization

Surgical excision of nonpalpable breast lesions using preoperative image-guided WL has been a cost-effective standard of care to assist surgical excision of nonpalpable breast cancer for several decades in the United States. Clear margins obtained with wire-guided excision are reported to be 70.8% to 87.4%.[8,18–22] Wires may be placed using mammography or ultrasound, and less commonly computed tomographic (CT) or MR guidance. Preoperative wires are placed on the same day of breast surgery and usually in the same building where surgery is scheduled. Multiple wires may be used to bracket lesions that measure 2 cm or greater or for satellite lesions.

Needle wire systems are packaged as a single-use sterilized wire. The semirigid localization wire is preloaded in a 3- to 15-cm length, 16- to 20-g needle introducer. The distal end of the semirigid localization wire varies by manufacturer and may include a barb, hook, or pigtail to anchor the wire at the intended target. The wire system is deployed when targeting is confirmed with needle/wire system at or adjacent to the target on imaging.[16,23] Once deployed, some wires may not be retracted, repositioned, or cut; such devices must be surgically removed.

Most often, the radiologist selects the image guidance modality used for imaging-guided WL based on the lesion visibility and patient's body habitus. Surgeons choose the wire system and communicate a preference whether the WL introducer needle should remain in place or be removed with only the wire left in place to mark the index lesion. The patient is transferred to the operating area with either the wire/needle system or the wire only. Because the wire must remain in position between the time of deployment and surgical excision, the WL requires patient compliance.

Various complications of the WL can adversely impact surgical success. Careful deployment of the WL parallel to the chest wall, securing the wire tail to the skin and minimizing breast

calcifications extending to the margins on the specimen radiograph are likely to correlate with residual tumor in the breast. Ultrasound of the specimen may be useful if the target lesion is mammographically occult but seen on ultrasound. A specimen radiograph may be used to document excision of the target CLIP for lesions that are visible only at MR imaging and preoperatively marked with a biopsy CLIP (**Fig. 1**).

Timely review and communication of specimen imaging findings directly to the surgeon impact the surgeon's decision whether to remove additional tissue. If the procedure radiologist is not available to review the specimen radiograph, a second radiologist should review the relevant needle biopsy results and radiology images to provide timely and accurate communication to the surgeon. The need for a second radiologist may occur more often when a non–wire localization device is placed 5 to 30 days before surgery.

594

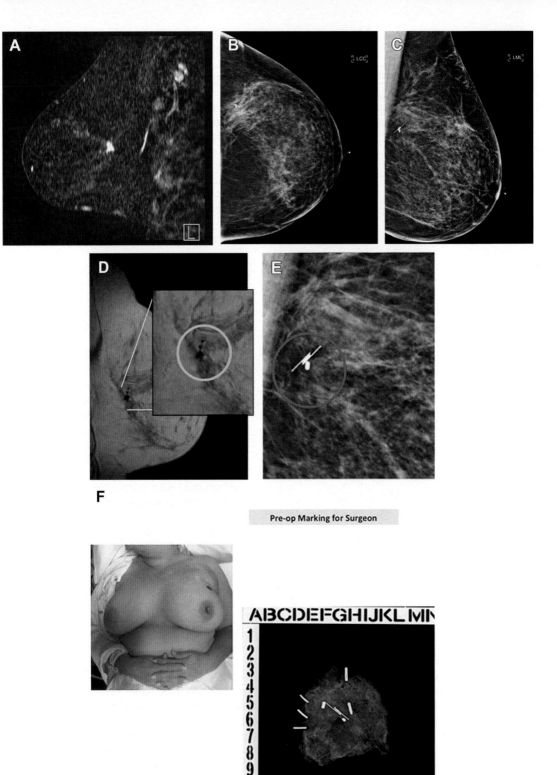

Fig. 1. A 50-year-old asymptomatic patient with mammographic and sonographic occult invasive ductal carcinoma (IDC) who presented with a 13-mm suspicious enhancing mass in the left breast (*A*). Stereotatically guided nonwire localization postprocedure mammogram confirms accurate deployment of the SCOUT at the bar clip in craniocaudal (CC) (*B*) and mediolateral (ML) (*C*) view. Sagittal MR with photographic enlargement of MR signal void (*yellow circle* in *D*) compares well with photographic enlargement of ML mammogram (*red circle* in *E*). T1-weighted non-fat-saturated MR image was acquired in the prone position and mammogram was acquired in the upright position. Photograph of patient in the supine operative position with skin marked over the lesion (*F*) can be saved to electronic chart. Specimen radiograph may be used to document excision of the target CLIP for lesions that are visible only at MR imaging and preoperatively marked with a biopsy CLIP.

movement, and shortest transit time to the OR can protect against unintended WL complications.[23] Because the wire should be placed immediately before surgery, logistical problems between the surgeon and radiology schedule can cause delays in surgical start time. In addition to the WL complication of wire migration, pneumothorax, site-specific pain, retention of wire fragments, hematoma, hemorrhage, bleeding, infection, adjacent tissue injury, hemoptysis, hemothorax, non–target tissue excision, organ or vessel perforation, and breast implant puncture can occur. Although wire migration typically involves locations within the breast, wire migration external to the breast (pericardium, pleural spaces, lung, mediastinum, neck muscles, axilla, and abdominal cavity) have also been reported.[23–25]

Retained wire fragments may occur if the wire is transected during surgery. Standard WL procedure specimen radiography provides documentation of excision of the entire wire. If the entire wire is not verified as expected, then the radiologist must notify the surgeon to search for and retrieve the missing wire fragments. Intraoperative radiograph imaging or postoperative chest CT or mammography may be needed. Rare cases of wire migration into the pleura or pericardium require thorascopic or open surgery to excise the retained wire fragment.[26]

The *mammographic* approach is performed under mild breast compression. The patient is commonly seated or standing upright but can also be positioned in the lateral recumbent or prone position. Mammographic guidance with 2-dimensional, stereotactic, or 3-dimensional (3D) imaging can be used. Stereotactic or 3D imaging aids in targeting lesions that are sonographically occult and can be imaged in one only mammographic projection; examples include high axillary tail lesions, including lymph nodes. Additional mammograms may be used to adjust needle wire placement.

The *sonographic* approach is performed with no breast compression. The patient is placed in the supine or supine oblique position, with the ipsilateral arm raised above the head. Ultrasound is performed using a high-frequency linear array transducer. The needle wire system is introduced at a skin entry site that is both nearest the lesion and allows a needle trajectory parallel to the chest wall. The transducer is oriented parallel to the needle trajectory for best visualization of wire deployment under real-time visualization.

The *CT* approach is performed using no breast compression with the patient in a supine or supine oblique position, with the ipsilateral arm raised above the head. A CT biopsy grid or fiducial marker on the skin provides a reference to determine the depth and trajectory angle for WL. After the needle wire is introduced, additional limited CT images may be obtained to direct needle wire adjustments.

The *MR* approach is performed using gentle breast immobilization. The patient is placed in the prone or prone oblique position with the patient's ipsilateral arm extended above the head. MR-guided wire localization for surgical excision is uncommon and is reserved for suspicious findings visible only at MR imaging.[23] All equipment/supplies used in the MR suite must be MR compatible. MR WL systems are MR conditional and can be scanned safely in a static magnetic field of 3-T or less and a spatial gradient field of 720 G/cm. MR breast biopsy coils with grid and pillar-post systems are placed at the planned lateral and/or medial approach site. A skin marker or fiducial serves as a reference for measuring the depth for needle wire lesion localization.

Gadolinium contrast intravenous bolus 0.1 mmol/kg with a 10- to 20-mL saline flush is followed by an abridged contrast-enhanced MR breast imaging protocol (localizer sequence, T1, T2, 2 time point postcontrast series, and a postprocedure T1 image to confirm accurate wire placement). This short protocol balances the competing demands of rapid acquisition of high-resolution images to offset the rapid contrast washout of some suspicious lesions. Computer-aided detection software may facilitate identification and targeting of the lesion. Simultaneous bilateral imaging can be performed for bilateral breast lesions. After the needle wire is introduced, any potential additional images for adjustment of needle/wire can result in contrast material washout and limit a visibility of the lesion. In addition, artifact from the localization wire may obscure the target. Therefore, a carefully planned approach that expedites efficiency will also optimize accuracy.

Localization Devices: Non–wire Localization

Although WL can be performed under mammographic, ultrasound, CT, or MR imaging guidance, none of the non–wire systems can be deployed under MR guidance at this time. Non–wire localization systems address some of the limitations of WL.[9–13,27,28]

Box 2 outlines some advantages of non–wire devices. The non–wire alternative devices use send-receive technology at a specific wavelength in the electromagnetic spectrum (**Fig. 2**), ranging from high frequency–high energy to low frequency–low energy: radioactive seed localization (RSL),[27–32] infrared radar (SCOUT),[9–11] magnetic susceptometry (MAGSEED),[12] and radiofrequency identification (RFID).[13]

Each non–wire system has 3 components: a single-use sterilized 5- to 12-mm-long device preloaded in a 12- to 18-g needle introducer, a reusable small console, and a dedicated handheld intraoperative probe (**Fig. 3**). The vendor may package the dedicated probe as a single-use sterilized probe or as a reusable probe with an appropriate sterile cover. Probes can detect the tag up to 4- to 6-cm depth, and the console emits real-time audio and numeric feedback to guide the surgeon during the excisional breast procedure.

Non–wire devices cannot be repositioned once deployed. More than one device may be used to bracket the full extent of disease in patients with large masses, satellite nodules, or extensive microcalcifications. Bracketing in the anterior-posterior plane is not advised because superimposed devices may be detected as only one device in the intraoperative supine patient. Marking the skin overlying the target lesion with the patient in the supine operative position and communicating skin-to-lesion depth can aid the surgeon during excision. Postlocalization preoperative orthogonal mammography is performed (**Fig. 4**).

In contrast to WL procedures that are scheduled with same-day surgery, the non–wire systems can be placed 5 to 30 days before surgery. This uncoupling of the radiology and surgery schedules allows for a more flexible, efficient, on-time procedure start in the OR. This flexibility enhances scheduling options for the patient, surgeon, radiologist, and OR teams.

Box 3 summarizes the common steps following localization with a non–wire device.

The radiologist who performs the localization procedure should prepare to interpret the specimen radiograph when possible. Because non–wire systems can be placed several days before surgery, or in a different facility, it is helpful to maintain an operative calendar for localization patients. In a multihospital setting, a shared localization calendar alert reminds the primary radiologist or alternate radiologist to review the patient imaging record and prepare for communication to the surgeon. Specimen radiographic image should be annotated to include direct OR contact number to facilitate timely communication between the radiologist and surgeon (see **Fig. 4**).

TYPES OF NON–WIRE DEVICES

Types of non–wire devices are compared in **Fig. 5**.

Radioactive Non–wire Device

The radioactive non–wire devices are active and contain an energy source. Radioactive device systems are constrained by nuclear regulatory rules for radioactive devices and therefore cannot be deployed in one facility and removed in another facility.

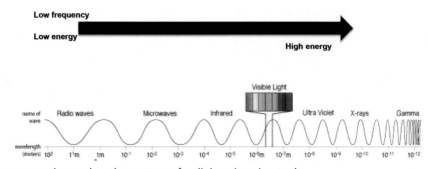

Fig. 2. Electromagnetic wavelength spectrum of radiology imaging tools.

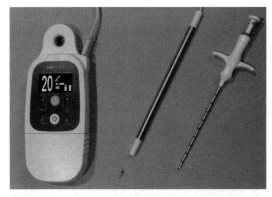

Fig. 3. Non–wire systems have 3 components: a single-use sterilized device preloaded in a needle introducer, a reusable console, and a dedicated handheld intraoperative probe. (*Courtesy of* Health Beacons, Inc, Concord, MA; with permission.)

Radioactive I125 Seed Localization

Since Gray and colleagues[27] first described RSL as an alternative to needle localization in 2001, dozens of peer-reviewed articles have compared RSL with WL[28–31] and reported noninferior breast cancer surgical outcomes including SM, re-excision and reoperation rates, specimen size, and cosmesis.

RSL is a 5-mm I125 pellet with a titanium shell. I125 has a 60-day half-life. Because radioactivity is low (0.100–0.200 mCi [3.7–7.4 MBq]), no special instructions need to be given to the patient, family, or the public when radioactive seeds are in place.[28]

Deployment of RSL procedure is similar to biopsy clip placement and can be performed 0 to 5 days before surgery. The surgeon uses an intraoperative gamma (γ) probe to identify and excise the target area and seed.

McGhan and colleagues[29] reviewed 1148 consecutive RSL procedures and reported 86% were localized with one seed with 76% placed 1 or more days before surgery. Pathologically negative margin rate was 97% of patients with invasive or in situ carcinoma (ductal carcinoma in situ, DCIS) at the first operation. Re-excision was performed in 9% of patients with invasive carcinoma and 19% of patients with DCIS for close (≤ 2 mm) margins. Reported adverse events included 3 seeds (0.3%) not deployed correctly on first attempt and 30 seeds (2.6%) displaced from the breast specimen during surgical excision of the target lesion. All seeds were retrieved, with no radiation safety concerns.

Because a sentinel lymph node biopsy using technetium-99m and RSL excision can use the intraoperative γ probe, both procedures can be performed at the same surgery, using the appropriate γ-probe settings (I125 seed emits 27 keV; technetium-99m emits 140 keV). Shin and colleagues[14] reported that targeted axillary dissection (TAD), selective removal of lymph nodes that were biopsy proven to contain metastasis and marked with a CLIP, may more accurately stage the axillary lymph nodes. TAD can be performed using RSL supplementary to SNL as a same-day breast or axillary surgical procedure.

Radioactive I125 Seed Localization Policies

A Nuclear Regulatory Commission (NRC) state license for medical use of radioactive materials is required for any facility that uses RSL. An authorized user at the facility must meet special training and experience requirements and be responsible for the safe use of radioactive material, compliance with all regulations, reporting adverse events, and ensuring staff education in radiation safety. Surgeons, pathologists, and nonauthorized radiologists implanting the seed sources work under the supervision of the authorized user and must complete approved safety training.

As such, the acquisition, implantation, excision, storage, transportation, and disposal of seeds must all fall under the same radioactive materials facility license (for radiology, surgery, pathology). The radioactive seed must be removed from the excised specimen before transport; otherwise, the Department of Transportation rules are invoked. The inventory of radioactive sources must be accounted for at all times and secured from unauthorized access or removal. Procedures must reflect location of the I125 source at any time. Loss, mishandling, or damage of a single I125 seed is reportable to the NRC.

Because the RSL gamma probe to detect extruded RSL seeds is not MR compatible, patients may not undergo MR imaging examination while the seed is in place. Lack of MRI compatibility may limit theoretic long-term RSL use for patients with breast cancer who have MR follow-up imaging in the neoadjuvant setting.

Because it is easy to learn and has noninferior surgical outcomes compared with WL, RSL is considered by some as the method of choice for localization of nonpalpable breast lesions. However, the use of radioactivity and its associated NRC safety precautions limited the widespread adoption of RSL.[9–11] Other nonradioactive, non–wire devices have recently become commercially available in Europe and the United States.

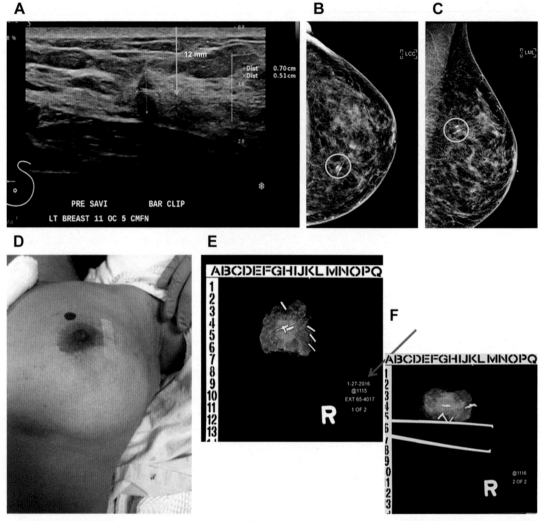

Fig. 4. Ultrasound-guided non–wire localization. Left breast ultrasound with 12-mm skin to lesion measurement (*yellow arrow, A*). Postlocalization, preoperative mammogram with SCOUT and CLIP *yellow circles* in CC (*B*) and ML (*C*) view. Photograph of the patient in the supine operative position with skin marked over the lesion (*D*) can be saved to electronic chart. Right breast specimen radiograph images of a separate patient are obtained in orthogonal projections and annotated to include direct OR contact number (*red arrow*) to facilitate timely communication between the radiologist and surgeon (*E, F*). Radiology-pathology concordance confirmed left IDC 5 × 7 × 5 mm, clear margins with both BAR CLIP + SCOUT in specimen.

NONRADIOACTIVE NON–WIRE DEVICES: SCOUT, MAGSEED, AND RFID

The nonradioactive non–wire devices are passive and contain no energy source. Nonradioactive device systems are not constrained by regulations for radioactive devices and therefore can be deployed in one facility and removed in another facility.

SCOUT RADAR DEVICE

SCOUT is a nonradioactive non–wire localization device that uses infrared light and radar technology. SCOUT was FDA cleared in August 2014 for localization of breast lesions. As of September 2016, SCOUT Radar has been used in more than 5000 patients in more than 75 US facilities.

The 12-mm SCOUT device is deployed via a 16-g needle introduced under imaging guidance 0 to 30 days before surgery. Retracting the release button, rather than pushing forward, to unsheathe the SCOUT, deploys the device.

The surgeon uses a dedicated intraoperative probe that emits infrared light to identify and excise the target area and SCOUT. SCOUT placed

Checklist postdeployment of non–wire localization procedure:

- Technologist includes all biopsy clips, and devices are included on preoperative final images
- Patient is placed in the supine or supine operative position and skin is marked
- Patient photograph with skin marking can be saved to electronic medical record to aid surgeon
- Patient discharged with instructions that include contact phone numbers and marking pen to maintain skin marking
- Shared preoperative non–wire calendar includes planned surgical facility and date

Checklist for day of surgery:

- Radiologist alerted to review preoperative patient imaging record
- OR technologist obtains specimen radiograph and notifies the radiologist
- Technologist annotates specimen radiograph images with direct OR contact number
- Radiologist communicates imaging results directly to surgeon

deeper than 4.5 cm may not produce a detectable signal through the skin. When the patient is in the supine surgical position, most lesions are within target depth (**Figs. 6 and 7**, Video 1).

Cox and colleagues[9,10] published the initial pilot study results of 50 patients and results from the prospective multicenter study of 153 patients (11 centers, 20 radiologists, and 16 surgeons). Successful surgery in 153/153 patients, successful device placement in 99.4%, and an overall 15.8% re-excision rate were reported.

In a separate feasibility study, Mango and colleagues[11] reported on a single-institution retrospective study that included one breast surgeon with 15/15 successful image-guided SCOUT placements in 13 patients. Final pathology of all (10 benign and 5 malignant) lesions had clear SMs with no re-excision or complications. Successful SCOUT device placement as measured on postprocedure mammogram averaged 0.2 cm (range, 0–1.0 cm) target-to-reflector distance, similar to RSL mean target-to-seed distance of 0.1 cm (range, 0–2.0 cm).[28,29] One significant SCOUT migration occurred in a postbiopsy hematoma. Hematoma may also limit infrared light

transmission and subsequent detection of SCOUT.

Because the SCOUT device is passive and has no significant MR compatibility or signal void artifact limitations, the patient may safely undergo MR (at 3 T or less) with the SCOUT in place. Since there is no inherent risk of reflector expiration in 30 days, theoretically the device could be placed longer term before surgery, before neoadjuvant chemotherapy response (see **Fig. 1**; **Fig. 8**).

The SCOUT system costs more than WL or RSL. The one-time initial purchase of the non–wire device system console and probe contributes to the cost. An institutional cost analysis may be helpful to assess the cost comparison of WL, RSL, and SCOUT. Non–wire devices have fewer OR start delays and cancellations; nonradioactive devices have lower administrative costs because there is no RSL NRC oversight needed. A non–wire nonradioactive method to localize and excise nonpalpable breast lesions may overcome many of the WL- and RSL-related limitations.

MAGSEED DEVICE

The MAGSEED device was FDA 510(k) cleared in March 2016 for the localization of breast lesions up to 30 days before surgery. Nonresearch, clinical use of MAGSEED has been commercially available in the US since August 2016. Two clinical studies are ongoing, one for lesion localization (NCT03020888) and one for localization of axillary lymph nodes (NCT03038152). MAGSEED is a metal marker which contains iron particles. The dedicated Sentimag probe uses MAGSEED to generate an alternating magnetic field that transiently magnetizes the iron in the MAGSEED. The tiny magnetic signature generated by MAGSEED is detected by the Sentimag probe (**Fig. 9**).

The MAGSEED device is 5 mm in length and is deployed under mammogram, ultrasound, or CT guidance. Deployment is similar to biopsy CLIP or RSL through a preloaded sterile18-g needle introducer. MAGSEED may not produce a detectable signal through the skin if placed greater than 4.0-cm depth. MAGSEED is MR conditional at 1.5 T and 3 T[12]; however, 4 to 6-cm signal void artifact due to the iron content (see **Fig. 8**) may limit diagnostic accuracy of breast MR imaging when MAGSEED is in place. Finally, non-magnetic tools (eg, titanium or polymer) need to be used with Sentimag while the probe is in use. Stainless steel surgical instruments, such as metal surgical retractors may not be compatible with MAGSEED. This may add separate per use fees in addition to the initial start-up OR supply costs for the dedicated console and probe.

	DEVICE (12–18 g)	WIRE	SEED	SAVI SCOUT	MAGSEED	RFID
DEVICE SIZE	3-15 CM	5 MM	12 MM	5 MM	9 MM
Hospital	☑	☑	☑	☑	☑
2nd Hospital or Outpatient Center		–	☑	☑	☑
same day	☑	☑	☑	☑	☑
0–5 d	–	☑	☑	☑	☑
0–30 d	–	–	☑	☑	☑
Deploy in US, MG, CT	☑	☑	☑	☑	☑
Deploy in MRI	☑	–	–	–	–
MRI Conditional	☑	–	☑	☑	☑
REPOSITION AFTER DEPLOYMENT	☑	–	–	–	–
SIGNAL DEPTH	☑	☑	4.5 CM	4 CM	6 CM
BRACKET	☑	☑	☑	☑	☑
U.S. TRIALS PUBLISHED	>30 Y	2001	2014	NONE	2014
AVAILABILE IN US	>30 Y	2001	2015	2016	Pending

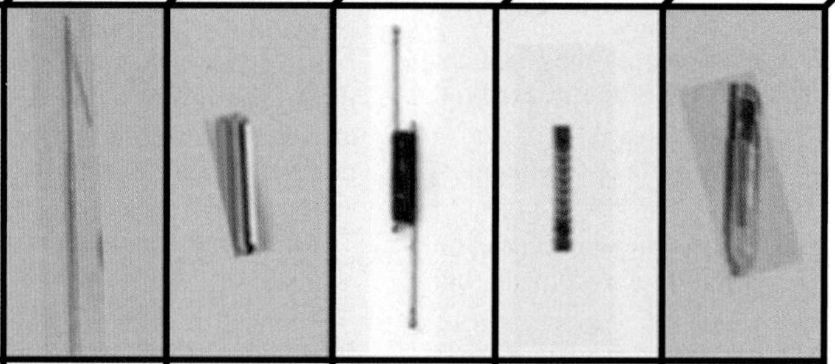

Fig. 5. Comparison of WL and non–wire localization devices.

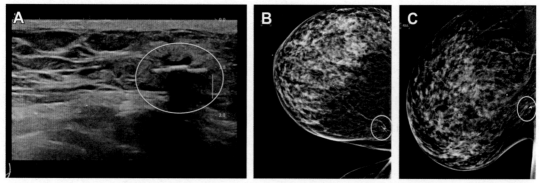

Fig. 6. IDC in posterior depth right breast at the 3:00 o'clock location would be difficult to localize with WL. Ultrasound localization documents non–wire SCOUT in the center of a hypoechoic mass with irregular margins (*yellow circle A*). Postlocalization mammogram confirms the posterior depth right at the 3:00 position (*yellow circles*) in the CC (*B*) and ML (*C*) view. This area would be difficult to localize with WL. Radiology-pathology concordance confirmed excision of a 14-mm IDC with clear margins. Receptors: estrogen receptor (ER) 100%; progesterone receptor (PR) 20%; and Her2 receptor negative.

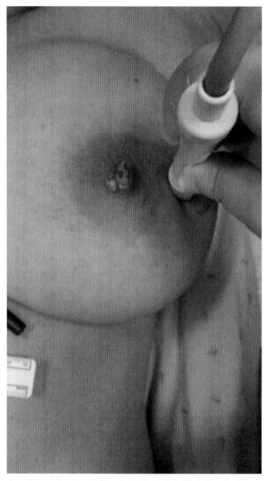

Fig. 7. Patient with non–wire localization. Photograph or video clip with audio that documents the skin marking over the lesion and probe angle with optimum audio signal can aid the surgeon.

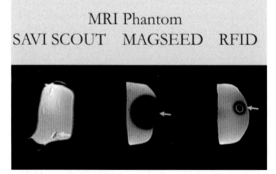

Fig. 8. MR images of a one-breast phantom with 3 non–wire devices. SCOUT (*yellow arrow*), MAGSEED (*blue arrow*), RFID (*orange arrow*) show varied signal void artifacts in noncontrast T1 non-fat-saturated MR sequences.

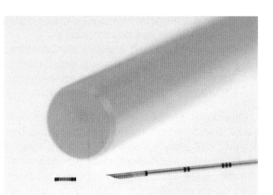

Fig. 9. Sentimag probe generates an alternating magnetic field to transiently magnetize the iron-containing MAGSEED. This signal is then detected by the Sentimag probe. (*Courtesy of* Endomag, Inc, Cambridge, United Kingdom; with permission.)

RADIOFREQUENCY IDENTIFICATION TAG

The FDA has approved implantation of radiofrequency tags in humans for the purposes of identification. RFID systems use radio waves to transfer information. A passive tag has no energy source and can communicate a range of information from one serial number to several pages of data. Pending FDA clearance, the 9-mm RFID tag can be deployed 0 to 30 days before surgery through a preloaded sterile 12-g needle similar to biopsy CLIP or RSL (see Fig. 3). When the patient is in the supine surgical position, the tag can be detected within 6 cm depth of the handheld loop probe at the skin surgance and 4 cm depth of the intraoperative surgical dedicated pencil probe.[13]

The RFID tag contains a ferrite rod wrapped with copper and a microprocessor. The RFID device is MR conditional. However, the ferrous and copper material in RFID creates a 2-cm signal void artifact that may limit diagnostic accuracy of breast MR imaging when the RFID is in place (see Fig. 8).

The FDA is not aware of any adverse events associated with RFID. The tags have a long history of use similar to those embedded in livestock and pets as a form of identification. FDA clearance is pending for intraoperative use of the RFID intraoperative pencil probe system. Clinical nonresearch use in the US breast patients is expected in 2017.

FUTURE OPPORTUNITIES

Future opportunities for non–wire, nonradioactive localization devices require large-scale multi-institutional studies in the United States. Areas for investigation and development may include the following:

- Longer-term placement in patients undergoing neoadjuvant treatment

- Placement in suspicious axillary lymph nodes
- MR-compatible needle introducers
- Comprehensive cost-analysis comparison to include device cost, start-up costs, institutional cost of OR delays and cancellations, administrative costs of NRC regulations

Patients who require neoadjuvant therapy, with suspicious axillary or intramammary lymph nodes, or those with lesions visible only with MR imaging could benefit from more accurate and cost-effective single-appointment localization. Streamlined single appointment could both mark the extent of disease and localize the surgical target before chemotherapeutic response.

Because non–wire device technology continues to evolve, the FDA monitors potential adverse events. Non–wire device transmitters could potentially cause interference or degrade the function of other implanted electronic medical devices, such as pacemakers, implantable defibrillators, and other electronic medical devices.

SUMMARY

The radiologist plays an important role in detection, diagnosis, localization, pathologic correlation, and follow-up management of patients with breast cancer. The preoperative breast localization devices used by the radiologist and the refined definitions of negative SMs impact the multidisciplinary treatment of breast cancer. This article has reviewed the wire and non–wire tools available for image-guided preoperative localization. Non–wire devices provide the benefits of improved efficiency with noninferior surgical results. Preoperative lesion localization up to 30 days before scheduled surgery may lead to other longer-term efficient and cost-effective applications for patients who require neoadjuvant treatment, patients who have suspicious lymph nodes for TAD, and those with lesions visible only at MR imaging.[32]

SUPPLEMENTARY DATA

Supplementary data related to this article can be found at http://dx.doi.org/10.1016/j.rcl.2016.12.012.

REFERENCES

1. Singletary S. Surgical margins in patients with early stage breast cancer treated with breast conservation therapy. Am J Surg 2002;184:383–93.
2. Fisher E, Anderson S, Redmond C, et al. Ipsilateral breast tumor recurrence and survival following lumpectomy and irradiation: pathological findings from NSABP protocol B-06. Semin Surg Oncol 1992;8:161–6.
3. Fisher B, Anderson S, Bryant J, et al. Twenty-year follow-up of a randomized trial comparing total mastectomy, lumpectomy, and lumpectomy plus irradiation for the treatment of invasive breast cancer. N Engl J Med 2002;347:1233–41.
4. Veronesi U, Cascinelli N, Mariani L, et al. Twenty-year follow-up of a randomized study comparing breast-conserving surgery with radical mastectomy for early breast cancer. N Engl J Med 2002;347:1227–32.
5. Houssami N, Macaskill P, Marinovichet ML, et al. Meta-analysis of the impact of surgical margins on local recurrence in women with early-stage invasive breast cancer treated with breast-conserving therapy. Eur J Cancer 2010;46:3219–32.
6. Morrow M, Harris JR, Schnitt SJ. Surgical margins in lumpectomy for breast cancer—bigger is not better. N Engl J Med 2012;367:79–82.
7. Fisher B, Dignam J, Bryant J, et al. Five versus more than five years of tamoxifen therapy for breast cancer patients with negative lymph nodes and estrogen receptor-positive tumors. J Natl Cancer Inst 1996;88:1529–42.
8. Corsi F, Sorrentino L, Bossi D, et al. Preoperative localization and surgical margins in conservative breast surgery. Int J Surg Oncol 2013;2013: 793819.
9. Cox CE, Garcia-Henriquez N, Glancy MJ, et al. Pilot study of a new nonradioactive surgical guidance technology for locating non-palpable breast lesions. Ann Surg Oncol 2016;23(6):1824–30.
10. Cox CE, Russel S, Prowler V, et al. A prospective, single arm, multi-site clinical evaluation of a nonradioactive surgical guidance technology for the location of nonpalpable breast lesions during excision. Ann Surg Oncol 2016;23(10):3168–74.
11. Mango V, Ha R, Gomberawalla A, et al. Evaluation of SAVI SCOUT surgical guidance system for localization and excision of nonpalpable breast lesions: a feasibility study. AJR Am J Roentgenol 2016;W1–4. http://dx.doi.org/10.2214/AJR.15.15962.
12. Magseed Indications for Use. Available at: http://us.endomag.com/sites/default/files/Magseed%20IFU_006USA_v40.pdf. Accessed November 23, 2016.
13. Dauphine C, Reicher JJ, Reicher MA, et al. A prospective clinical study to evaluate the safety and performance of wireless localization of nonpalpable breast lesions using radiofrequency identification technology. AJR Am J Roentgenol 2015;204(6):W720–3.
14. Shin K, Caudle A, Kuerer HM, et al. Clinical Perspective. Radiologic mapping for targeted axillary dissection: needle biopsy to excision. AJR Am J Roentgenol 2016;207:1372–9.
15. Landercasper J, Attai D, Atisha D, et al. Toolbox to reduce lumpectomy reoperations and improve cosmetic outcome in breast cancer patients: The American Society of Breast Surgeons Consensus Conference. Ann Surg Oncol 2015;22:3174–83.

16. American College of Radiology. ACR practice parameter for the imaging management of DCIS and invasive breast carcinoma. 2013; Available at: https://www.acr.org/~/media/ACR/Documents/PGTS/guidelines/DCIS_Invasive_Breast_Carcinoma.pdf. Accessed November 1, 2016.

17. Hayes M. National Consortium of Breast Centers. Poster presentation 2015; Available at: https://www.researchgate.net/publication/281243161_Breast_Biopsy_Marker_Placement_Accuracy.pdf. Accessed November 1, 2016.

18. Homer MJ, Pile-Spellman ER. Needle localization of occult breast lesions with a curved-end retractable wire: technique and pitfalls. Radiology 1986;161:547–8.

19. Kopans DB, Swann CA. Preoperative imaging-guided needle placement and localization of clinically occult breast lesions. AJR Am J Roentgenol 1989;152:1–9.

20. Kopans DB, Meyer JE, Lindfors KK, et al. Breast sonography to guide cyst aspiration and wire localization of occult solid lesions. AJR Am J Roentgenol 1984;143:489–92.

21. Silverstein M, Lagios M, Groshen S, et al. The influence of margin width on local control of ductal carcinoma in situ of the breast. N Engl J Med 1999;340:1455–61.

22. Moy L, Newell M, Mahoney M, et al. ACR appropriateness criteria stage I breast cancer. J Appl Commun Res 2014;11:1160–8.

23. Mahoney M, Newell M, Bailey L, et al. ACR practice parameter for the performance of magnetic resonance imaging-guided breast interventional procedures. 2014; ACR.org/Quality-Safety Standards. Available at: https://www.acr.org/~/media/ACR/Documents/PGTS/guidelines/MRI_Guided_Breast.pdf?la=en. Accessed February 17, 2017.

24. Mahoney M, Ingram D. Breast emergencies: types, imaging features, and management. AJR Am J Roentgenol 1989;202:1–9.

25. Homer MJ. Transection of the localization hooked wire during breast biopsy. AJR Am J Roentgenol 1983;141:929–30.

26. Azoury F, Sayad P, Rizk A. Thoracoscopic management of a pericardial migration of breast biopsy localization wire. Ann Thorac Surg 2009;87:1937–9.

27. Gray RJ, Salud C, Nguyen K, et al. Randomized prospective evaluation of a novel technique for biopsy or lumpectomy of nonpalpable breast lesions: radioactive seed versus wire localization. Ann Surg Oncol 2001;8:711–5.

28. Jakub J, Gray R, Degnim A, et al. Current status of radioactive seed for localization of nonpalpable breast lesions. Am J Surg 2010;199(4):522–8.

29. McGhan L, McKeever S, Pockaj B, et al. Radioactive seed localization for nonpalpable breast lesions: review of 1,000 consecutive procedures at a single institution. Ann Surg Oncol 2011;18(11):3096–101.

30. Hughes J, Mason M, Gray R, et al. A multi-site validation trial of radioactive seed localization as an alternative to wire localization. Breast J 2008;14(2):153–7.

31. Sharek D, Zuley ML, Zhang JY, et al. Radioactive seed localization versus wire localization for lumpectomies: a comparison of outcomes. AJR Am J Roentgenol 2015;204:872–7.

32. Caudle A, Yang W, Mittendorf E. Selective surgical localization of axillary lymph nodes containing metastases in patients with breast cancer: a prospective feasibility trial. JAMA Surg 2015;150(2):137–43.

Index

Note: Page numbers of article titles are in **boldface** type.